Cerebrotendinous Xanthomatosis

Antonio Federico • Andrea E. DeBarber
Tzipora C. Falik-Zaccai
Hidde H. Huidekoper • Robert D. Steiner
Editors

Cerebrotendinous Xanthomatosis

A Treatable Rare Neurometabolic Disorder

Springer

Editors
Antonio Federico
Department of Medicine, Surgery and Neurosciences, University of Siena
Siena, Italy

Andrea E. DeBarber
School of Medicine
Oregon Health and Science University
Portland, OR, USA

Tzipora C. Falik-Zaccai
Genetic Department
Azrieli Faculty of Medicine
Safed, Israel

Hidde H. Huidekoper
Department of Pediatrics
Center for Lysosomal and Metabolic Diseases, Erasmus MC University Medical Center
Rotterdam, The Netherlands

Robert D. Steiner
Division of Genetics and Metabolism
University of Wisconsin School of Medicine and Public Health
Madison, WI, USA

ISBN 978-3-031-92525-2 ISBN 978-3-031-92526-9 (eBook)
https://doi.org/10.1007/978-3-031-92526-9

This Springer imprint is published by the registered company Springer Nature Switzerland AG
The registered company address is: Gewerbestrasse 11, 6330 Cham, Switzerland

This book is dedicated to Prof. Vladimir Berginer, who passed away at the age of 94 years, on May 7, 2024, while this book was under preparation, after a long life devoted to the research and the care of patients with Cerebrotendinous Xanthomatosis.
The Editors

Preface

Two years ago, in association with the CTX Alliance, we decided to organize an international workshop on Cerebrotendinous Xanthomatosis (CTX), an ultrarare metabolic condition of lipid metabolism involving liver, brain, eyes, bone, peripheral nerves, tendons, hearth, etc., due to a primary genetic defect in *CYP27A1*.

In order to celebrate and give special recognition to Professor Vladimir Berginer for his important role in the research and care of CTX for many years, and also his pioneering treatment of CTX patients with chenodeoxycholic acid substitution therapy, we desired to have the meeting in the beautiful city of Jerusalem, Israel, as a satellite workshop of the 2023 annual symposium of the International Society for the Study of Inborn Errors of Metabolism (SSIEM) (Fig. 1).

The meeting held from August 27 to 29, 2023, included more than 109 in-person participants from many countries, with also the presence of 19 patients with CTX/ patient advocates. Many others attended the meeting online.

This was a unique occasion during which a large number of experts on CTX from all parts of the world shared old and new insights on the disease, from the clinical experiences in different countries, unresolved issues in research and therapy, basic insights in pathophysiology, innovative potential treatments including gene therapy, to the general organization of clinical care.

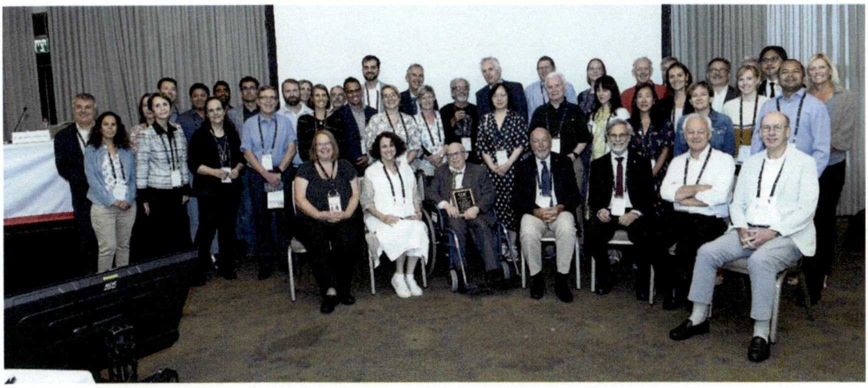

Fig. 1 Group picture of the invited speakers and some participants in the 2023 CTX International Scientific Meeting with Prof. V. Berginer after his award ceremony

It also gave the possibility to discuss collaborative studies and projects, including setting up an international CTX patient registry and putting together this book. This book collects the presentations of the invited speakers during the scientific sessions, and provides a general overview on the past, present, and future directions of research in CTX, a multi-systemic treatable disorder, representing an interesting model of metabolic interaction between the liver and brain. With the presence of symptoms involving eyes (cataracts), brain (dementia), peripheral nerves (neuropathy), bone (osteoporosis), and other symptoms typically evident in aged persons, CTX may also represent an interesting model of a treatable premature aging disorder.

As doctors, allied health professionals, and scientists, we will continue our efforts for better understanding the intriguing pathogenic mechanisms underlying CTX, to help patients in our care and to support families. We hope this book can contribute to these efforts.

Editors
Siena, Italy — Antonio Federico
Portland, OR, USA — Andrea E. DeBarber
Safed, Israel — Tzipora C. Falik-Zaccai
Rotterdam, The Netherlands — Hidde H. Huidekoper
Madison, WI, USA — Robert D. Steiner
Marshfield, WI, USA

Meeting Co-organizer and Author
Kulpsville, USA, *CTX Alliance* — Jean Pickford

Contents

About the Editors

Antonio Federico, MD, PhD Specialist in Mental and Nervous Diseases, is Emeritus Professor of Neurology at University of Siena, Siena, Italy, where he was full professor of Neurology; director of Dept. Neurological Sciences, of the Unit of Neurology and Neurometabolic Diseases, of the PhD program in Clinical Neurosciences, and of the Postgraduate School of Neurology; and vice-Rector of the University. He was President of the Italian Society of Neurology and Chairman of the Scientific Committee of the European Academy of Neurology (EAN) and of the EAN Panel on Rare Neurologic Diseases. Actually he chairs the Specialist Group on Rare Neurologic Diseases of the World Federation of Neurology. He was Editor-in-Chief of Neurological Sciences, Springer-Verlag, Editor for more than 10 years; he is in the editorial board of many journals and has published more than 600 articles in the main international journals. He is also author of many books. Finally he received two Honoris Causa Degrees in Medicine and Pharmacy in the Universities of Bucharest and Cluj-Napoca. His main interest is Clinical Neurology, with particular regard to Neurodegenerative diseases, Parkinson's diseases, and other movement disorders, myopathies, and neuropathies, white matter diseases, rare neurologic disorders, and neurometabolic diseases. He published more than 50 articles on cerebrotendinous xanthomatosis (CTX), a disorder which was one of his main research topics from 1980.

Andrea E. DeBarber, PhD is a Research Associate Professor at Oregon Health & Science University (OHSU) Portland, Oregon, where she oversees the OHSU Sterol Analysis Laboratory, which performs biochemical diagnostic testing for CTX. Her research focuses on developing improved biochemical testing for rare genetic disorders of sterol and bile acid synthesis. Over the last decades, she has identified multiple blood and urine biomarkers that are useful both for diagnosis and to monitor the efficacy of therapy for CTX. Her combination of expertise in bioanalytical techniques and deep research experience in CTX marks her as a distinguished scientist in the field. She has published more than 25 articles on CTX, a disorder that has been one of her main research topics for the last two decades. In addition, she serves as Co-Chair of the Medical & Scientific Advisory Board for the CTX Alliance patient advocacy group and is leading a taskforce to nominate CTX for consideration for addition to the US Recommended Uniform Screening Panel of disorders screened for in newborns. In 2025, for her service and commitment to the lives of people with CTX and their families, she was awarded the Dr. Hugo Moser service award by the United Leukodystrophy Foundation.

Hidde H. Huidekoper, MD, PhD was trained as a pediatrician specialized in inherited metabolic diseases at the Amsterdam University Medical Center, Amsterdam, the Netherlands, where he also obtained his PhD on the subject "In vivo kinetic studies in inborn errors of metabolism." Since 2015 he is affiliated to the Center for Lysosomal and Metabolic Diseases at the Erasmus MC University Medical Center in Rotterdam, the Netherlands. In his current position he is treating and following children over the whole spectrum of inherited metabolic diseases. He has a special research interest in CTX and classic late-infantile neuronal ceroid lipofuscinosis (CLN2 disease) for which he is leading the clinical and research program in the Netherlands. Together with Dr. Frederic Vaz, Amsterdam University Medical Center, he has been working on the development of a method for and implementation of newborn screening for CTX. He also co-coordinates the subnetwork for lysosomal storage disorders of the European Reference Network for Hereditary Metabolic Disorders (MetabERN) and is leader of the work package on clinical outcome research and board member within the United for Metabolic Diseases research consortium in the Netherlands. In 2025 he was appointed Head of the Division of Inherited Metabolic Diseases, Department of Pediatrics, and Chair of the Center for Lysosomal and Metabolic Diseases at the Erasmus MC University Medical Center, Rotterdam, The Netherlands.

Tzipora C. Falik-Zaccai, MD is a Full Professor of Medical Genetics, Metabolism, and Pediatrics at the Azrieli Faculty of Medicine, Bar-Ilan University, where she serves as Head of the Department of Genetics. She is the founding director and Director Emeritus of the Institute of Human Genetics at the Galilee Medical Center. In addition, Prof. Falik-Zaccai previously held the position of Vice Dean for Medical Research and was instrumental in establishing the MD-PhD program, which she led until recently, aimed at fostering excellence among outstanding students.

As a physician-scientist, Prof. Falik-Zaccai's research interests focus on neurogenetic diseases, inherited metabolic disorders, cardiogenetic conditions, genetic testing, and the development of innovative approaches to genetic counseling. Her clinical and research endeavors have long centered on rare genetic disorders, including CTX, osteogenesis imperfecta, and DNA repair-related diseases such as Xeroderma Pigmentosum and Cockayne Syndrome. She has dedicated significant efforts to the identification of causative genes for rare genetic disorders and has pioneered tailored genetic counseling models for ethnically diverse populations at high risk for genetic conditions and congenital anomalies. These initiatives aim to enhance education, prevention, and the reduction of the personal and societal burden associated with genetic disorders in various communities across Israel.

Prof. Falik-Zaccai is the founder of a national center for CTX, where patients benefit from comprehensive diagnostic and follow-up care provided by a multidisciplinary team. She has developed screening programs targeting populations at risk for CTX and has led investigations into multiple aspects of the disease, including the development of newborn screening protocols in collaboration with Dr. Andrea DeBarber, studies on pregnant women with CTX, and research on the natural history of the disease.

As an accomplished researcher, Prof. Falik-Zaccai has served as Principal Investigator on more than a dozen research projects that have resulted in the identification of novel causative genes for rare diseases. Her work has been published in leading international peer-reviewed journals in the fields of Pediatrics, Medical Genetics, and Molecular Genetics.

Robert D. Steiner, MD is a Clinical Professor of Genetics and Metabolism at the University of Wisconsin School of Medicine and Public Health. He is Medical Director for Newborn Screening for Wisconsin's Department of Health Services. Nationally, he serves as Editor-in-Chief of *Genetics in Medicine*, an official journal of the American College of Medical Genetics and Genomics (ACMG); he also serves on the ACMG board of directors.

Dr. Steiner is a physician-scientist interested in inherited metabolic diseases, metabolic bone diseases, genetic testing, and newborn screening. He has longstanding clinical and research interests in CTX, Smith-Lemli-Opitz syndrome (SLOS), phenylketonuria (PKU), and lysosomal storage diseases (LSD). He is also part of a research team that is a member of the NIH-funded Impact of Genomic Variation on Function (IGVF) Consortium, and co-principal investigator of an NIH-funded study of treatment for infantile neuronal ceroid lipofuscinosis. He is an accomplished researcher, having served as Principal Investigator for more than a dozen clinical trials/clinical research studies on CTX, SLOS, Osteogenesis Imperfecta, PKU, LSDs, and others. He has authored or co-authored over 190 peer-reviewed original research articles as well as nearly 100 reviews, book chapters, and letters on genetic diseases, genetic testing, and related topics.

Part I

Clinical Experience and Disease Spectrum for International Cerebrotendinous Xanthomatosis (CTX) Patient Cohorts

Cerebrotendinous Xanthomatosis (CTX): General Review and History of the Research on Its Pathogenesis and Therapy

1

Antonio Federico

Introduction

Cerebrotendinous xanthomatosis (CTX) is a rare autosomal recessive disease with usually the first clinical symptoms appearing in early infantile period, with diarrhoea, cataracts, followed later by tendon xanthomas, abnormalities in the central nervous system (especially pyramidal and cerebellar systems), mental deterioration until dementia, behavioural changes, severe psychiatric syndrome, peripheral neuropathy, osteoporosis and early atherosclerosis. Biochemically it is characterized by an increase of the cholestanol and other sterols concentrations in plasma and all tissues, especially in the tendons and central nervous system. The primary biochemical defect in the synthesis of bile acids is due to a deficiency of a hepatic mitochondrial enzyme (C27-steroid-26-hydrolase) belonging to the cytochrome P 450 family. Many mutations have recently been identified on the gene located on chromosome 2 in families from different ethnic groups [1].

The administration of chenodeoxycholic acid (CDCA) reduces the neosynthesis of cholestanol and normalizes the synthesis of bile acids, with consequent improvement in some symptoms and slowing their further evolution [2].

We here report the history of the research in these disorders, from the description of the first families to the main contributions in the discovery of the pathogenetic mechanisms and therapy.

A. Federico (✉)
Department of Medicine, Surgery and Neurosciences, Medical School, University of Siena, Siena, Italy
e-mail: federico@unisi.it

A. Federico et al. (eds.), *Cerebrotendinous Xanthomatosis*,
https://doi.org/10.1007/978-3-031-92526-9_1

The Clinical Presentation

CTX in Childhood

Even if the full clinical presentation occurs mostly in youth/adulthood, the first clinical manifestations are often reported already in childhood, starting with diarrhoea and cataracts [3–5] followed by mild and slowly progressive mental retardation and subclinical pyramidal and cerebellar signs [6].

Their early recognition and the correct diagnosis are important for therapy and prevention. Recent data on childhood presentation are reported in this volume [7].

In 1998, van Heijst et al. reported neurophysiologic and neuroimaging analyses in 5 CTX children and reviewed 13 other cases from the literature: the main clinical signs were associated with EEG abnormalities (theta background activity with episodic high voltage delta and theta discharges in the absence of epileptic seizures), with no changes in electromyography, conduction velocity, evoked potentials; neuroimaging analyses showed small hypodensities in the supratentorial white matter [8].

CYP27A1 mutations have been also reported in infants with neonatal cholestatic jaundice [6] or severe hepatitis [9], conditions in which CTX diagnosis has to be considered in order to facilitate the correct diagnosis. The early recognition, in fact, and the correct diagnosis are important for an early therapy and prevention. Recent data on childhood presentation are reported in this volume [7]. Table 1.1 summarizes the main clinical CTX presentation in childhood. The neurologic and psychiatric symptoms may be very mild at this age, and xanthomas may be not yet evident appearing in the following years.

CTX in Adulthood

The main clinical features in adults include juvenile cataracts, tendon xanthomas (especially in the Achilles tendons), systemic signs (premature atherosclerosis, osteoporosis, respiratory failure, cardiovascular disease, endocrine and hepatic

Table 1.1 Clinical CTX presentation in childhood

Neonatal cholestatic jaundice
Severe hepatitis
Neonatal or early diarrhoea
Infantile cataracts
Mental retardation
Behavioural abnormalities
Some pyramidal and cerebellar involvement

abnormalities), neurological signs (dementia, cerebellar syndrome, pyramidal syndrome, bulbar paralysis, epilepsy, extrapyramidal signs and peripheral neuropathy) and psychiatric disorders. Cataracts, atherosclerosis, osteoporosis and dementia are clinical manifestations, suggesting a premature ageing [10] (Table 1.2).

Ocular Findings

Cataracts are often the first symptom [3, 4]: in 75% of cases, they appear in the first decade of life and in 25% later (even after the age of 40); the early onset of cataracts in CTX patients has been related to higher cholestanol levels in the lens [11]. In an experimental model, Inoue et al. in 2000 [12] reported that cholestanol induces apoptosis of corneal endothelial and lens epithelial cells similarly to what previously reported in cerebellar neurons [13]. Rarer ophthalmic manifestations are eyelid xanthelasmas [14–18], optic nerve atrophy [19] and proptosis [20]. Pikuleva [21] reports in this volume more detailed data on cholestanol accumulation in the brain and eye in CTX.

Dotti et al. [20] described the ocular changes of 13 CTX patients, reporting that cataracts were constantly present in all patients; other signs include paleness of the optic disc and signs of premature ageing of the retina as sclerosis of the retinal vessels and cholesterol-like deposits.

More recently several reports have evaluated the prevalence of CTX mutations in patients with juvenile cataracts: Fox et al. [22] reported that out of 347 enrolled patients, 74 pathogenic and 69 likely pathogenic variants have been identified. Atilla et al. [23] investigated the prevalence of CTX in patients with idiopathic bilateral juvenile cataract in a Turkish cohort and reported that CTX was present in 7 out of 452 patients (1.55%). Similar data have also been reported in other patients cohorts from Spain [24] by Fernandez-Eulate et al. and in USA by Freedman et al. [25]. Mignarri et al. [26] in the suspicion index score for CTX diagnosis include early cataracts within one of the higher score indicators for CTX diagnosis.

Table 1.2 The main clinical CTX signs in adults

Cataracts and other ocular changes
Tendon xanthomas
Chronic diarrhoea
Hepatic abnormalities
Endocrine changes
Cardiovascular diseases and premature atherosclerosis
Respiratory failure
Neurologic signs (cerebellar and pyramidal syndrome; mental deterioration and dementia; extrapyramidal signs; peripheral neuropathy; epilepsy)
Psychiatric disorders (behavioural abnormalities, autistic spectrum disorders, hallucinations, etc.)
Osteoporosis and bone fractures

Xanthomas

Tendon xanthomas (Fig. 1.1) are typical of CTX, appearing in the second or third decade of life [20]; sometimes they may be absent [6]. In addition to the classic localization on the Achilles tendons, they have been observed in the extensor tendons of the elbow and hand, the patellar tendons, in the lungs, bones and CNS, especially in the cerebellum. Histologically, xanthomas are characterized by birefringent crystalline storage material surrounded by numerous multinucleated giant cells with foamy cytoplasm [27, 28].

Cardiovascular System

A possible CTX complication is premature atherosclerosis with involvement of the coronary arteries and cardiac ischemic complications [18, 29–33].

Shore et al. in 1981 [34] observed that in CTX patients, low serum HDL levels and a low concentration of apolipoprotein B-bound cholesterol are present.

Cohen et al. [35] in 2022 have reported higher cardiovascular risk factors and premature vascular changes in ten young CTX patients associated also with increased intima carotid media thickness, suggesting that a proper assessment

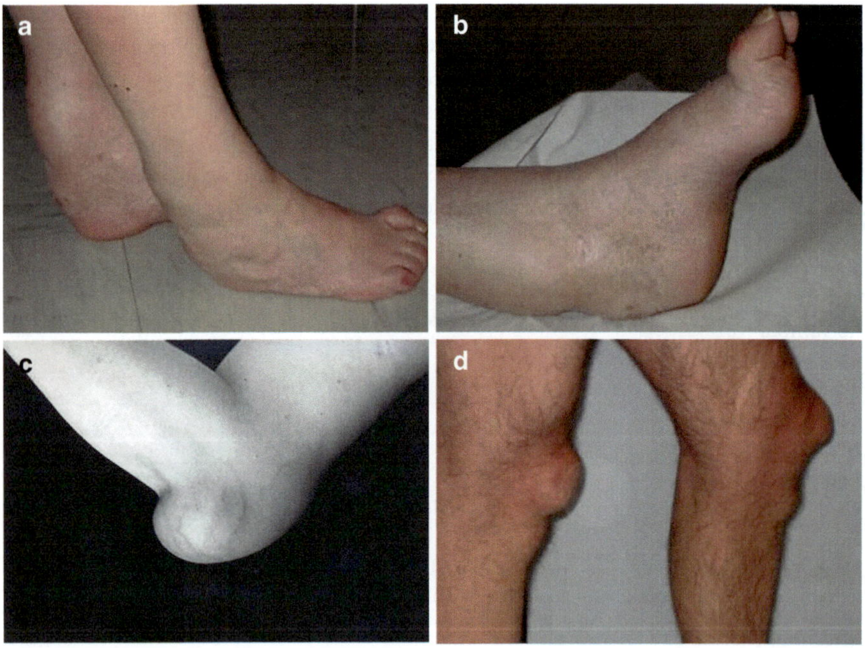

Fig. 1.1 Achille's (**a**, **b**), elbow extensor's (**c**) and patellar tendons' xanthomas (**d**) in CTX patients

should be implemented with preventive measures to reduce the risk of atherosclerotic cardiovascular disease. The pathophysiology of these changes has been recently described by a review of literature particularly discussing the relationship between cholestanol increase and cholesterol levels [36].

Dotti et al. [37] in 1998 observed lipomatous hypertrophy of the atrial septum in four CTX patients, which may explain some sudden death in these patients.

Pulmonary Manifestations

Kabawata et al. [38] in 1998 described giant foam cells (due to intracellular accumulation of sterols) in bronchoalveolar lavage fluid (where cholestanol levels were increased) and in lung biopsy findings of five patients without any lung symptom; these data could explain the presence of chronic cough in many cases.

Pulmonary lymphangioleiomyomatosis has been also reported in association with a CTX case by Dormans et al. in 1997 [39].

Enterohepatic System Involvement

Chronic diarrhoea is common in CTX, usually presenting in childhood: Cruysberg et al. in 1991 [3] observed a history of chronic diarrhoea in three children with CTX and suggested that this clinical finding may represent the first evident manifestation of the disease together with progressive bilateral cataracts. Diarrhoea improves after CDCA replacement therapy.

Cases of CTX with biliary tract stones have been reported [40–42].

Neonatal cholestasis may be a severe isolate onset signs, which may be fatal if not correctly diagnosed and treated [43–45].

Skeleton Changes

Van Bogaert et al. [14] described in the first CTX patient granulomatous lesions in the lumbar vertebrae and femur. Berginer et al. [46] in 1993 highlighted the presence of osteoporosis and bone fractures. Federico et al. [47] in the same year observed in CTX patients a reduction in bone density (osteopenia) and in intestinal absorption of radiocalcium, with normal levels of vitamin D and its metabolites; the increase in bone mineral density following CDCA therapy correlated with the normalization of bile acids serum levels, suggesting that the abnormal bile acids composition may influence the intestinal transport of calcium, causing osteopenia.

The higher risk of fractures has been reported more recently by Wejjakul et al. [48] in 2017.

Nephrolithiasis and Nephrocalcinosis

They have been reported in three CTX patients who also showed clinical features of an incomplete form of type 1 renal tubular acidosis by Chang and Cheng in 1995 [49].

Endocrine Abnormalities

Cases of hypothyroidism have been occasionally described [17, 50].

Neurological Signs

Mental Retardation or Deterioration (Dementia)

Some patients show mental retardation in early childhood, but in the majority of cases intellectual abilities are normal or slightly impaired until puberty. Slow mental deterioration starting in the second/third decade is common with a progressive evolution until dementia [51]. CDCA therapy can slow it down or even stop it. Sugama et al. [52] and Chun et al. [53] described a CTX mutated case with progressive behavioural symptoms of fronto-temporal dementia. In the spinal CTX variant. [54] Verrips et al. report that intellectual abilities are almost always normal or very mildly impaired.

Psychiatric Symptoms

They include behavioural changes, hallucinations, agitation, aggression, depression, suicide attempts—findings that sometimes characterize the onset of the disease [55, 56]. Stelten et al. in 2018 [57] out of a cohort of 77 CTX patients, 10 of them (13%; nine paediatric and one adult cases) showed autistic spectrum disorder.

All symptoms may be stabilized or improved after CDCA therapy. Mental deterioration or dementia can frequently mask psychiatric manifestations.

Pyramidal Syndrome

Signs of involvement of the pyramidal system are almost always present, characterized by hyperactive deep tendon reflexes, parapareto-spastic gait and Babinski sign, often associated with significant ataxic symptoms and severe walking impairment.

A CTX form, mainly characterized by symptoms and signs related to the involvement of the cortico-spinal tracts and medullary dorsal columns in the absence of cerebellar signs, dementia, peripheral neuropathy and xanthomas at the time of clinical presentation, was firstly described by Van Bogaert [16] in 1965; it was further characterized from a clinical, laboratory, neuropathological and neuroradiological point of view by Verrips et al. [54] in 1999 in seven patients. This form (the so-called spinal variant) should be included in the differential diagnosis of chronic progressive spastic paraparesis mainly when symptoms are preceded by bilateral cataracts and diarrhoea.

Cerebellar Syndrome

The involvement of the cerebellum can present as ataxia, hypotonia, dysarthria and dysmetria: cerebellar signs are very frequent in patients with CTX and can sometimes represent the predominant clinical feature [58]. The specific neuroimaging changes of dentate nuclei (see later) may explain these symptoms.

Extrapyramidal Manifestations

They are not rare and include dystonia and atypical parkinsonism [59–63]. Stelten et al. [64] in 2019 reported that 23% of patients with CTX show movement disorders, including parkinsonism. Recently Yu et al. [65] have published that the levels of serum cholestanol in patients with sporadic PD are higher than controls. They also reported that cholestanol activates the asparagine endopeptidase protease (AEP) inducing the fragmentation of α-synuclein (α-syn) and its aggregation. Furthermore, in a mouse model, cholestanol has been shown to promote the spreading of α-syn pathology induced by intrastriatal injection of α-syn fibrils [65].

The presence of palatal myoclonus was firstly reported by Van Bogaert et al. and by Philippart and Van Bogaert [14, 17].

Seizures

They are rare in children but may occur in 50% of adult patients [10, 66–68].

Nonspecific EEG alterations (increased slow waves with polymorphic delta and theta activity in the absence of focal pathology) have been found in patients who had never presented seizures [68, 69] .

Peripheral Neuropathy

Several electrophysiological [70–74] and morphological studies [75–83] have documented the presence of a peripheral neuropathy in almost all patients with CTX, associated with distal muscular atrophy and pes cavus.

Muscle Abnormalities

Federico et al. in 1991 [84] observed signs of a mild myopathy (increased variability of fibre calibre with the presence of randomly distributed atrophic fibres) and mitochondrial ultrastructural anomalies; mitochondrial alterations with decreased activity of mitochondrial respiratory chain enzymes were confirmed by Dotti et al. [85], who also found increased serum lactate and pyruvate levels.

Verrips et al. [86] observed no signs of myopathy or mitochondrial dysfunction and concluded that muscle damage is not considered characteristic of CTX.

Neuroimaging

The first computed tomography (CT) and magnetic resonance imaging (MRI) studies in CTX patients were those of Berginer et al. in 1981 and Waterreus et al. 1987 [87, 88], showing widespread cerebral and cerebellar white matter lesions. Subsequently Fiorelli et al. [59] in one case and Hokezu et al. [89] in seven cases described focal cerebral and cerebellar lesions and observed the presence of mild cerebral atrophy in all patients.

Bencze et al. [90] in 1990 first analysed MR images of the spinal cord of a patient with CTX, reporting a moderate cervical cord atrophy.

Berginer et al. [91] and Dotti et al. [91] in 1994 in a MR study showed the presence of cerebral and cerebellar atrophy in almost all examined patients, often associated with atrophy of the corpus callosum (frequently evident in many neurometabolic diseases) and of the brainstem; furthermore, bilateral focal lesions were identified in the cerebellar dentate nuclei, associated with white matter alterations (leukoencephalopathy) described in the majority of patients, without correlation of the cholestanol level and without atrophy or other changes in the spinal cord.

Barkhof et al. [92] from the Verrip's group described CT and MR images of 24 CTX patients in which cerebral atrophy was present in 58% of cases, hyperintensities in T2-weighted images, at the level of the periventricular white matter in 100%, in the globus pallidus in 63%, the cerebral peduncles in 67%, in the dentate nuclei in 79% and the cerebellar white matter (42%); five patients with spinal variant of the disease showed increased signal intensity in the lateral and dorsal cords; the neuroimaging alterations were more marked in the oldest patients with a longer disease duration, while in patients under 20 years of age only mild or moderate hyperintensities were identified in the periventricular white matter. A clear link between the severity of the lesions and clinical disability was not identified, and correlations between the severity of the neuroradiological picture and serum cholestanol levels or genotype were excluded.

De Stefano et al. [93] demonstrated that dentate nuclei lesions, clearly evident on conventional MRI in many but not all patients (9 out of 12), are better highlighted with FLAIR-type sequences (fluid-attenuated inversion recovery), suggesting that these changes could be considered a specific and constant neuroradiological feature of CTX and an important diagnostic marker in patients with incomplete clinical manifestations or in the initial stage of the disease.

De Stefano et al. [93] in a magnetic resonance spectroscopy investigation (RMS) highlighted a decrease in N-acetylaspartate (NAA) and an increase in lactate (La) at the cerebral and cerebellar level in 12 patients: the first data suggest widespread axonal damage (in agreement with the neuropathological study of Soffer et al. in 1995 [94]), and the second could indicate a cerebral mitochondrial dysfunction (in agreement with the previous observations by Federico et al. in 1991 and Dotti et al. in 1995 [84, 85]). The quantification of brain imaging with other MR techniques has been more recently confirmed by Inglese et al. in 2003 [95].

Mignarri et al. in 2017 [96] investigated a cohort of 38 patients, describing both supratentorial and infratentorial abnormalities at MRI, the latter being related to clinical disability and including a wide spectrum of dentate nuclei alterations. The presence of cerebellar vacuolation may be regarded as a useful biomarker of disease progression and response to therapy. On the other hand, the absence of dentate nuclei signal alteration should be considered an indicator of better prognosis.

The dentate changes in CTX have been also recently utilized to investigate the role of dentate nucleus in human oculomotor control [97] .

Specific articles on MRI and CTX are reported in this book [98, 99] .

Electrophysiology

The first electrophysiological study in CTX subjects [70] using electromyography (EMG) and analysis of peripheral nerve conduction reported in all the four patients investigated a decrease in peripheral conduction velocities, more marked in the oldest subjects, with more severe symptoms.

Ugawa et al. in 1988 [71] evaluated central motor and sensory conduction velocities, motor-evoked potentials (MEPs) and somatosensory-evoked potentials (SEPs): central motor (CMCT) and somatosensory conduction times (SSCT) were increased in all the four patients. The authors attributed these alterations to the axonal degeneration of the cortico-spinal tract and the posterior columns.

Tokimura et al. in 1992 [69] in seven CTX patients detected a decrease in peripheral conduction velocity (PCV) in 28.6% of cases and alterations in somatosensory (SEPs), acoustic (AEPs/BAEPs) and visual-evoked potentials (VEPs) in 100%, 42.9% and 57.1% of cases, respectively; a correlation was identified between the cholestanol/cholesterol ratio and the alteration of some parameters, but no significant changes were observed after 1 year of therapy (CDCA) with reduction in serum cholestanol and the cholestanol/cholesterol ratio.

Mondelli et al. (1992) [72] analysed the evoked potentials of ten patients in which a reduction of peripheral motor (MEPs) and sensory (SEPs) conduction velocity has been reported in 80% of cases; the SEPs analysis showed a delay of N9 (compatible with peripheral neuropathy) in 50% of cases and a prolongation of the latencies between the N13 and N20 peaks (IPL, interpeak latencies) in 40% of cases (prolongation of the central conduction); the study of BAEPs (brain-stem auditory evoked potentials) revealed a prolongation of the IPL between I and III and between I and V in 50% of cases (conduction delay along the auditory nerve); the VEPs were altered (delay and temporal dispersion) in 86% of the patients studied (this alteration did not seem related to the presence of cataract); MEPs from transcranial magnetic stimulation showed altered latencies and a marked increase in central motor conduction time (CMCT) in all examined patients, especially in the lower limbs, even in some individuals without clinical signs of pyramidal dysfunction. Treatment with CDCA 750 mg/day for at least 2 years improved CV, SEPs and VEPs; BAEPs remained unchanged, but baseline values were normal or slightly abnormal, and MEPs were not reassessed.

Restuccia et al. [73] observed that the MEPs and SEPs of two CTX patients showed an increase in central motor and sensory conduction times, respectively: these data suggested the presence of axonal degeneration of the long transmission pathways of the CNS, the involvement of which was not furthermore highlighted by magnetic resonance imaging of the brain and medulla; one of the two patients was studied after 6 and 12 months of therapy with CDCA and an improvement in the neurophysiological data (especially the CMCT) was found, suggesting that an early therapy may reverse the initial axonal/myelin damage when treatment is started early.

In 2001 Mondelli et al. [74] published the results of the electrophysiological follow-up of five patients with CTX treated for 11 years with CDCA at a dose of 750 mg/day. The main results are reported in Table 1.3.

According to the authors, the alterations of the SEPs and MEPs could be due to a distal central axonopathy (degeneration of the large diameter axons that constitute the long transmission pathways of the CNS) rather than to widespread degeneration

Table 1.3 The main results of CDCA therapy in 5 CTX patients following for 11 years [74]

The plasma concentration of cholestanol, elevated in all patients at time 0 (T0), normalized after 2 months of therapy, remaining within the normal range thereafter
The therapy reduced the size of the xanthomas in some cases and apparently stabilized the clinical picture of all patients
Nerve Conduction Velocities, abnormally low in 3 patients at T0, normalized after 4 months of therapy and remained normal over the 11 years of observation
The VEPs, markedly altered at T0 with increased P100 latency in 4 cases, clearly improved after 2 years of therapy and remained normal thereafter
BAEP, which showed increased IPL I–III and I–V in two patients at T0, normalized in one of the patients after 2 years of therapy
The SEPs, which even after 3 years of therapy showed an increase in IPL N24-P40 in the lower limbs, remained abnormal in 3 patients after 11 years of therapy, showing a slight and slow improvement
The MEPs, which showed a marked increase in CMCT in all five patients studied even after 2 years of therapy, improved in all patients after 8 years of therapy despite absence of any clinical improvement: this finding can be explained by the fact that other motor pathways, in addition to the cortico-spinal tract studied by MEPs, are involved in spasticity.

of the supratentorial sensory and motor pathways; this hypothesis seems to be in agreement with the neuroradiological [91, 100] and neuropathological studies [76, 94] .

The Clinical Heterogeneity

Marked variability in signs and symptoms, severity and age of onset between patients is present in CTX [101] even in patients within the same family, suggesting that other biomolecular changes may regulate the clinical presentation. An interesting family has been recently reported by Guenzel et al. [102] in 2021 who described two siblings, one with the spinal form and the second with a very mild form (minor tendon xanthomatosis and gastrointestinal complaints). Both carried compound heterozygous variants in CYP27A1: NM_000784.3: c.410G > A (p.Arg137Gln) and c.1183C > T (p.Arg395Cys). However, biochemical analysis of these patients revealed normal levels of serum cholestanol and relatively mild elevations of the bile acid precursors 7α-hydroxy-4-cholesten-3-one and 7α,12α-dihydroxy-4-cholesten-3-one, showing that also cholestanol elevation may not be constantly increased in CTX patients.

Genetics and Molecular Biology

CTX (OMIM 213700) is an autosomal recessive disease caused by mutations in the CYP27A1 gene: this gene, isolated by Cali et al. [103] in 1991 and located on the long arm of chromosome 2, more precisely on the 2q35-qter locus [104], encodes the mitochondrial enzyme sterol 27-hydroxylase, a member of the cytochrome P450 superfamily, which is responsible for the degradation of the cholesterol side chain in the pathway of bile acids synthesis.

The structure of the human CYP27A1 gene was elucidated by Leitersdorf et al. in 1993 [105]. The mRNA contains 1966 base pairs and encodes a protein of 531 amino acids; the latter consists of the mature enzyme of 498 amino acids and a mitochondrial signal sequence of 33 amino acids [103].

Many different mutations of the CYP27A1 gene have been described in patients with CTX of different ethnicities and geographical origins. About 50% of the mutations can be found in the region of exons 6–8; furthermore, most of these mutations are amino acid substitutions. No specific correlation between genotype and phenotype has been established [101, 103–113], suggesting the presence of other factors capable of modifying the phenotype, which can be extremely variable even within the same family.

Molecular genetic analysis in patients is an important step for the CTX diagnostic algorithm also in all family members of affected patients since it allows the diagnosis in a pre-symptomatic stage of a treatable pathology and the identification of heterozygous subjects, with the consequent possibility of genetic counselling and prenatal diagnosis [113].

Biochemical Pathogenesis

Biosynthesis of Bile Acids

The primary bile acids, cholic acid (CA) and chenodeoxycholic acid (CDCA), are synthesized in the liver starting from cholesterol, requiring the involvement of 10–15 enzymes such as hydroxylases, oxidoreductases, reductases, ligases, oxidases, thiolases and transferases [114–118].

The classical pathway of conversion of cholesterol to bile acids begins with the 7α-hydroxylation of cholesterol exclusively occurring in the liver, which is responsible for the synthesis of more than 50% of bile acids under normal conditions. The activity of the enzyme cholesterol 7α-hydroxylase (CYP7A1) is regulated with a negative feedback mechanism by bile acids reabsorbed from the intestine, returning thereafter to the liver via the portal venous system (enterohepatic recirculation) [114–121].

An overview on the role of bile acid pathway intermediates in CTX is reported by Griffiths et al. in this volume [121].

Metabolic Alterations in CTX

In 1968 Menkes et al. [28] found high quantities of cholestanol (a metabolite of cholesterol normally present only in low amounts) in the blood, in the cerebellum and in the brain of two CTX patients; subsequently increased levels of cholestanol have been observed in many tissues (tendons, lungs etc.). In 1971 Salen demonstrated that the bile acid pattern of CTX patients was altered, with very low levels of chenodeoxycholic acid [122]; Salen and Grundy (1973) confirmed an increase in cholestanol synthesis in CTX patients compared to controls (60 mg per day versus 14 mg per day) [123].

Setoguchi et al. [124] firstly reported a block in the metabolic pathway of bile acid synthesis consisting of an incomplete oxidation of the cholesterol side chain to carboxylic acid.

Salen et al. [29, 125–129] suggested that the CTX-specific enzymatic defect was localized at the level of microsomal 24β-hydroxylation of 5β-cholestan-3α-7α-12α-tetrol; subsequently other studies clearly indicated that the primary metabolic defect of CTX is the deficiency of the mitochondrial enzyme sterol C27-hydroxylase [42, 130–132].

In healthy subjects, approximately 80% of bile acids are equally divided between cholic and chenodeoxycholic acid; the other bile acids, deoxycholic (20%) and lithocholic (2–4%), derive from the metabolism of the intestinal bacterial flora. In CTX patients, cholic acid is 80% of the total amount of bile acids and only small quantities of chenodeoxycholic acid are detectable; other bile acids (deoxycholic and lithocholic) are almost absent [128].

Björkhem and Boberg (1995) [117] confirmed that in CTX an excess of cholestanol (5α-cholestan-3β-ol) is present in the brain, in xanthomas, in plasma (ten times higher than in healthy subjects) and in the bile.

The metabolic pathway for the formation of cholestanol is controversial. Salen et al. [126–128] hypothesized that the activity of the enzyme involved in the normal cholestanol synthesis, the microsomal 3β-hydroxysteroid dehydrogenase, was increased in CTX patients. It has been suggested that the increased levels of cholestanol could derive from the intermediate bile acid pathway starting from 7α-hydroxycholesterol [42, 132, 133]; this hypothesis is currently the most reliable, supported by experimental data and also by the effects of different treatments on the synthesis of cholestanol: therapy with chenodeoxycholic acid (CDCA), in fact, causes inhibition of the enzyme cholesterol 7α-hydroxylase with consequent reduction of cholestanol precursors, such as 7α-hydroxy-4-cholesten-3-one and cholesta-4,6-dien-3-one [134].

Shore et al. (1981) found low serum HDL cholesterol concentrations and normal or decreased LDL and total cholesterol levels in CTX patients, probably due to increased conversion of cholesterol to bile acids followed by increased LDL receptor activity [34].

Neuropathology

Van Bogaert et al. [14] described CNS white matter lesions as areas of demyelination; subsequent studies [17, 18, 135, 136] have supported this hypothesis. Menkes [28] provided a detailed description of the pathology of the spinal cord and brain in CTX, describing in the spinal cord demyelination of the pyramidal tracts and posterior columns with occasional areas of fibrillar gliosis and microcystic degeneration; in the brain, he reported demyelination of the pyramidal tracts and deposits of amorphous neutral lipids and sterol crystals in the red nucleus and the substantia nigra, and in the cerebellum a severe dentate nuclei lesion and extensive demyelination of the white matter. These lesions have been considered as neurodegenerative findings by Derby et al. [136] and Pop et al. [76] who concluded that the damage is related to neuroaxonal degeneration and not to primary demyelination. The data described by Barkhof et al. [92] in two patients showed accumulations of lipid crystals and perivascular macrophages in correspondence with the lesions, loss of neurons, demyelination, fibrosis and reactive astrocytosis, as well as deposition of hemosiderin and calcifications in the dentate nuclei.

The results of anatomopathological studies concerning the peripheral nervous system are also conflicting, with the description of normal findings by Van Bogaert et al. [14, 15] and Philippart and Van Bogaert [17], demyelinating findings [74, 78, 81, 83]; axonal/demyelinating findings [79, 80, 82]; axonal changes [76] and also nerve abnormality secondary to a vascular/compressive causes [77].

Soffer et al. in 1995 [94] in a neuropathological study of a CTX patient tried to clarify the pathogenesis of neurological damage as reported in Table 1.4.

Table 1.4 The main neuropathologic findings in CTX according to Soffer et al. [94]

(a) The damage of brain cells seems to involve mainly the white matter
(b) Significant loss of fibres in the centrum semiovale; minor changes in the subcortical white matter, with little or no changes in the commissures and other tracts
(c) Extensive degeneration of some parts of the brain, spinal cord and optic pathway associated with massive deposition of lipid products, gliosis and occasional axonal spheroids
(d) Involvement of the cerebellar white matter with the formation of xanthomas in some areas mainly in the dentate

The authors found no signs of demyelination or evidences supporting the hypothesis of abnormal myelin composition and suggested that the main pathological mechanism could be neuroaxonal degeneration: the accumulation of neurotoxic metabolites in the CNS could alter the metabolic apparatus of neurons with consequent 'dying-back' axonal degeneration due to impairment of the functional integrity of the neuron.

The study of the PNS also highlighted the presence of a predominantly distal axonal peripheral neuropathy.

More recently Kapas et al. (2014) [137] described a premature age-associated limbic tauopathy in a genetically confirmed CTX case.

Mechanism of Cerebral Accumulation of Cholestanol

Menkes et al. in 1968 [28] first noted that large quantities of cholestanol were accumulated in the brain of a patient with CTX; similar observations were reported by Muckenhausen et al. in 1969 [138] in two patients and by Philippart and Van Bogaert in 1969 [17] in a member of the first CTX family.

Salen in 1971 [122] evaluated plasma and tissue concentrations of cholestanol in six patients with CTX and reported a ten-fold increase in serum cholestanol concentrations and a 10- to 100-fold cholestanol content in 15 tissues, in which a significant increase (30%) in cholesterol levels was also observed.

Buchmann and Clausen in 1986 [139] showed that rabbits fed a cholestanol-enriched diet for eight weeks had twice as much brain cholestanol as controls; similar observations were reported in mice by Byun et al. [140]. Salen et al. in 1987 [141] observed increased concentrations of cholestanol and apolipoprotein B in the cerebrospinal fluid of six patients with CTX and suggested the presence of an alteration in the permeability of the blood-brain barrier (BBB). CDCA therapy re-established the selective permeability of the BBB and reduced the CSF concentrations of cholestanol, apolipoprotein B, apolipoprotein AI and albumin.

Bhattacharyya et al. in 2007 [142] found that the BBB of two patients with CTX was intact and that there was no transfer of cholesterol and cholestanol into the brain despite the presence of a high synthesis of cholestanol (evidenced by increased serum levels) and a high content of cholestanol in the nervous system: it was hypothesized that cholestanol could be synthesized in the brain starting from cholesterol or from a circulating precursor of chenodeoxycholic acid, which is capable of crossing the BBB.

Panzenboeck et al. [143], using experimental models, demonstrated that 7α-hydroxy-4-cholesten-3-one, a precursor of cholestanol whose plasma levels are increased 50–250 times in CTX, is able to cross the BBB extremely easily (transport is approximately 100 times more efficient than cholestanol) and can be converted into cholestanol by neuronal and glial cells and by macrophages derived from monocytes: the accumulation of cholestanol at the brain level could therefore occur secondarily to the intracellular conversion of a precursor able of rapidly crossing the BBB; this hypothesis is in agreement with the observation that CDCA treatment, normalizing the levels of bile acid precursors, is able to decrease the size of cholestanol-containing xanthomas also in the CNS [2, 29, 119] .

Pathogenesis of Neurological Damage

Inoue et al. in 1999 [13] in a histopathological study of the cerebellum of mice with hypercholestanolemia (fed with cholestanol) reported that cholestanol induces apoptosis of cerebellar neuronal Purkinje cells by activating the interleukin-1B converting enzyme (ICE) and the CPP32 protease: this mechanism could be the basis of the cerebellar ataxia typical of patients with CTX; the same group [12] in 2000 showed that cholestanol also induces apoptosis of corneal endothelial cells (corneal opacities) and of lens epithelial cells (cataracts). When cholesterol is partially replaced by cholestanol in the cell membrane, the fluidity of the membrane is reduced and the regulation of calcium channels is altered.

A second pathogenetic hypothesis is based on the toxicity of oxysterols, oxygenated derivatives of cholesterol, which could accumulate due to the lack of 27-hydroxylase. Lizard et al. in 1999 [144] observed that at the level of the vessel walls, 7β-hydroxycholesterol and 7-ketocholesterol play an important role in the apoptosis processes of endothelial and muscle cells and in the necrosis of fibroblasts. Miguet-Alfonsi et al. [145] demonstrated that oxysterols, and in particular 7β-hydroxycholesterol and 7-ketocholesterol, cause oxidative stress due to the increased production of superoxide anion and other ROS (toxic products of oxygen metabolism): the increased production of ROS is associated with lipid peroxidation inducing the apoptotic process, data confirmed by Ryan et al. in 2004 [146].

Some Numbers on the Development of CTX Research in the International Scientific Literature

Like many other rare diseases, also for CTX, an increased interest was reflected in the recent years by an increased number of international publications.

Figure 1.2 shows the increase within the years of the scientific publications as reported by PubMed from 1957 (only 1) to 2023 [26] for a total of more than 800 articles.

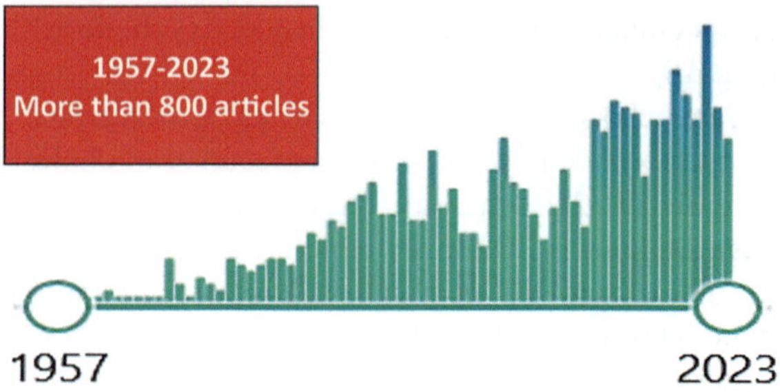

Fig. 1.2 Scientific publication on CTX as reported by PubMed from 1957 to 2023

Table 1.5 Scientists with more than 19 articles reported in PubMed until 2023

Name	Number	Years
Salen G.	63	(1971–2018)
Bjorkhem I	47	(1980–2022)
Federico A	41	(1990–2022)
Verrips A	29	(1996–2023)
Wavers RA	28	(1991–2023)
Berginer V	25	(1979–2009)
Debarber A	19	(2010–2023)

The authors who mainly contributed to the CTX research are reported in Table 1.5. The most active scientist on the topic was G. Salen with 63 papers which were mainly dedicated to clarifying the basic metabolism of bile acids and its role in the CTX pathogenesis.

The countries more involved in the CTX research are reported in Table 1.6, with the number of publications and the years. The USA and Japan had the highest number of publications, followed by Italy and the Netherlands and by many other countries.

CTX patients have been reported worldwide (USA, Israel, Italy, Japan, the Netherlands, Belgium, Brazil, Canada, France, Iran, India, Norway, Tunisia, Spain, China, Sweden and others), with clusters of patients in some geographic areas; see CTX at https://www.ncbi.nlm.nih.gov/books/NBK1409/, but prevalence of the disease is considered to be underestimated [147].

Pilo-de-la-Fuente et al. estimated a minimum prevalence of 1/18,000,000 individuals in Spain [148].

A recent genetic epidemiological study based on the Exome Aggregation Consortium (ExAC) cohort, a large cohort of over 60,000 unrelated subjects, evaluated the allele frequency of 57 known and 29 predicted CTX-causing variants and

Table 1.6 The number of articles in PubMed (23.11.23) published in the different countries on CTX

Country	Numbers	Years
USA	75	(1974–2023)
Japan	73	(1986–2023)
Italy	54	(1990–2023)
The Netherlands	52	(1988–2023)
India	43	(1994–2023)
China	33	(2000–2023)
Germany	33	(1996–2023)
France	26	(1995–2023)
Sweden	26	(1994–2023)
Israel	21	(1981–2022)
Spain	19	(2000–2023)

estimated the incidence of CTX to be 1:134,970–1:461,358 in Europeans, 1:263,222–1:468,624 in Africans, 1:71,677–1:148,914 in Americans, 1:64,247–1:64,712 in East Asians and 1:36,072–1:75,601 in South Asians [149].

More recently allelic prevalence and geographic distribution of CTX has been reported [150, 151], also providing a geographic map of estimated disease distribution.

Prevalence among Jews of Moroccan origin and the Druze in Israel has been reported to be particularly high [152, 153] .

Notes on the Pioneers of the CTX Research

The First CTX Families and the Role of the Ludo van Bogaert's Group

Ludo Van Bogaert (1897–1989) was one of the most prominent personality in Neurology in the past-century. He was the founder and head of the Born-Bunke Institute in Antwerpen, where my mentor and director, prof. GC Guazzi (with whom I collaborated for many years and substituted him in Siena as full professor of Neurology) was the head of the Neuropathology laboratory in Antwerpen for more than 10 years. I consider as a 'scientific genetic background' the fact that I was involved in the study of many genetic diseases in which prof. Van Bogaert was a pioneer (CTX, CADASIL, several metabolic diseases, etc.) (Fig. 1.3).

He was born in a noble Belgian family, in which the father and other relatives were MD. He was graduated at Bruxelles Libre University, collaborated with prof. Pierre Marie in France at La Salpetriere and with prof. Spatz and prof. Hallervorden in Germany; he founded and became director of the Born-Bunke Institute in Antwerpen, one of the most important centre of research in neuropathology. He founded the World Federation of Neurology, becoming president for 4 years (1957–1961). He published more than 730 articles, giving an important contribution

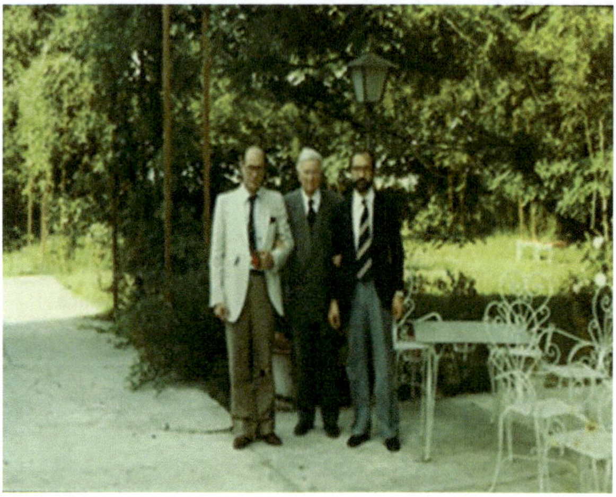

Fig. 1.3 Prof. Ludo van Bogaert with prof. G.C. Guazzi and myself in Siena, where he received honoris causa degree in Medicine in 1982

to the knowledge of the neuropathologic basis of many hereditary and metabolic diseases. He was also an important expert and collector of paintings and fine arts objects, which he donated to the Royal Museum of Fine Arts at Antwerp, while his library was donated to the Royal Library Albert I at Brussels.

His role in CTX was the description of the first patient who was a woman with dementia, ataxia, pyramidal syndrome, bulbar paralysis, xanthomas of the Achilles tendons and cataracts: the name cerebrotendinous xanthomatosis was chosen due to the unusual presence of xanthomas in the tendons, in the brain and in other tissues despite normal serum cholesterol levels [14] (Fig. 1.4).

Other cases were reported by Van Bogaert et al. [15] in 1937. In 1965, he described the spinal form [16].

In 1968, Menkes et al. [28] observed that the central nervous system of two patients with CTX contained increased levels of cholestanol, data subsequently confirmed by other collaborators and in particular by Philippart [17, 154] (Fig. 1.5).

Prof. Vladimir Berginer, the Pioneer Who Introduced CDCA Therapy in CTX Patients (Fig. 1.6)

Prof. V. Berginer is Professor Emeritus, Faculty of Health Sciences, Ben-Gurion University of the Negev, Beer-Sheva, Israel

He was born on 1929 in Kishinev (USSR) where he was educated and received the degree in Medicine and residency in Neurology. From 1957 to 1973, he was chairman of the Neurology Department in Kishinev and professor in this University. In 1973, he immigrated in Israel with his family. They settled first in Beer Sheva and then moved to Omer.

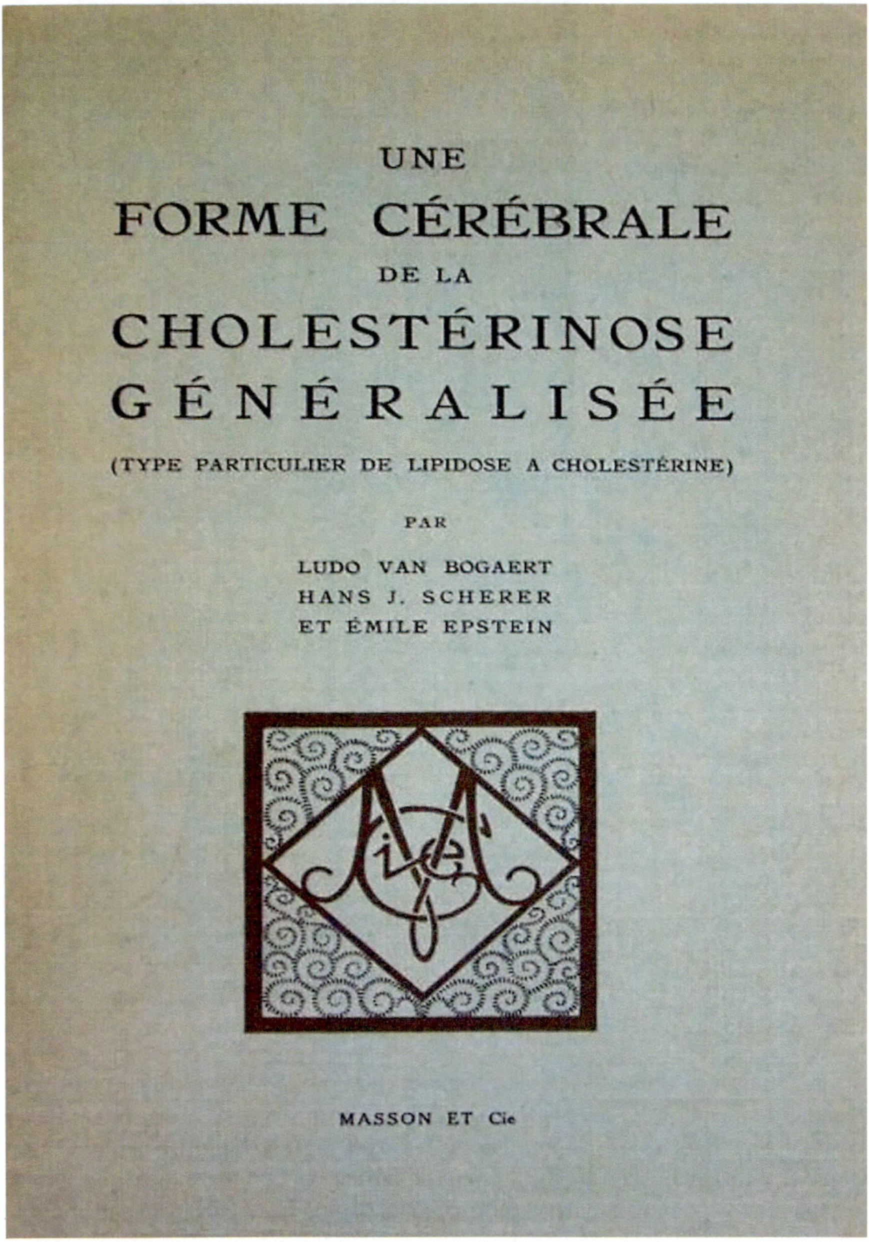

Fig. 1.4 Frontpage of the first publication on the first CTX case. "Une forme cérébrale de la colesterinose generalisée. Type particulier de lipidose a cholesterine", by L. Van Bogaert, HJ. Scherer end E.Epstein. Masson (1937) [14]

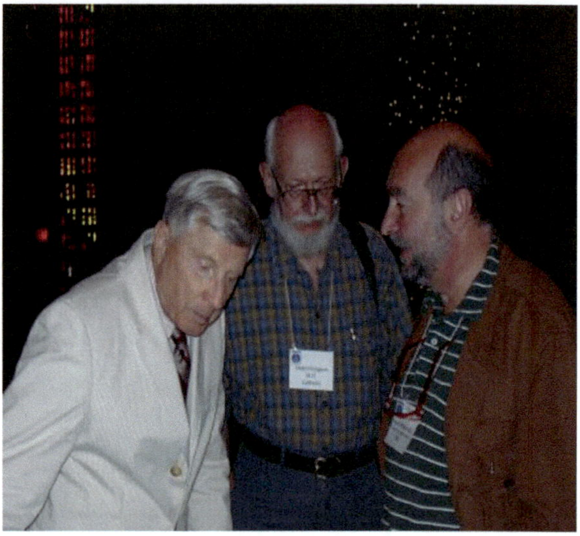

Fig. 1.5 Prof. M. Philippart with prof. Austin (who was the first to study metachromatic leucodystrophy) and myself in a Leucodystrophy meeting

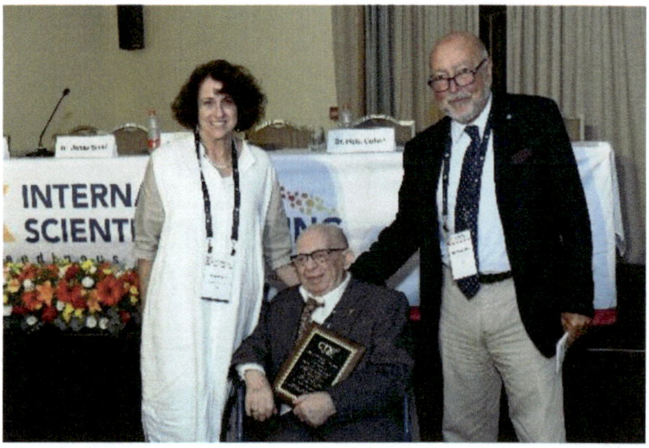

Fig. 1.6 Prof. V. Berginer, at this meeting, receiving the CTX Award

Prof. Berginer worked as a neurologist in the Soroka Medical Center where he became the head of the neuro-vascular unit. He also served as a consultant in the Yoseftal Medical Center in Eilat. He received his professorship from Ben Gurion University and published more than 200 scientific papers. He studied intensively this disorder becoming a real pioneer in understanding the mechanism and possible cure for CTX. In Israel, the patients and their families wrote: 'The Era of CTX is divided into two periods. The first part from 1936 to 1984 is recognized by studying CTX as a fatal disease. From 1984 and up to date CTX is recognized as a treatable disease'. A huge difference that was made possible thanks to the research and devotion of prof. Berginer to understanding the disease and helping patients and families worldwide.

I report here a letter of prof. Amos Korncyn, professor emeritus of Neurology in Tel Aviv University, who firstly accepted prof. Berginer in Beer Sheba Hospital after his arrival in Israel.

Dear Antonio,

Vladimir Berginer told me about the conference you are organizing In Jerusalem next month in which you will honor him, and asked me to write a few words describing him, including facets you are probably unaware of.

Please find it here:

Vladimir Berginer immigrated to Israel from the USSR in 1973 after completing his doctoral thesis in Moscow. Coming to Israel presented several challenges to a neurologist: new country, language, medical system etc. A few weeks later he was brought to the Beer Sheba Hospital and introduced to me, the chairman (and only member) of the neurology unit there at the time. Despite the difficulties, Vladimir was devoted to the mission of excelling in clinical practice.

I presented him an exceptional case of a young man whose diagnosis was unknown to me. It took Vladimir less than one week to come back, telling me it's CTX, a hardly known entity at the time. But he went further, to concentrate on this disease, its epidemiology, clinical manifestations and therapy. The rest is history, evidenced by his many articles on the subject.

An unknown part of Vladimir's biography was the fact that he was invited, in 1978, to serve as a psychological consultant to Viktor Korchnoi in the world match for the title of World Chess Championship against Karpov which took place in the Philippines.

Later on Vladimir developed an interesting and controversial theory, that of the David and Goliath match, in which he suggested that the physical height of Goliath was in fact an expression of his acromegaly due to a pituitary adenoma, which caused him to develop temporal hemianopia, which David used in their famous duel.

Vladimir is an excellent clinical neurologist, but with a scope of interests beyond medicine. He is much liked by his many friends in the neurology community in Israel and much appreciated by colleagues worldwide.

Professor emeritus Amos D Korczyn
CONy President
Department of Neurology, Tel Aviv University

The main articles of prof. Berginer contributing to the knowledge of the CTX are reported in Table 1.7.

With G. Salen, he firstly suggested the therapy with chenodeoxycholic acid in this disorder [2], showing evidences of the improvement in many clinical signs, treatment that became the basic therapy of this disorder as recently reported by Stelten et al. [155] .

The Contribution by Gerald Salen's Group, as Pioneer in the Investigation the CTX Pathogenesis and the Role of Bile Acids (see Figs. 1.6 and 1.7)

He was born in Philadelphia, on 1935 from a family emigrated in the USA from the Eastern Poland/Ukraine at the end of the nineteenth century. After receiving the bachelor of science degree in Pharmacy and after the MD degree and residency in

Table 1.7 The main articles by prof. V. Berginer on CTX

Peripheral neuropathy in cerebrotendinous xanthomatosis. Kuritzky A, Berginer VM, Korczyn AD. Neurology. 1979; 29(6):880–1.
Genetics of cerebrotendinous xanthomatosis (CTX): an autosomal recessive trait with high gene frequency in Sephardim of Moroccan origin. Berginer VM, Abeliovich D. Am J Med Genet. 1981;10(2):151–7.
Computed tomography in cerebrotendinous xanthomatosis. Berginer VM, Berginer J, Salen G, Shefer S, Zimmerman RD. Neurology. 1981; 31(11):1463–5.
EEG in cerebrotendinous xanthomatosis (CTX). Berginer VM, Radwan H, Korczyn AD, Kott E, Salen G, Shefer S. Clin Electroencephalogr. 1982; 13(2):89–96.
Pregnancy in women with cerebrotendinous xanthomatosis (CTX): high risk condition for fetus and newborn infant? Berginer VM, Carmi R, Salen G. Am J Med Genet. 1988; 31(1):11–6.
Psychiatric disorders in patients with cerebrotendinous xanthomatosis. Berginer VM, Foster NL, Sadowsky M, Townsend JA 3rd, Siegel GJ, Salen. G. Am J Psychiatry. 1988; 145(3):354–7.
Epileptic seizure as a presenting symptom of cerebrotendinous xanthomatosis. A Arlazorof, B Roitberg, E Werber, R Shidlo, V M Berginer. Epilepsia. 1991; 32(5):657–61.
Biochemical abnormalities in cerebrotendinous xanthomatosis. G Salen, S Shefer, V Berginer. Dev Neurosci. 1991; 13(4–5):363–70.
Osteoporosis and increased bone fractures in cerebrotendinous xanthomatosis. V M Berginer, S Shany, D Alkalay, J Berginer, S Dekel, G Salen, G S Tint, D Gazit. Metabolism. 1993; 42(1):69.
Magnetic resonance imaging in cerebrotendinous xanthomatosis: a prospective clinical and neuroradiological study. V M Berginer, J Berginer, A D Korczyn, R Tadmor. J Neurol Sci.1994; 122(1):102–8.
Cerebrotendinous xanthomatosis in the Israeli Druze: Molecular Genetics and Phenotypic Characteristics. E Leitersdorf, R Safadi, V Meiner, A Reshef, I Bjorkhem,Y Friedlander, S Morkos, and V M. Berginer. Am.J. Hum. Genet. 1994; 55:907–915
Molecular genetics of cerebrotendinous xanthomatosis in Jews of north African origin. A Reshef, V Meiner, V M Berginer, E Leitersdorf. J Lipid Res. 1994; 35(3):478–83.
The neuropathology of cerebrotendinous xanthomatosis revisited: a case report and review of the literature. D. Soffer, D Benharroch, V Berginer. Acta Neuropathol. 1995; 90(2):213–20.
Historical aspects of CTX. V. Berginer. Hist Neurosci 1995; 4: 127–131

Gastroenterology in Philadelphia, he was appointed at Rockefeller University, where he started to work on the cholesterol, bile acids and related sterols metabolism in the laboratory of Edward Ahren in 1966, mainly on the metabolism of non-cholesterol sterols, sitosterol and cholestanol, in normal conditions and in two disorders, which represented his special interest for five decades of life, cerebrotendinous xanthomatosis and sitosterolemia.

By 1969, he was affiliated in the New York Veterans Hospital (section Gastroenterology) and the Dept Medicine, New York University Medical Center. After he moved to New Jersy Medical School, Newark, where he became the Director of the Dept. Gastroenterology and developed basic research on the

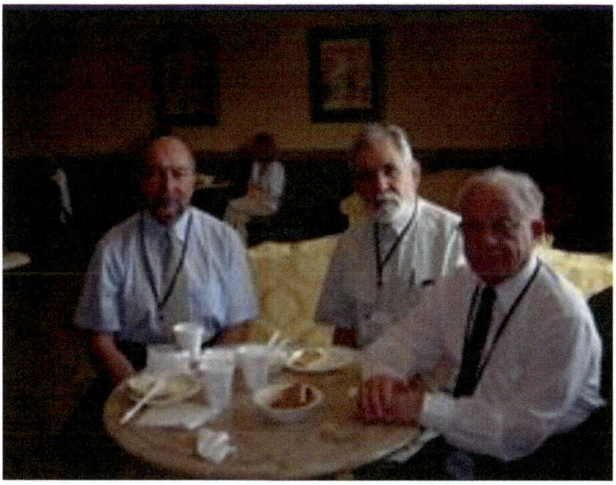

Fig. 1.7 Prof. G. Salen with prof. Berginer and myself at a leucodystrophy meeting in the USA

pathophysiology of CTX, with the evidence that the loss of chenodeoxycholic acid and abnormalities in bile acids were on the basis of the cell abnormalities and the cell degeneration with particular regards to CNS, with alteration of brain-blood barriers, and that a supplementation with CDCA may preserve these changes.

He published more than 60 articles on the different aspects of the CTX pathophysiology, with particular regards to the clinical and the biochemical aspects of bile acids abnormalities.

In 1971, Salen noticed that the composition of the bile of CTX patients was altered, with very low concentrations of chenodeoxycholic acid and the presence of bile acid precursors [122] .

In 1974, Setoguchi et al. from his group demonstrated that patients with CTX have a defect in bile acid biosynthesis that leads to the excretion of large amounts of bile alcohols in the bile, faeces, and urine [124].

The most important articles are reported in Table 1.8.

He completely dedicated his life to patients, also helping them when CDCA was no more available in the market before his approval for its use in CTX. In that period, we collaborated to increase the awareness of the medical and scientific society in different ways, participating both to the international debate on the availability of CDCA for CTX patients and to help patients supplying them with drug produced in my hospital without any cost for them [156–158].

He died on 2020, but his research remains basic for the further development of the knowledge of the pathogenesis and therapy of both CTX and sitosterolemia.

Table 1.8 Some of the most important articles by prof. G. Salen on CTX

Cholestanol deposition in cerebrotendinous xanthomatosis. A possible mechanism. Salen G. Ann Intern Med. 1971; 75(6):843–51.
Biosynthesis of 5 -cholestan-3 -ol in cerebrotendinous xanthomatosis. Salen G, Polito A. J Clin Invest. 1972; 51(1):134–40.
The metabolism of cholestanol, cholesterol, and bile acids in cerebrotendinous xanthomatosis. Salen G, Grundy SM. J Clin Invest. 1973; 52(11):2822–35.
Chenodeoxycholic acid inhibits increased cholesterol and cholestanol synthesis in patients with cerebrotendinous xanthomatosis. Salen G, Meriwether TW, Nicolau G. Biochem Med. 1975; 14(1):57–74.
Identification of pentahydroxy bile alcohols in cerebrotendinous xanthomatosis: characterization of 5beta-cholestane-3alpha, 7alpha, 12alpha, 24xi, 25-pentol and 5beta-cholestane-3alpha, 7alpha, 12alpha, 23xi, 25-pentol. Shefer S, Dayal B, Tint GS, Salen G, Mosbach EH. J Lipid Res. 1975; 16(4):280–6.
Bile alcohol metabolism in man. Conversion of 5beta-cholestane-3alpha, 7alpha, 12alpha, 25-tetrol to cholic acid. Salen G, Shefer S, Setoguchi T, Mosbach EH. J Clin Invest. 1975; 56(1):226–31.
Transformation of 5 alpha-cholest-7-en-3 beta-ol to cholesterol and cholestanol in cerebrotendinous xanthomatosis. Tint GS, Salen G. J Lipid Res. 1974; 15(3):256–62.
A biochemical abnormality in cerebrotendinous xanthomatosis. Impairment of bile acid biosynthesis associated with incomplete degradation of the cholesterol side chain. Setoguchi T, Salen G, Tint GS, Mosbach EH. J Clin Invest. 1974; 53(5):1393–401.
Plasma esterification of cholestanol, normally and in cerebrotendinous xanthomatosis. Skrede S, Stokke KT. Scand J Clin Lab Invest. 1974; 33(2):97–100.
Increased formation of ursodeoxycholic acid in patients treated with chenodeoxycholic acid. Salen G, Tint GS, Eliav B, Deering N, Mosbach EH. J Clin Invest. 1974; 53(2):612–21.

Conclusions

In the recent years, we learned a lot by studying the pathophysiology of CTX; the disease became more easily clinically recognizable and diagnosed also with molecular genetic tests, and new therapies have been investigated, all topics that are reported in the following articles in this book. The disease, thanks to the efforts of all the pioneers and all the other scientists involved in the research of the CTX pathogenesis and clinics, is less orphan of therapy and care: it is possible now an early and also a prenatal diagnosis and new born screening program [159], and an early therapy seems to be able to prevent the presentation of dramatic clinical evolution. Also new genetic therapies are developing and reported in this book [160]. Finally the organization of a patient network of family associations in the world will help the patient to feel not isolated but to collaborate with the scientists and doctor to improve their clinical conditions [161, 162].

I hope that research, culture, collaboration within the groups and harmony between the different peoples will be stronger than individualisms, causing abuses, abnormal social behaviours and aggression, freedom deprivation and wars—phenomena increased in the recent years in the world, greatly decreasing our general wellbeing and happiness These issues limits the resources dedicated to research for a better life to money transfer involved in destruction and death.

Acknowledgements I thanks all people who collaborated with me for many years on CTX, coauthors of many articles (particularly Dr. Mignarri who collected the CTX registry of our cohort and in his PhD thesis many data on the old literature) and all CTX patients and families who have been followed for many years by our group. I thank also prof. Falic Zaccai and prof. Korczyn from Israel who gave me some more information on the biography of prof. Berginer.

References

1. Gallus GN, Federico A. Cerebrotendinous xanthomatosis. In: Adam MP, Feldman J, Mirzaa GM, Pagon RA, Wallace SE, Bean LJH, Gripp KW, Amemiya A, editors. GeneReviews, 2003 Jul 16 (updated 2022 Mar 17). Seattle (WA): University of Washington, Seattle; 1993–2023.
2. Berginer VM, Salen G, Shefer SN. Long-term treatment of cerebrotendinous xanthomatosis with chenodeoxycholic acid. N Engl J Med. 1984;311(26):1649–52.
3. Cruysberg JR, Wevers RA, Tolboom JJ. Juvenile cataract associated with chronic diarrhea in pediatric cerebrotendinous xanthomatosis. Am J Ophthalmol. 1991;112:606–7.
4. Cruysberg JR, Wevers RA, van Engelen BG, Pinckers A, van Spreeken A, Tolboom JJ. Ocular and systemic manifestations of cerebrotendinous xanthomatosis. Am J Ophthalmol. 1995;120:597–604.
5. Bindl L, Lütjohann D, Lentze MJ, von Bergmann K. Cerebrotendinous xanthomatosis presenting as "cholognic diarrhoea". Acta Paediatr. 2001;90:828–9.
6. Verrips A, van Engelen BG, Wevers RA, van Geel BM, Cruysberg JR, van den Heuvel LP, Keyser A, Gabreels FJ. Presence of diarrhea and absence of tendon xanthomas in patients with cerebrotendinous xanthomatosis. Arch Neurol. 2000;57:520–4.
7. Zubariogly T, Kiykim E, Akouglu-Zeybek C. CTX pediatric presentation. In: Federico A, et al., editors. Cerebrotendinous xanthomatosis: a treatable rare neurometabolic disorder. Cham: Springer. This volume, In preparation.
8. van Heijst AF, Verrips A, Wevers RA, Cruysberg JR, Renier WO, Tolboom JJ. Treatment and follow-up of children with cerebrotendinous xanthomatosis. Eur J Pediatr. 1998;157:313–6.
9. Clayton PT, Verrips A, Sistermans E, Mann A, Mieli-Vergani G, Wevers R. Mutations in the sterol 27-hydroxylase gene (CYP27A) cause hepatitis of infancy as well as cerebrotendinous xanthomatosis. J Inherit Metab Dis. 2002;25:501–13.
10. Dotti MT, Salen G, Federico A. Cerebrotendinous xanthomatosis as a multisystem disease mimicking premature ageing. Dev Neurosci. 1991;13(4–5):371–6.
11. McKenna P, Morgan SJ, Bosanquet RC, Laker MF. A case of cerebrotendinous xanthomatosis. II: the sterol content of a cataractous lens. Br J Ophthalmol. 1990;74:629–30.
12. Inoue K, Kubota S, Tsuru T, Araie M, Seyama Y. Cholestanol induces apoptosis of corneal endothelial and lens epithelial cells. Invest Ophthalmol Vis Sci. 2000;41:991–7.
13. Inoue K, Kubota S, Seyama Y. Cholestanol induces apoptosis of cerebellar neuronal cells. Biochem Biophys Res Commun. 1999;256:198–203.
14. Van Bogaert L, Scherer HJ, Epstein E. Une forme cerebrale de la cholesterinose generalisee. Paris: Masson et Cie; 1937.
15. Bogaert L, Scherer H, Froehlich A, Epstein E. Une deuxieme observation de cholestérinose tendineuse symmetrique avec symptomes cérébraux. Ann Med Interne. 1937;42:69–101.
16. Van Bogaert L. Spinal cholesterinosis. Brain. 1965;88:687–96.
17. Philippart M, Van Bogaert L. Cholestanolosis (cerebrotendinous xanthomatosis). A follow-up study on the original family. Arch Neurol. 1969;21:603–10.
18. Schimschock JR, Alvord EC Jr, Swanson PD. Cerebrotendinous xanthomatosis. Clinical and pathological studies. Arch Neurol. 1968;18:688–98.
19. Morgan SJ, McKenna P, Bosanquet RC. Case of cerebrotendinous xanthomatosis. I: unusual ophthalmic features. Br J Ophthalmol. 1989;73:1011–4.

20. Dotti MT, Rufa A, Federico A. Cerebrotendinous xanthomatosis: heterogeneity of clinical phenotype with evidence of previously undescribed ophthalmological findings. J Inherit Metab Dis. 2001;24:696–706.
21. Pikuleva IA. Cholestanol accumulation in the brain and eye in CTX. In: Federico A, et al., editors. Cerebrotendinous xanthomatosis: a treatable rare neurometabolic disorder. Cham: Springer. This volume, Springer, 2025.
22. Fox JC, Dutta R, Nihalani BR, Ponte A, Talsness DM, VanderVeen DK, Steiner RD, Freedman SF. Identification of pathogenic genetic variants in patients with acquired early-onset bilateral cataracts using next-generation sequencing. J AAPOS. 2024;10:103808. https://doi.org/10.1016/j.jaapos.2023.11.011.
23. Atilla H, Coskun T, Elibol B, Kadayifcilar S, Altinel S, GEN-EYE-I Working Group. Prevalence of cerebrotendinous xanthomatosis in cases with idiopathic bilateral juvenile cataract in ophthalmology clinics in Turkey. J AAPOS. 2021;25(5):269.e1–6.
24. Fernández-Eulate G, Martin GC, Dureau P, Speeg-Spatz C, Brassier A, Gillard P, Bremond-Gignac D, Thouvenin D, Pagan C, Lamari F, Nadjar Y. Prospective cholestanol screening of cerebrotendinous xanthomatosis among patients with juvenile-onset unexplained bilateral cataracts. Orphanet J Rare Dis. 2022;17(1):434.
25. Freedman SF, Brennand C, Chiang J, DeBarber A, Del Monte MA, Duell PB, Fiorito J, Marshall R. Prevalence of cerebrotendinous xanthomatosis among patients diagnosed with acquired juvenile-onset idiopathic bilateral cataracts. JAMA Ophthalmol. 2019;137(11):1312–6.
26. Mignarri A, Gallus GN, Dotti MT, Federico A. A suspicion index for early diagnosis and treatment of cerebrotendinous xanthomatosis. J Inherit Metab Dis. 2014;37(3):421–9.
27. Menkes JH. Cerebrotendinous xanthomatosis. In: Vinken PJ, Bruyn GW, editors. Handbook of clinical neurology, vol. 10. Amsterdam: North Holland Pubbl Co; 1970. p. 532–41.
28. Menkes JH, Shimshock JR, Swanson PD. Cerebrotendinous xanthomatosis. The storage of cholestanol within the nervous system. Arch Neurol. 1968;19:47–53.
29. Salen G, Shefer S, Berginer VM. Familial diseases with storage of sterols other than cholesterol: cerebrotendinous xanthomatosis and sitosterolemia with xanthomatosis. In: Stanbury JB, Wyngarden JB, Frederickson DS, Brown MS, Goldstein JL, editors. The metabolic basis of inherited disease. 5ª ed. New York: McGraw-Hill; 1983. p. 713–30.
30. Fujiyama J, Kuriyama M, Arima S, Shibata Y, Nagata K, Takenaga S, Tanaka H, Osame M. Atherogenic risk factors in cerebrotendinous xanthomatosis. Clin Chim Acta. 1991;200:1–11.
31. Kerleau JM, Lefebvre H, Houdent C, Wolf LM. L'atherome coronien precoce. Une complicance peu connue de la xanthomatose cerebrotendineuse (letter). Presse Med. 1993;22:1460.
32. Valdivielso P, Calandra S, Duran JC, Garuti R, Herrera E, Gonzalez P. Coronary heart disease in a patient with cerebrotendinous xanthomatosis. J Intern Med. 2004;255:680–3.
33. Frih-Ayed M, Boughammoura-Bouatay A, Ben Hamda K, Chebel S, Ben Farhat M. Hypertrophy of the atrial septum in the cerebrotendinous xanthomatosis. Rev Med Interne. 2005;26:992–3.
34. Shore V, Salen G, Cheng FW, Forte T, Shefer S, Tint GS, Lindgren FT. Abnormal high density lipoproteins in cerebrotendinous xanthomatosis. J Clin Invest. 1981;68:1295–304.
35. Cohen H, Hassin-Baer S, Shaish A. Features of the metabolic syndrome and subclinical atherosclerosis in patients with cerebrotendinous xanthomatosis: an augmented risk for premature cardiovascular disease. Front Genet. 2022;13:997069.
36. Ribeiro RM, Vasconcelos SC, Lima PLGSB, Coelho EF, Oliveira AMN, Gomes EABM, Mota LA, Radtke LS, Carvalho MDS, Araújo DABS, Pinheiro MSN, Gama VCV, Júnior RMM, Braga Neto P, Nóbrega PR. Pathophysiology and treatment of lipid abnormalities in cerebrotendinous xanthomatosis: an integrative review. Brain Sci. 2023;13(7):979.
37. Dotti MT, Mondillo S, Plewnia K, Agricola E, Federico A. Cerebrotendinous xanthomatosis: evidence of lipomatous hypertrophy of the atrial septum. J Neurol. 1998;245:723–6.
38. Kawabata M, Kuriyama M, Mori S, Sakashita I, Osame M. Pulmunary manifestations in cerebrotendinous xanthomatosis. Intern Med. 1998;37:922–6.

39. Dormans TP, Verrips A, Bulten J, Cox N. Pulmonary lymphangioleiomyomatosis and cerebrotendinous xanthomatosis: is there a link? Chest. 1997;112(1):273–4.
40. Canelas HM, Quintao EC, Scaff M, Vasconcelos KS, Brotto MW. Cerebrotendinous xanthomatosis: clinical and laboratory study of 2 cases. Acta Neurol Scand. 1983;67:305–11.
41. Bouwes Bavinck JN, Vermeer BJ, Gevers Leuven JA, Koopman BJ, Wolthers BG. Capillary gas chromatography of urine samples in diagnosing cerebrotendinous xanthomatosis. Arch Dermatol. 1986;122:1269–72.
42. Skrede S, Björkhem I, Kvittingen EA, Buchmann MS, Lie SO, East C, Grundy S. Demonstration of 26-hydroxylation of C27-steroids in human skin fibroblasts, and a deficiency of this activity in cerebrotendinous xanthomatosis. J Clin Invest. 1986;78:729–35.
43. Zhang P, Zhao J, Peng XM, Qian YY, Zhao XM, Zhou WH, Wang JS, Wu BB, Wang HJ. Cholestasis as a dominating symptom of patients with CYP27A1 mutations: an analysis of 17 Chinese infants. J Clin Lipidol. 2021;15(1):116–23.
44. Pietrobattista A, Spada M, Candusso M, Boenzi S, Dionisi-Vici C, Francalanci P, Morrone A, Ferri L, Indolfi G, Agolini E, Giordano G, Monti L, Maggiore G, Knisely AS. Liver transplantation in an infant with cerebrotendinous xanthomatosis, cholestasis, and rapid evolution of liver failure. Pediatr Transplant. 2022;26(6):e14318.
45. Degrassi I, Amoruso C, Giordano G, Del Puppo M, Mignarri A, Dotti MT, Naturale M, Nebbia G. Case report: early treatment with chenodeoxycholic acid in cerebrotendinous xanthomatosis presenting as neonatal cholestasis. Front Pediatr. 2020;8:382.
46. Berginer VM, Shany S, Alkalay D, Berginer J, Dekel S, Salen G, Tint GS, Gazit D. Osteoporosis and increased bone fractures in cerebrotendinous xanthomatosis. Metabolism. 1993;42:69–74.
47. Federico A, Dotti MT, Loré F, Nuti R. Cerebrotendinous xanthomatosis: pathophysiological study on bone metabolism. J Neurol Sci. 1993;115:67–70.
48. Wejjakul W, Chatmaitri S, Wattanarojanaporn T, Pongkunakorn A, Ittiwut C, Shotelersuk V. Bilateral femoral neck fractures in cerebrotendinous xanthomatosis treated by hip arthroplasties: the first case report and literature review. J Orthop Case Rep. 2017;7(5):54–8.
49. Chang WN, Cheng YF. Nephrolithiasis and nephrocalcinisis in cerebrotendinous xanthomatosis: report of three siblings. Eur Neurol. 1995;1995(35):55–7.
50. Idouji K, Kuriyama M, Fujiyama J, Osame M, Hoshita T. Hypothyroidism with increased serum levels of cholestanol and bile alcohol — analogous symptoms to cerebrotendinous xanthomatosis. Rinsho Shinkeigaku. 1991;31:402–6.
51. Verrips A, Hoefsloot LH, Steenbergen GC, Theelen JP, Wevers RA, Gabreels FJ, van Engelen BG, van den Heuvel LP. Clinical and molecular genetic characteristics of patients with cerebrotendinous xanthomatosis. Brain. 2000;23:908–19.
52. Sugama S, Kimura A, Chen W, Kubota S, Seyama Y, Taira N, Eto Y. Frontal lobe dementia with abnormal cholesterol metabolism and heterozygous mutation in sterol 27-hydroxylase gene (CYP27). J Inherit Metab Dis. 2001;24:379–92.
53. Chun MY, Heo NJ, Seo SW, Jang H, Suh YL, Jang JH, Kim YE, Kim EJ, Moon SY, Jung NY, Lee SM, Kim HJ. Case report: cerebrotendinous xanthomatosis with a novel mutation in the *CYP27A1* gene mimicking behavioral variant frontotemporal dementia. Front Neurol. 2023;14:1131888.
54. Verrips A, Nijeholt GJ, Barkhof F, Van Engelen BG, Wesseling P, Luyten JA, Wevers RA, Stam J, Wokke JH, van den Heuvel LP, Keyser A, Gabreels FJ. Spinal xanthomatosis: a variant of cerebrotendinous xanthomatosis. Brain. 1999;122:1589–95.
55. Shapiro S. Depression in a patient with dementia secondary to cerebrotendinous xanthomatosis. J Nerv Ment Dis. 1983;171:568–71.
56. Berginer VM, Foster NL, Sadowsky M, Townsend JA, Siegel GJ, Salen G. Psychiatric disorders in patients with cerebrotendinous xanthomatosis. Am J Psychiatry. 1988;145:354–7.
57. Stelten BML, Bonnot O, Huidekoper HH, van Spronsen FJ, van Hasselt PM, Kluijtmans LAJ, Wevers RA, Verrips A. Autism spectrum disorder: an early and frequent feature in cerebrotendinous xanthomatosis. J Inherit Metab Dis. 2018;41(4):641–6.

58. Okuma H, Kitagawa Y, Tokuoka K, Takagi S. Cerebrotendinous xanthomatosis with cerebellar ataxia as the chief symptom. Intern Med. 2007;46:1259–61.
59. Fiorelli M, Di Piero V, Bastianello S, Bozzao L, Federico A. Cerebrotendinous xanthomatosis: clinical and MRI study (a case report). J Neurol Neurosurg Psychiatry. 1990;53:76–8.
60. Rogelet P, Gerard JM, Michotte A, Masingue M, Destee A. Cerebrotendinous xanthomatosis. 2 cases with magnetic resonance imaging. Rev Neurol (Paris). 1992;148:541–5.
61. Dotti MT, Federico A, Garuti R, Calandra S. Cerebrotendinous xanthomatosis with predominant parkinsonian syndrome: further confirmation of the clinical heterogeneity. Mov Disord. 2000;15:1017–9.
62. Ohno T, Kobayashi S, Hayashi M, Sakurai M, Kanazawa I. Diphenylpyraline-responsive parkinsonism in cerebrotendinous xanthomatosis: long-term follow up of three patients. J Neurol Sci. 2001;182:95–7.
63. Grandas F, Martin-Moro M, Garcia-Munozguren S, Anaya F. Early-onset parkinsonism in cerebrotendinous xanthomatosis. Mov Disord. 2002;17:1396–7.
64. Stelten BML, Bart PC, van de Warrenburg BPC, Wevers RA, Verrips A. Movement disorders in cerebrotendinous xanthomatosis. Parkinsonism Relat Disord. 2019;58:12–6.
65. Yu T, Nie S, Bu L, Liu M, He J, Niu X, Feng H, Guo J, Tang B, Zhang Z, Ye K, Jiang H, Chen L, Zhang Z. Cholestanol accelerates α-synuclein aggregation and spreading by activating asparagine endopeptidase. JCI Insight. 2023;8(21):e165841.
66. Matsumuro K, Takahashi K, Matsumoto H, Okatsu Y, Kuriyama M. A case of cerebrotendinous xanthomatosis with convulsive seizures. Rinsho Shinkeigaku. 1990;30:207–9.
67. Arlazoroff A, Roitberg B, Werber E, Shidlo R, Berginer VM. Epileptic seizure as a presenting symptom of cerebrotendinous xanthomatosis. Epilepsia. 1991;32:657–61.
68. Berginer VM, Radwan H, Korczyn AD, Kott E, Salen G, Shefer S. EEG in cerebrotendinous xanthomatosis (CTX). Clin Electroencephalogr. 1982;13:89–96.
69. Tokimura Y, Kuriyama M, Arimura K, Fujiyama J, Osame M. Electrophysiological studies in cerebrotendinous xanthomatosis. J Neurol Neurosurg Psychiatry. 1992;55:52–5.
70. Kuritzky A, Berginer VM, Korczyn AD. Peripheral neuropathy in cerebrotendinous xanthomatosis. Neurology. 1979;29:880–1.
71. Ugawa Y, Kohara N, Shimpo T, Mannen T. Central motor and sensory conduction in adrenoleukomyeloneuropathy, cerebrotendinous xanthomatosis, HTLV-1-associated myelopathy and tabes dorsalis. J Neurol Neurosurg Psychiatry. 1988;51:1069–74.
72. Mondelli M, Rossi A, Scarpini C, Dotti MT, Federico A. Evoked potentials in cerebrotendinous xanthomatosis and effect induced by chenodeoxycholic acid. Arch Neurol. 1992;49:469–75.
73. Restuccia D, Di Lazzaro V, Servidei S, Colosimo C, Tonali P. Somatosensory and motor evoked potentials in the assessment of cerebrotendinous xanthomatosis before and after treatment with chenodeoxycholic acid: a preliminary study. J Neurol Sci. 1992;112:139–46.
74. Mondelli M, Sicurelli F, Scarpini C, Dotti MT, Federico A. Cerebrotendinous xanthomatosis: 11-year treatment with chenodeoxycholic acid in five patients. An electrophysiological study. J Neurol Sci. 2001;190:29–33.
75. Ohnishi A, Yamashita Y, Goto I, Kuroiwa Y, Murakami S, Ikeda M. De- and remyelination and onion bulb in cerebrotendinous xanthomatosis. Acta Neuropathol (Berl). 1979;45:43–5.
76. Pop PH, Joosten E, van Spreeken A, Gabreëls-Festen A, Jaspar H, ter Laak H, Vos A. Neuroaxonal pathology of central and peripheral nervous systems in cerebrotendinous xanthomatosis (CTX). Acta Neuropathol. 1984;64:259–64.
77. Katz DA, Scheinberg L, Horoupian DS, Salen G. Peripheral neuropathy in cerebrotendinous xanthomatosis. Arch Neurol. 1985;42:1008–10.
78. Argov Z, Soffer D, Eisenberg S, Zimmerman Y. Chronic demyelinating peripheral neuropathy in cerebrotendinous xanthomatosis. Ann Neurol. 1986;20:89–91.
79. Federico A, Palmeri S, Ciacci G, Rossi A, Malandrini A, Alessandrini C, Salen G, Guazzi GC. Peripheral neuropathy in CTX: seven cases in two families. Neurology. 1987;37(Suppl 1):360.

80. Voiculescu V, Alexianu M, Popescu-Tismana G, Pastia M, Petrovici A, Dan A. Polyneuropathy with lipid deposits in Schwann cells and axonal degeneration in cerebrotendinous xanthomatosis. J Neurol Sci. 1987;82:89–99.
81. Amiel H, Gherardi R, Kanaan HY, Buisson J, Genthon R, Zinszner J, Giroux C, Delaporte P, Salama J. Cerebrotendinous xanthomatosis. Apropos of a case using magnetic resonance study of the brain and nerve biopsy. Ann Med Interne (Paris). 1989;140:525–7.
82. Donaghy M, King RH, McKeran RO, Schwartz MS, Thomas PK. Cerebrotendinous xanthomatosis: clinical, electrophysiological and nerve biopsy findings, and response to treatment with chenodeoxycholic acid. J Neurol. 1990;237:216–9.
83. Ben Hamida M, Chabbi N, Ben Hamida C, Mhiri C, Kallel R. Peripheral neuropathy in a sporadic case of cerebrotendinous xanthomatosis. Rev Neurol (Paris). 1991;147:385–8.
84. Federico A, Dotti MT, Volpi N. Muscle mitochondrial changes in cerebrotendinous xanthomatosis. Ann Neurol. 1991;30:734–5.
85. Dotti MT, Manneschi L, Federico A. Mitochondrial enzyme deficiency in cerebrotendinous xanthomatosis. J Neurol Sci. 1995;129:106–8.
86. Verrips A, van Engelen BG, ter Laak H, Gabreels-Festen A, Janssen A, Zwarts M, Wevers RA, Gabreels FJ. Cerebrotendinous xanthomatosis. Controversies about nerve and muscle: observations in ten patients. Neuromuscul Disord. 2000;10:407–14.
87. Berginer VM, Berginer J, Salen G, Shefer S, Zimmerman RD. Computed tomography in cerebrotendinous xanthomatosis. Neurology. 1981;31:1463–5.
88. Waterreus RJ, Koopman BJ, Wolthers BG, Oosterhuis HJ. Cerebrotendinous xanthomatosis (CTX): a clinical survey of the patient population in The Netherlands. Clin Neurol Neurosurg. 1987;89:169–75.
89. Hokezu Y, Kuriyama M, Kubota R, Nakagawa M, Fujiyama J, Osame M. Cerebrotendinous xanthomatosis: cranial CT and MRI studies in eight patients. Neuroradiology. 1992;34:308–12.
90. Bencze KS, Vande Polder DR, Prockop LD. Magnetic resonance imaging of the brain and spinal cord in cerebrotendinous xanthomatosis. J Neurol Neurosurg Psychiatry. 1990;53:166–7.
91. Berginer VM, Berginer J, Korczyn AD, Tadmor R. Magnetic resonance imaging in cerebrotendinous xanthomatosis: a prospective clinical and neuroradiological study. J Neurol Sci. 1994;122:102–8.
92. Barkhof F, Verrips A, Wesseling P, van der Knaap M, van Engelen BG, Gabreëls FJ, Keyser A, Wevers RA, Valk J. Cerebrotendinous xanthomatosis: the spectrum of imaging findings and the correlation with neuropathologic findings. Radiology. 2000;217:869–76.
93. De Stefano N, Dotti MT, Mortilla M, Federico A. Magnetic resonance imaging and spectroscopic changes in brains of patients with cerebrotendinous xanthomatosis. Brain. 2001;124:121–31.
94. Soffer D, Benharroch D, Berginer VM. The neuropathology of cerebrotendinous xanthomatosis revisited: a case report and review of the literature. Acta Neuropathol. 1995;1995(90):213–20.
95. Inglese M, De Stefano N, Pagani E, Dotti MT, Comi G, Federico A, Filippi M. Quantification of brain damage in cerebrotendinous xanthomatosis with magnetization transfer MR imaging. AJNR Am J Neuroradiol. 2003;2003(24):495–500.
96. Mignarri A, Dotti MT, Federico A, De Stefano N, Battaglini M, Grazzini I, Galluzzi P, Monti L. The spectrum of magnetic resonance findings in cerebrotendinous xanthomatosis: redefinition and evidence of new markers of disease progression. J Neurol. 2017;264(5):862–74.
97. Rosini F, Pretegiani E, Mignarri A, Optican LM, Serchi V, De Stefano N, Battaglini M, Monti L, Dotti MT, Federico A, Rufa A. The role of dentate nuclei in human oculomotor control: insights from cerebrotendinous xanthomatosis. J Physiol. 2017;595(11):3607–20.
98. Cortese R, Manco C, De Stefano N. Overview of neuroimaging in CTX diagnosis. In: Federico A, et al., editors. Cerebrotendinous xanthomatosis: a treatable rare neurometabolic disorder. Cham: Springer. This volume, In preparation.
99. Mochel F. Novel neuroimaging tool to monitor Cerebrotendinous Xanthomatosis (CTX) . In Cerebrotendinous Xanthomatosis. A treatable neurometabolic disorder. Federico et al Edts. Springer, 2025. This volume.

100. Dotti MT, Federico A, Signorini E, Caputo N, Venturi C, Filosomi G, Guazzi GC. Cerebrotendinous xanthomatosis (van Bogaert-Scherer-Epstein disease): CT and MR findings. AJNR Am J Neuroradiol. 1994;15:1721–6.
101. Salen G, Steiner RD. Epidemiology, diagnosis, and treatment of cerebrotendinous xanthomatosis (CTX). J Inherit Metab Dis. 2017;40(6):771–81.
102. Guenzel AJ, DeBarber A, Raymond K, Dhamija R. Familial variability of cerebrotendinous xanthomatosis lacking typical biochemical findings. JIMD Rep. 2021;59(1):3–9.
103. Cali JJ, Hsieh CL, Francke U, Russell DW. Mutations in the bile acid biosynthetic enzyme sterol 27-hydroxylase underlie cerebrotendinous xanthomatosis. J Biol Chem. 1991;266:7779–83.
104. Lee MH, Hazard S, Carpten JD, Yi S, Cohen J, Gerhardt GT, Salen G, Patel SB. Fine-mapping, mutation analysis, and structural mapping of cerebrotendinous xanthomatosis in U.S. pedigrees. J Lipid Res. 2001;42:159–69.
105. Leitersdorf E, Reshef A, Meiner V, Levitzki R, Schwartz SP, Dann EJ, Berkman N, Cali JJ, Klapholz L, Berginer VM. Frameshift and splice-junction mutations in the sterol 27-hydroxylase gene cause cerebrotendinous xanthomatosis in Jews of Moroccan origin. J Clin Invest. 1993;91:2488–96.
106. Leitersdorf E, Safadi R, Meiner V, Reshef A, Bjorkhem I, Friedlander Y, Morkos S, Berginer VM. Cerebrotendinous xanthomatosis in the Israeli Druze: molecular genetics and phenotypic characteristics. Am J Hum Genet. 1994;55:907–15.
107. Dotti MT, Garuti R, Calandra S, Federico A. Clinical and genetic variability of CTX (Abstract). Eur J Neurol. 1996;3(Suppl 5):12.
108. Björkhem I, Leitersdorf E. Sterol 27-hydroxylase deficiency: a rare cause of xanthomas in normocholesterolemic humans. Trends Endocrinol Metab. 2000;11:180–3.
109. Gallus GN, Dotti MT, Federico A. Clinical and molecular diagnosis of cerebrotendinous xanthomatosis with a review of the mutations in the CYP27A1 gene. Neurol Sci. 2006;27:143–9.
110. Garuti R, Croce MA, Tiozzo R, Dotti MT, Federico A, Bertolini S, Calandra S. Four novel mutations of sterol 27-hydroxylase gene in Italian patients with cerebrotendinous xanthomatosis. J Lipid Res. 1997;38:2322–34.
111. Garuti R, Lelli N, Barozzini M, Dotti MT, Federico A, Bertolini S, Calandra S. Partial deletion of the gene encoding sterol 27-hydroxylase in a subject with cerebrotendinous xanthomatosis. J Lipid Res. 1996;37:662–72.
112. Garuti R, Lelli N, Barozzini M, Tiozzo R, Dotti MT, Federico A, Ottomano AM, Croce A, Bertolini S, Calandra S. Cerebrotendinous xanthomatosis caused by two new mutations of the sterol-27-hydroxylase gene that disrupt mRNA splicing. J Lipid Res. 1996;37:1459–67.
113. Meiner V, Meiner Z, Reshef A, Bjorkhem I, Leitersdorf E. Cerebrotendinous xanthomatosis: molecular diagnosis enables presymptomatic detection of a treatable disease. Neurology. 1994;44:288–90.
114. Björkhem I. Mechanism of bile acid biosynthesis in mammalian liver. In: Danielsson H, Sjövall J, editors. Comprehensive biochemistry. Amsterdam: Elsevier Scientific Publishing Company; 1985. p. 231–78.
115. Björkhem I, Eggertsen G. Genes involved in initial steps of bile acids synthesis. Curr Opin Lipidol. 2001;12:97–103.
116. Princen HM, Post SM, Twisk J. Regulation of bile acid synthesis. Curr Pharm Des. 1997;1997(3):59–84.
117. Björkhem I, Boberg KM. Inborn errors in bile acid biosynthesis and storage of sterols other than cholesterol. In: Scriver CR, Beaudet AL, Sly WS, Valle D, editors. The metabolic and molecular basis of inherited disease. 7ª ed. New York: McGraw-Hill; 1995. p. 2073–99.
118. Björkhem I, Boberg KM, Leitersdorf E. Inborn errors in bile acid biosynthesis and storage of sterols other than cholesterol. In: Scriver CR, Beaudet AL, Sly WS, Valle D, editors. The metabolic and molecular basis of inherited disease. 8ª ed. New York: McGraw-Hill; 2001. p. 2961–88.
119. Björkhem I, Diczfalusy U, Lütjohann D. Removal of cholesterol from extrahepatic sources by oxidative mechanisms. Curr Opin Lipidol. 1999;10:161–5.

120. Lütjohann D, Breuer O, Ahlborg G, Nennesmo I, Sidén A, Diczfalusy U, Björkhem I. Cholesterol homeostasis in human brain: evidence for an age-dependent flux of 24S-hydroxycholesterol from the brain into the circulation. Proc Natl Acad Sci USA. 1996;93:9799–804.
121. Griffiths W, Yutur E, Ali Asgar M, Wang Y. Role of bile acid pathway intermediates in pathology of CTX. In: Federico A, et al., editors. Cerebrotendinous xanthomatosis: a treatable rare neurometabolic disorder. Springer. 2025. This volume.
122. Salen G. Cholestanol deposition in cerebrotendinous xanthomatosis. A possible mechanism. Ann Intern Med. 1971;75:843–5.
123. Salen G, Grundy SM. The metabolism of cholestanol, cholesterol, and bile acids in cerebrotendinous xanthomatosis. J Clin Invest. 1973;52:2822–35.
124. Setoguchi T, Salen G, Tint GS, Mosbach EH. A biochemical abnormality in cerebrotendinous xanthomatosis. Impairment of bile acid biosynthesis associated with incomplete degradation of the cholesterol side chain. J Clin Invest. 1974;53:1393–401.
125. Salen G, Meriwether TW, Nicolau G. Chenodeoxycholic acid inhibits increased cholesterol and cholestanol synthesis in patients with cerebrotendinous xanthomatosis. Biochem Med. 1975;14:57–74.
126. Salen G, Shefer S, Setoguchi T, Mosbach EH. Bile alcohol metabolism in man. Conversion of 5beta-cholestane-3alpha, 7alpha, 12alpha, 25-tetrol to cholic acid. J Clin Invest. 1975;56:226–31.
127. Salen G, Shefer S, Tint GS. Transformation of 4-cholesten-3-one and 7 alpha-hydroxy-4-cholesten-3-one into cholestanol and bile acids in cerebrotendinous xanthomatosis. Gastroenterology. 1984;87:276–83.
128. Salen G, Shefer S, Tint GS, Nicolau G, Dayal B, Batta AK. Biosynthesis of bile acids in cerebrotendinous xanthomatosis. Relationship of bile acid pool sizes and synthesis rates to hydroxylations at C-12, C-25, and C-26. J Clin Invest. 1985;76:744–51.
129. Salen G, Zaki FG, Sabesin S, Boehme D, Shefer S, Mosbach EH. Intrahepatic pigment and crystal forms in patients with cerebrotendinous xanthomatosis (CTX). Gastroenterology. 1978;74:82–9.
130. Oftebro H, Björkhem I, Skrede S, Schreiner A, Pederson JI. Cerebrotendinous xanthomatosis: a defect in mitochondrial 26-hydroxylation required for normal biosynthesis of cholic acid. J Clin Invest. 1980;65:1418–30.
131. Björkhem I, Fausa O, Hopen G, Oftebro H, Pedersen JI, Skrede S. Role of the 26-hydroxylase in the biosynthesis of bile acids in the normal state and in cerebrotendinous xanthomatosis. An in vivo study. J Clin Invest. 1983;71:142–8.
132. Skrede S, Björkhem I, Buchmann MS, Hopen G, Fausa O. A novel pathway for biosynthesis of cholestanol with 7 alpha-hydroxylated C27-steroids as intermediates, and its importance for the accumulation of cholestanol in cerebrotendinous xanthomatosis. J Clin Invest. 1985;5:448–55.
133. Buchmann MS, Björkhem I, Lund AM, Skrede S. On the mechanism of byosinthesis of cholestanol from 7α-hydroxycholesterol. Scand J Clin Lab Invest. 1986;46(Suppl 184):41–6.
134. Reihnér E, Björkhem I, Angelin B, Ewerth S, Einarsson K. Bile acid synthesis in humans: regulation of hepatic microsomal cholesterol 7α-hydroxylase activity. Gastroenterology. 1989;97:1498–505.
135. Elleder M, Michalec C, Jirásek A, Khun K, Havlová M, Ranný M. Membranocystic lesion in the brain in cerebrotendinous xanthomatosis. Histochemical and ultrastructural study with evidence of its ceroid nature. Virchows Arch B Cell Pathol Incl Mol Pathol. 1989;57:367–74.
136. Derby BM, Pogacar S, Mueckenhausen C, Moser HW. Cerebrotendinous xanthomatosis: a clinicopathological biochemical and metabolic study (abstract). J Neuropathol Exp Neurol. 1970;29:139.
137. Kapás I, Katkó M, Harangi M, Paragh G, Balogh I, Kóczi Z, Regelsberger G, Molnár MJ, Kovacs GG. Cerebrotendinous xanthomatosis with the c.379C>T (p.R127W) mutation in the CYP27A1 gene associated with premature age-associated limbic tauopathy. Neuropathol Appl Neurobiol. 2014;40(3):345–50.

138. Muckenhausen C, Derby DM, Moser HW. Conversion of 14-cholesterol to cholestanol in cerebrotendinous xanthomatosis (abstract). Fed Proc. 1969;28:882.
139. Buchmann MS, Clausen OP. Effects of cholestanol feeding and cholestyramine treatment on the tissue sterols in the rabbit. Lipids. 1986;21:738–43.
140. Byun DS, Kasama T, Shimizu T, Yorifuji H, Seyama Y. Effect of cholestanol feeding on sterol concentrations in the serum, liver, and cerebellum of mice. J Biochem. 1988;103:375–9.
141. Salen G, Berginer V, Shore V, Horak I, Horak E, Tint GS, Shefer S. Increased concentrations of cholestanol and apolipoprotein B in the cerebrospinal fluid of patients with cerebrotendinous xanthomatosis. Effect of Chenodeoxycholic acid. N Engl J Med. 1987;316:1233–8.
142. Bhattacheryya AK, Lin DS, Connor WE. Cholestanol metabolism in patients with cerebrotendinous xanthomatosis: absorption, turnover and tissue deposition. J Lipid Res. 2007;48:185–92.
143. Panzenboeck U, Anderson U, Hansson M, Sattler W, Meaney S, Björkhem I. On the mechanism of cerebral accumulation of cholestanol in patients with cerebrotendinous xanthomatosis. J Lipid Res. 2007;48:1167–74.
144. Lizard G, Monier S, Cordelet C, Gesquière L, Deckert V, Gueldry S, Lagrost L, Gambert P. Characterization and comparison of the mode of cell death, apoptosis versus necrosis, induced by 7β-hydroxycholesterol and 7-ketocholesterol in the cells of the vascular wall. Arterioscler Thromb Vasc Biol. 1999;19:1190–200.
145. Miguet-Alfonsi C, Prunet C, Monier S, Bessède G, Lemaire-Ewing S, Berthier A, Ménétrier F, Néel D, Gambert P, Lizard G. Analysis of oxidative processes and of myelin figures formation before and after the loss of mitochondrial transmembrane potential during 7beta-hydroxycholesterol and 7-ketocholesterol-induced apoptosis: comparison with various pro-apoptotic chemicals. Biochem Pharmacol. 2002;64:527–41.
146. Ryan L, O'Callaghan YC, O'Brien NM. Comparison of the apoptotic processes induced by the oxysterols 7beta-hydroxycholesterol and cholesterol-5beta, 6beta-epoxide. Cell Biol Toxicol. 2004;20:313–23.
147. Lorincz MT, Rainier S, Thomas D, Fink JK. Cerebrotendinous xanthomatosis: possible higher prevalence than previously recognized. Arch Neurol. 2005;62:1459–63.
148. Pilo-de-la-Fuente B, Jimenez-Escrig A, Lorenzo JR, Pardo J, Arias M, Ares-Luque A, Duarte J, Muñiz-Pérez S, Sobrido MJ. Cerebrotendinous xanthomatosis in Spain: clinical, prognostic, and genetic survey. Eur J Neurol. 2011;18(10):1203–11.
149. Appadurai V, DeBarber A, Chiang PW, Patel SB, Steiner RD, Tyler C, Bonnen PE. Apparent underdiagnosis of Cerebrotendinous Xanthomatosis revealed by analysis of ~60,000 human exomes. Mol Genet Metab. 2015;116(4):298–304.
150. Pramparo T, Steiner RD, Rodems S, Jenkinson C. Allelic prevalence and geographic distribution of cerebrotendinous xanthomatosis. Orphanet J Rare Dis. 2023;18(1):13.
151. Pramparo T, Jenkinson C. Epidemiology of CTX. In: Federico A, et al., editors. Cerebrotendinous xanthomatosis: a treatable rare neurometabolic disorder. Springer. This volume.
152. Berginer VM, Abeliovich D. Genetics of cerebrotendinous xanthomatosis (CTX): an autosomal recessive trait with high gene frequency in Sephardim of Moroccan origin. Am J Med Genet. 1981;10:151–7.
153. Falik-Zaccai TC, Kfir N, Frenkel P, Cohen C, Tanus M, Mandel H, Shihab S, Morkos S, Aaref S, Summar ML, Khayat M. Population screening in a Druze community: the challenge and the reward. Genet Med. 2008;10:903–9.
154. Menkes JH, Philippart M. Cholestanol storage in the nervous system of two patients with cerebrotendinous xanthomatosis. Trans Am Neurol Assoc. 1968;93:66–9.
155. Stelten BML, Dotti MT, Verrips A, Elibol B, Falik-Zaccai TC, Hanman K, Mignarri A, Sithole B, Steiner RD, Verma S, Yahalom G, Zubarioglu T, Mochel F, Federico A. Expert opinion on diagnosing, treating and managing patients with cerebrotendinous xanthomatosis (CTX): a modified Delphi study. Orphanet J Rare Dis. 2021;16(1):353.
156. Samenuk P, Koffeman BM. Cgenodeoxycholic treatment of cerebrotendinous xanthomatosis. Neurology. 2001;56:695.

157. Salen G. Chenodeoxycholic acid treatment of cerebrotendinous xanthomatosis. Neurology. 2001;56:695–6.
158. Federico A, Dotti MT. Chenodeoxycholic acid treatment in Cerebrotendinous xanthomatosis in Italy. Neurology. 2001;57:1743.
159. DeBarber AE, Kalfon L, Fedida A, Fleisher Sheffer V, Ben Haroush S, Chasnyk N, Shuster Biton E, Mandel H, Jeffries K, Shinwell ES, Falik-Zaccai TC. Newborn screening for cerebrotendinous xanthomatosis is the solution for early identification and treatment. J Lipid Res. 2018;59(11):2214–22.
160. Hernandez-Alcouba R, Molina A, Gonzales-Aseguinolaza G. Gene therapy for CTX. In: Federico A, et al., editors. Cerebrotendinous xanthomatosis: a treatable rare neurometabolic disorder. Springer. This volume.
161. Huidekoper H. CTX remaining challenges and the need for international collaboration. In: Federico A, et al., editors. Cerebrotendinous xanthomatosis: a treatable rare neurometabolic disorder. Springer. This volume.
162. Steiner RD, DeBarber A, Larson A, Blanchard B, Laurie S, Odedara N, Rosengrant H, Dutta R. Living with cerebrotendinous xanthomatosis: patient, caregiver, and expert perspectives. Adv Ther. 2024;41(2):467–75.

Cerebrotendinous Xanthomatosis (CTX) in Italy

2

Antonio Federico, Gian Nicola Gallus, Andrea Mignarri, Maria Teresa Dotti, and Alessandra Rufa

Introduction

Here we report the experience with CTX in Italy, started in the 1980s following the first family with three adult sisters affected by progressive cognitive deterioration, cataracts, xanthomas and all other classical CTX symptoms. We developed a diagnostic methodology for diagnosis, a working group in collaboration with molecular geneticists, ophthalmologists, neurophysiologists, neuroimaging experts, cardiologists, biochemists, experts in osteoporosis and calcium metabolism, etc., creating in Siena a Reference Center for this disorder as well as for other neurometabolic diseases and developing research in the area, with many publications on the topic during the following years.

Distribution of Our CTX Patient Cohort in Italy

Figure 2.1 shows the geographical distribution of the CTX patients in the Italian regions. Within the years 1985 to 2015, we regularly followed 60 patients from almost all the Italian regions (Fig. 2.1).

Patients received regular annual observation and follow-up and were treated by chenodeoxycholic acid therapy [1].

A. Federico (✉) · G. N. Gallus · A. Mignarri · M. T. Dotti · A. Rufa
Department of Medicine, Surgery and Neurosciences, Medical School, University of Siena, Siena, Italy
e-mail: antonio.federico@unisi.it

A. Federico et al. (eds.), *Cerebrotendinous Xanthomatosis*,
https://doi.org/10.1007/978-3-031-92526-9_2

Fig. 2.1 Regional distribution of CTX patients followed by our group (1985–2015)

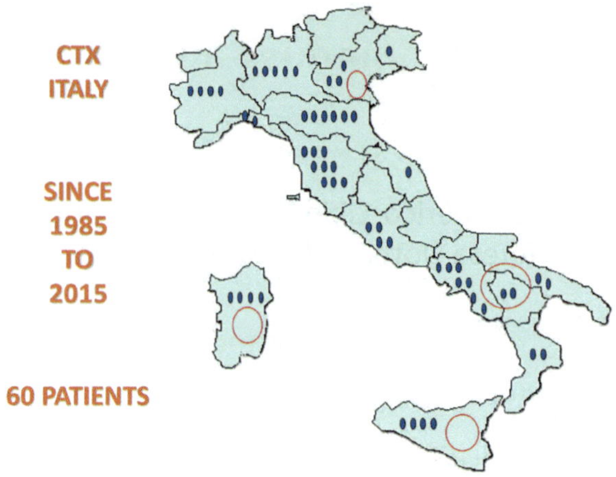

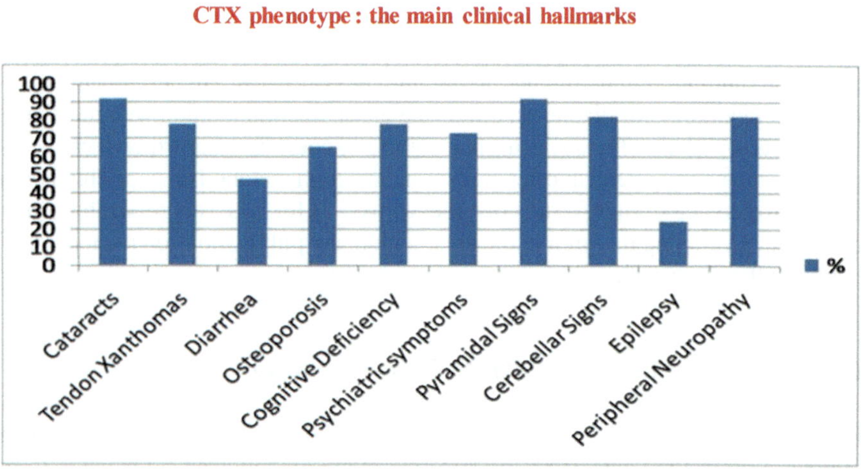

Fig. 2.2 Symptoms in the cohort of patients (% of total patients)

CTX Symptoms

Our patient cohort is mainly characterized by adult patients, in which the diagnosis has been made several years after the onset of signs and symptoms. The mean age is 35.5 ± 11.8. The symptoms are reported in Fig. 2.2, showing that cataracts, pyramidal signs and peripheral neuropathy were the main symptoms, followed by tendon xanthomas, cognitive deficiency, cerebellar signs and psychiatric symptoms. Osteoporosis was evident in more than 60% of cases. Chronic diarrhoea reported by patients by memory in childhood was described in 45% of our cohort. Epilepsy is present in 23% of cases. We had four patients without xanthomas and four with late onset cataracts.

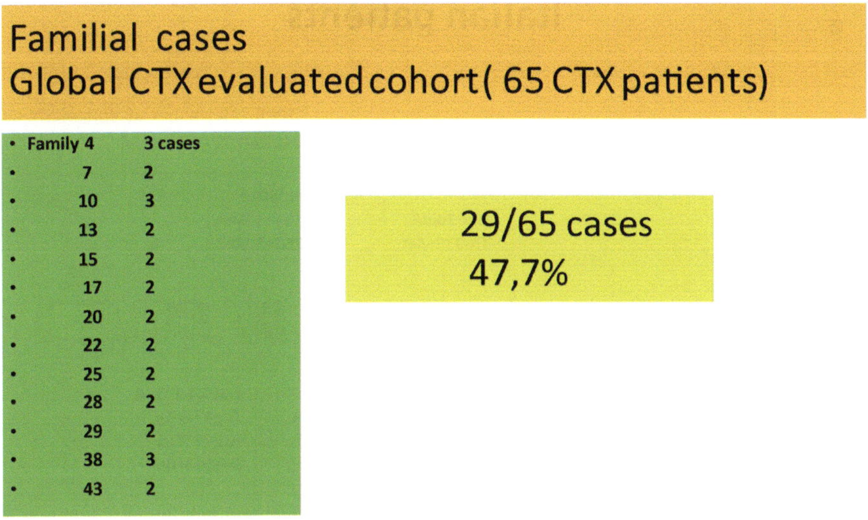

Fig. 2.3 Families with more than one affected individual

The patient cohort we have followed consist of 49 families (35 families with one affected subject, 11 families with two and 3 families with three affected individuals). Consanguinity was present in a few families. Families with more than one affected subject were 28.6% and familial patients were 47.7% of the total cohort (Fig. 2.3).

The delay of diagnosis has changed over the years in Italy. In the 1980s–1990s, our patients were mainly adults with 20–40 years of signs of the disease. With better knowledge of the disease by general neurologists and paediatricians in the following years, we diagnosed also juvenile patients and some neonates. However, the majority of patients are young adults with the full clinical symptomatology, and a final diagnosis was obtained 20–30 years after the onset of the first signs or symptoms.

The patients were annually followed in our Center with a follow-up including neurologic and neuropsychologic examinations, brain MRI evaluation, neurophysiologic and ophthalmologic examinations, bone mineral densitometry, cardiologic evaluation, general biochemical examinations, serum cholestanol and bile acids, urinary bile alcohols and mineral and vitamin D analyses.

Molecular Genetic Analyses

All patients have been genetically investigated by previously reported methods [2] and the results are reported in Fig. 2.4a, b.

The different pathogenic variants generally showed no geographic predilection; the pathogenic variant p.Arg479Cys *CYP27A1* has been found with a higher prevalence in Sardinia [3] .

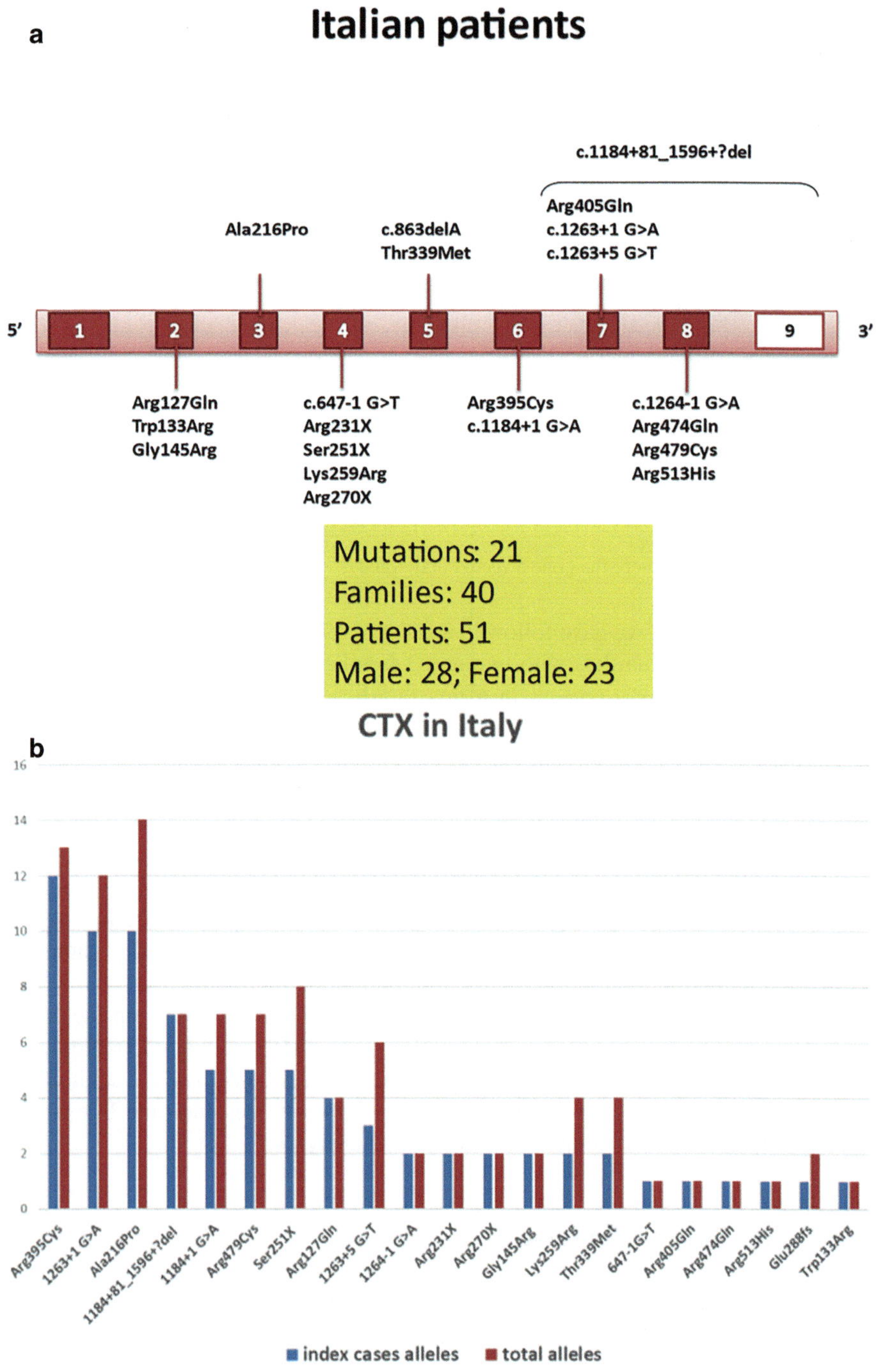

Fig. 2.4 (**a**) Distribution of pathogenic variants along the *CYP27A1* gene in 51 Italian CTX patients. (**b**) The frequency of pathogenic variants in Italian CTX patients

Therapeutic Approach

All patients have been treated with Chenodeoxycholic acid (CDCA) initially as an off-label prescription, followed after 2001 by a generic product, and after the EMA (European Medicine Agency) approval, by commercial CDCA, 250 mg orally three times daily with few side effects.

After the CDCA became temporarily unavailable in 2000 due to cessation of production of this drug by pharmaceutical companies (the drug was initially approved for treatment of gallstones but is no longer used for this purpose), patients remained therapeutic orphans. In collaboration with our Hospital Pharmacy after a few months, we produced a generic CDCA product, which was supplied to all patients at no cost, until the regulatory approval of commercial CDCA for CTX therapy by the EMA and in Italy by the AIFA (Italian Drug Agency, Agenzia Italiana del Farmaco) was achieved [4, 5].

In 2023, 47 CTX patients are under CDCA therapy in the different centres within the Italian Rare Disease Network. The majority are adult patients; the majority of them continuously receive CDCA (250 mg three times/day).

One patient, in which a neonatal diagnosis has been made followed by CDCA therapy, remained without any CTX symptoms over nearly 15 years follow-up. The child presented with neonatal cholestasis was diagnosed with CTX at the age of 2 months. The diagnosis was confirmed by demonstration of elevated cholestanol in serum and the molecular genetic analysis of the *CYP27A1* gene with homozygosity for a deletion of 1.9 Kb with loss of exons 7,8,9. CDCA therapy was immediately started with normalization of biochemical parameters after 2 months therapy and normal growth and development up to the age of 15 years: cholestanol before therapy was 3140 ± 55 μg/dl, normal controls 470 ± 87 μg/dl; after 14 months of therapy (10 mg/kg/day for 2 months, followed by 15 mg/kg/day for 5 years and after 100 mg × 3/day) cholestanol decreased to 600 μg/dl and after 2 years, it was completely normal [6].

In another case, combined therapy with simvastatin, CDCA, and plasmapheresis was utilized. Despite the consistent reduction of cholestanol to normal or even subnormal levels, a definite improvement of clinical symptoms was not noted [7].

Recently, in another Center in Italy, liver transplantation has been performed in a 4-month child with severe cholestasis, in which a CTX diagnosis was performed. He is free of any neurologic symptom over 2-year follow-up [8].

The CTX Suspicion Index

In 2014, we reported a CTX suspicion index, composed of weighted scores assigned to indicators such as family history characteristics and common systemic and neurological features, on the basis of a pooled analysis of selected international CTX series. The indicators were classified for suspicion for CTX as very strong (score 100), strong (50) or moderate (25). The suspicion index was then applied retrospectively to our CTX population. Early systemic signs such as cataract, diarrhoea and neonatal cholestatic jaundice were considered strong indicators, together with neurological features such as intellectual impairment, psychiatric disturbances, ataxia, spastic paraparesis and dentate nuclei abnormalities at MRI. Tendon xanthomas were regarded as very strong indicators, as was an affected sibling. A total score ≥100 warranted serum cholestanol assessment. Elevated cholestanol or a total score ≥200, with one very strong or four strong indicators, warranted *CYP27A1* gene analysis. In our patient cohort, age at diagnosis was 35.5 ± 11.8 years (mean ± standard deviation), whereas with the application of the diagnostic tool, the age of diagnosis, controlling the symptoms in the clinical history, became retrospectively possible at 10.6 ± 9.8 years ($p < 0.01$), theoretically allowing diagnosis and treatment of CTX before neurological disability occurred [9].

Peculiar Clinical Findings in Our Cohort

Muscle mitochondrial changes histochemically and electron microscopically [10] and biochemically detected with mitochondrial enzyme deficiency [11] have been reported in three and one, respectively, CTX patients who received muscle biopsy. However, serum and brain lactate (via MR brain spectroscopy) [12] was slightly elevated in many patients.

Evidence of lipomatous hypertrophy of the atrial septum has been reported in 4/9 CTX cases after transthoracic echocardiography, suggesting that careful cardiac examination should be considered, even in the absence of clinical manifestations [13].

Extensive investigations on bone metabolism have been reported, with abnormalities in vitamin D adsorption and improvement after CDCA therapy [14, 15].

In 13 patients, the second most frequent ocular abnormality after cataracts, which were found in all subjects, was optic disc paleness in 6 patients, signs of premature retinal senescence as retinal vessel sclerosis in 4, cholesterol like deposits and myelinated nerve fibres in 2 [16]. A thorough eye movement investigation was performed in 19 CTX patients and the data were compared with the neuroimaging findings, with particular regards to dentate atrophy: the most severe saccadic changes were evident in patients with more severe dentate nucleus abnormalities at MRI, confirming the important role of this cerebellar nucleus in involuntary eye movement control [17].

Extensive neuroimaging studies have been performed and those findings are reported in another article of this book [12].

CTX Care in Italy

The main centres for CTX diagnosis and care in Italy are Milan, Siena, Rome and Naples with a complete diagnostic set-up from the clinical, neurophysiological, neuroimaging, neurophthalmologic, biochemical and molecular genetic facilities. Siena for years was the unique centre involved in the CTX diagnosis and therapy. With the regulatory approval of CDCA therapy for CTX by AIFA, patients now may receive the drug approved by the local Health Service, through the local hospital, and usually are followed by their general practitioners and neurologists.

Italian Rare Diseases Program and Orphanet list 39 Italian certified centres for CTX therapy prescription. Four centres have all facilities for full diagnostic tests and are considered Reference Centers, which usually have an annual or biannual control of the patients they follow.

The therapy is completely covered by the National Health System for patients with a prescription performed by a Certified CTX Center within the Regional Rare Diseases Network. The actual cost of 100 capsules is more than 23,000 euros.

CTX Research in Italy

The main centres involved in CTX research are Siena (our centre, 31 publications), Milan (3 publications), Rome (6 publications) and Naples (6 publications).

PubMed reports 54 CTX publications in Italy within the years 1990–2023 (Table 2.1), indicating a great interest for the scientific community in the research of clinical and pathogenetic aspects of this disease.

Table 2.1 CTX publications reported by PubMed

Global publication	(1957–2023)	809
USA	(1974–2023)	77
Italy	(1990–2023)	54
The Netherlands	(1987–2023)	50
Germany	(1996–2023)	32
Israel	(1981–2023)	31
France	(1995–2023)	26
Sweden	(1994–2023)	26
Spain	(2000–2023)	20
Great Britain	(1996–2023)	12

Conclusions

CTX was extensively investigated in Italy over the last 40 years, with the goals of early clinical recognition followed by timely diagnosis and therapy. Patients receive a regular follow-up by multi-specialist teams in which neurologists or paediatricians are the leaders. Therapies are fully supported by the National Health Service. Some difficulties, however, are present for long-term neurorehabilitation as is the case for many chronic neurodegenerative diseases.

In Italy, a patient advocacy group has not yet formed and we hope that it will be created in the near future in order to support families, patients, research and care facilities, including the CTX neonatal screening programme.

Acknowledgements We thank all the members of the Unit of Neurometabolic and Clinical Neurology, University of Siena and of other Hospital and University Departments for their collaboration in this area. We are grateful to all patients, learning a lot from them about their disease, which was important for our research.

References

1. Federico A. Chenodeoxycholic acid therapy. In: Federico A, et al., editors. Cerebrotendinous xanthomatosis: a treatable rare neurometabolic disorder. Cham: Springer; 2025. This volume.
2. Gallus GN, Dotti MT, Federico A. Clinical and molecular diagnosis of cerebrotendinous xanthomatosis with a review of the mutations in the CYP27A1 gene. Neurol Sci. 2006;27(2):143–9.
3. Mandrile G, Gallus GN, Mura G, Di Sapio A, Sotgiu MA, Montella A, Giachino DF, Dotti MT, Ulgheri L, Federico A. Cerebrotendinous xanthomatosis: recurrence of the CYP27A1 mutation p.Arg479Cys in Sardinia. Neurol Sci. 2014;35(8):1303–5.
4. Federico A, Dotti MT. Treatment of cerebrotendinous xanthomatosis. Neurology. 1994;44(11):2218.
5. Federico A, Dotti MT. Chenodeoxycholic acid treatment in cerebrotendinous xanthomatosis in Italy. Neurology. 2001;157:1743.
6. Degrassi I, Amoruso C, Giordano G, Del Puppo M, Mignarri A, Dotti MT, Naturale M, Nebbia N. Case report: early treatment with chenodeoxycholic acid in cerebrotendinous xanthomatosis presenting as neonatal cholestasis. Front Pediatr. 2020;8:382.
7. Dotti MT, Lütjohann D, von Bergmann K, Federico A. Normalisation of serum cholestanol concentration in a patient with cerebrotendinous xanthomatosis by combined treatment with chenodeoxycholic acid, simvastatin and LDL apheresis. Neurol Sci. 2004;25(4):185–91.
8. Pietrobattista A, Spada M, Candusso M, Boenzi S, Dionisi-Vici C, Francalanci P, Morrone A, Ferri L, Indolfi G, Agolini E, Giordano G, Monti L, Maggiore G, Knisely AS. Liver transplantation in an infant with cerebrotendinous xanthomatosis, cholestasis, and rapid evolution of liver failure. Pediatr Transplant. 2022;26(6):e14318.
9. Mignarri A, Gallus GN, Dotti MT, Federico A. A suspicion index for early diagnosis and treatment of cerebrotendinous xanthomatosis. J Inherit Metab Dis. 2014;37(3):421–9.
10. Federico A, Dotti MT, Volpi N. Muscle mitochondrial changes in cerebrotendinous xanthomatosis. Ann Neurol. 1991;30(5):734–5.
11. Dotti MT, Manneschi L, Federico A. Mitochondrial enzyme deficiency in cerebrotendinous xanthomatosis. J Neurol Sci. 1995;129(2):106–8.

12. Cortese R, Manco C, De Stefano N. Overview of neuroimaging in cerebrotendinous xanthomatosis. In: Federico A, et al., editors. Cerebrotendinous xanthomatosis: a treatable rare neurometabolic disorder. Cham: Springer. This Volume.
13. Dotti MT, Mondillo S, Plewnia K, Agricola E, Federico A. Cerebrotendinous xanthomatosis: evidence of lipomatous hypertrophy of the atrial septum. J Neurol. 1998;245(11):723–6.
14. Federico A, Dotti MT, Loré F, Nuti R. Cerebrotendinous xanthomatosis: pathophysiological study on bone metabolism. J Neurol Sci. 1993;115(1):67–70.
15. Martini G, Mignarri A, Ruvio M, Valenti R, Franci B, Del Puppo M, Federico A, Nuti R, Dotti MT. Long-term bone density evaluation in cerebrotendinous xanthomatosis: evidence of improvement after chenodeoxycholic acid treatment. Calcif Tissue Int. 2013;92(3):282–6.
16. Dotti MT, Rufa A, Federico A. CTX: heterogeneity of clinical phenotype with evidence of undescribed ophthalmologic finding and premature aging. J Inherit Metab Dis. 2001;24:696–706.
17. Rosini F, Pretegiani E, Mignarri A, Optican LM, Serchi V, De Stefano N, Battaglini M, Monti L, Dotti MT, Federico A, Rufa A. The role of dentate nuclei in human oculomotor control: insights from cerebrotendinous xanthomatosis. J Physiol. 2017;595(11):3607–20.

Cerebrotendinous Xanthomatosis (CTX) in the Netherlands

3

Bianca M. L. Stelten, Hanka Dekker, and Aad Verrips

Introduction and History

Cerebrotendinous xanthomatosis (CTX) (OMIM #213700) was first described by the Belgian neurologist Ludo van Bogaert (1897–1989) who was a world-renowned neurologist and neuropathologist [1]. Initially, this disease was called van Bogaert-Scherer-Epstein disease, later to be replaced by an adequate but equally tongue twisting description of the main symptoms: Cerebrotendinous xanthomatosis. After the first description of the disease, it took several decades before the metabolic and genetic causes became clearer. CTX results from the deficiency of the enzyme sterol 27-hydroxylase, encoded by the *CYP27A1* gene [2]. The sequence of the human sterol 27-hydroxylase cDNA was first described in 1991 [3], and over time more than 120 different genetic variants have been reported. The classic symptomatology in CTX patients includes neonatal cholestasis, infantile-onset diarrhoea, juvenile-onset cataract, young adult-onset tendon xanthomas, and a variety of neurological and psychiatric manifestations in adult patients. The symptomatology can vary from nearly asymptomatic up to severe disability.

Figure 3.1 shows the bile acid synthesis in patients with CTX. Deficiency of the enzyme sterol 27-hydroxylase results in a shortage of the primary bile acids cholic acid (CA) and in particular chenodeoxycholic acid (CDCA). The absence of the negative feedback of CDCA results in increased activity of the enzyme 7α-hydroxylase (*CYP7A1*), the accumulation of bile acid precursors, cholestanol, bile alcohols and abnormal bile acids. Most of the cholestanol accumulation in patients with CTX derives from 7α-hydroxylated metabolites of cholesterol.

B. M. L. Stelten · H. Dekker · A. Verrips (✉)
Canisius-Wilhelmina Hospital, Department of Neurology, Nijmegen, The Netherlands
e-mail: a.verrips@cwz.nl

A. Federico et al. (eds.), *Cerebrotendinous Xanthomatosis*,
https://doi.org/10.1007/978-3-031-92526-9_3

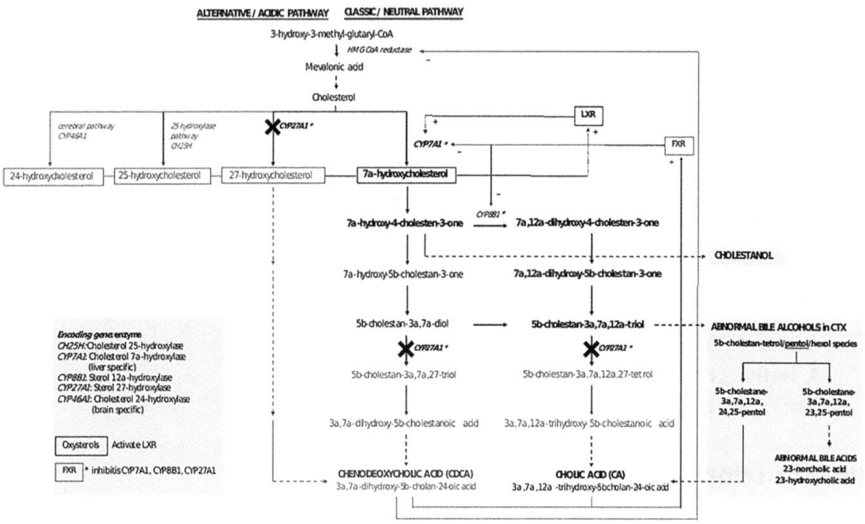

Fig. 3.1 Bile acid synthesis in patients with CTX (simplified version of a complex metabolic pathway) [4, 7–13]

The production of cholestanol from the bile acid precursor 7α-hydroxy-4-cholesten-3-one is of major importance for the accumulation of cholestanol in patients with CTX [4, 5].

Currently, the standard treatment is oral administration of CDCA, inhibiting *CYP7A1* via FXR, and HMG-CoA reductase, restoring the feedback inhibition. CDCA has been used as a therapy for CTX since 1975 [6]. CDCA was originally developed for the treatment of gallstones. Though no more than 100 patients with CTX, worldwide, were diagnosed at that time, off-label prescription of CDCA was followed and adapted worldwide by medical specialists who had patients with CTX in their care.

Expertise in the Netherlands

In the Netherlands, interest in Inborn Errors of Metabolism and in rare neurological diseases is usually present in university hospitals. The specific biochemical expertise in neurometabolic disorders like CTX was historically especially present in the Radboud university in Nijmegen. This university has a specific research institute for neurocognitive research called the Donders Institute, but also the translational metabolic laboratory in the children's hospital of the university, contributed to mapping symptoms with biochemical and genetical abnormalities. Furthermore, ophthalmologist prof. Dr. J.R.M. Cruysberg had a keen eye for diagnosing CTX in patients with cataracts in combination with chronic diarrhoea.

The study on CTX patients in the Netherlands started with the thesis of Dr. B.J. Koopman in Groningen in 1987: 'Cerebrotendinous xanthomatosis (CTX) and other inborn errors of metabolism in bile acid synthesis'. This was followed in 2000 by the thesis of Dr. A. Verrips in Nijmegen, 'Cerebrotendinous xanthomatosis. Some clinical, radiological, genetic and pathophysiological aspects'. At that time, there were 58 patients out of 32 unrelated families followed and treated with CDCA in the Netherlands that were described. Currently, the Canisius Wilhelmina Hospital in Nijmegen is the acknowledged reference- and expertise centre for CTX in the Netherlands. In 2023, Dr. B.M.L. Stelten finished a thesis on CTX, 'Cerebrotendinous xanthomatosis. A treatable error of metabolism'. The aim of this thesis was to expand the knowledge about the phenotypic heterogeneity in CTX, hopefully leading to a better and earlier recognition of this disease in clinical practice. A further aim was to describe the long-term follow-up treatment effects in the Dutch CTX cohort of 79 patients (56 patients with long-term follow-up data), the biggest cohort of CTX patients described so far.

The Dutch CTX Cohort

Diagnosis of CTX is often delayed by many years, losing a window of opportunity to start early treatment, preventing irreversible symptoms and shortening the diagnostic odyssey for patients and families. Research in the Netherlands focusses on expanding the knowledge about the phenotypic heterogeneity in CTX, as a strategy to improve awareness. Implementation of routine testing in patients who present with classic signs of CTX is the first strategy to improve detection.

There is considerable phenotypic heterogeneity in CTX and there is no clear genotype-phenotype correlation. 'Spinal xanthomatosis' is a clinical and radiological separate entity of CTX [14]. Our Dutch CTX cohort also showed that autism spectrum disorder (ASD) is an early and probably underestimated frequent feature in CTX [15]. Screening for CTX should be performed in patients with ASD, especially when accompanied by neonatal cholestasis, diarrhoea, intellectual disability, juvenile cataract and/or neurological involvement. Movement disorders represent a rare clinical feature in CTX but should be considered, particularly in case of early onset, and when associated with other neurological features and/or with systemic features (diarrhoea, cataract and tendon xanthomas). Parkinsonism seems to be a treatment-resistant feature in CTX patients [16]. While neurological symptoms are considered to be a clinical hallmark of untreated adult CTX patients, we observed untreated adult patients without neurological involvement, highlighting the existence of a 'milder phenotype', in which adult CTX patients may present with tendon xanthomas as the only or predominant feature [17]. In the Netherlands, there is also a shift in making a diagnosis of CTX, with whole exome sequencing as an important tool. Another strategy to improve the diagnosis of CTX is to incorporate the *CYP27A1* gene into diagnostic targeted gene panels. Unfortunately, in the Netherlands, there is no uniformity in gene panel content. One of the upcoming and promising developments to improve detection is newborn screening.

In chapter "Treatment During Pregnancy in Women with Cerebrotendinous Xanthomatosis (CTX)", the largest retrospective study reporting clinical long-term

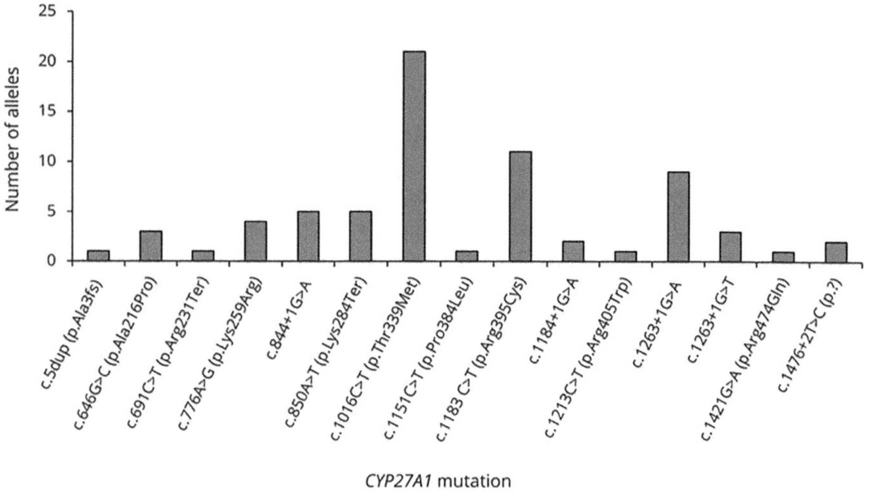

Fig. 3.2 Allele frequencies of *CYP27A1* variants in 54 Dutch patients with CTX (35 families, total of 70 alleles; in 2 siblings no genetic testing was done)

follow-up and MRI characteristics of Dutch patients with CTX is discussed [18, 19]. Figure 3.2 shows the allele frequencies of the *CYP27A1* variants found in this cohort in the Netherlands.

The Insurance System in the Netherlands

To fully understand the availability of CDCA for CTX patients, we must explain a little how the health insurance system in the Netherlands changed after the political decision to reform it from a public system (driven by governmental institutions) to a hybrid system (driven by private insurers, only partly under the responsibility of the government).

Curative medicine in the Netherlands is provided for every citizen under a single Health Insurance Act, which replaced a number of separate public and private health insurance types in 2006. Roughly 60% of the total healthcare budget is allocated towards services provided under the Health Insurance Act.

The Dutch health insurance system combines elements of public and private insurance. The central government is directly involved in implementing the Health Insurance Act and sets a number of public requirements which guarantee the social nature of the health insurance:

- Private individuals are required to purchase basic health insurance and are free to choose their own insurer.
- Health insurers are required to accept these private individuals under their policy, irrespective of their health condition.

- The premiums for a policy offered are equal for all policyholders, regardless of their health condition, age or background.
- Health insurers have a duty of care: they must guarantee that healthcare is available in the basic package for all their policyholders.
- The contents of the insured basic health insurance package are provided for under the law.

The central government is not directly involved in the actual implementation of the Health Insurance Act: the procedures involved are determined by healthcare providers, health insurers and insured parties. This structure ensures that healthcare providers have a great deal of freedom, while competition and market forces presumably create the incentives required to work efficiently and at a high quality level. The contents of the basic health insurance package (which has to be available for all) are determined by the government after advice of the National Healthcare Institute (Zorginstituut).

Availability of CDCA in the Netherlands

Historically in the Netherlands, it has not always been easy to get the prescribed CDCA treatment to CTX patients. In the early years, due to the rarity of the disease and the lack of diagnostic expertise, patients were often diagnosed late into the disease course. Delay in diagnosis from onset of symptoms was later reported to be between 15 and 25 years. If patients after diagnosis were prescribed CDCA, the actual access was most of the time up to the institutions where they were treated because of their neurologic problems and mental disability.

Until 2009, Chenofalk (CDCA) was available in the Netherlands, primarily used for the treatment of gallstones. In 1991, Ursodeoxycholic acid (UDCA) was deemed to be more effective by clinical specialists to treat gallstones than Chenodeoxycholic acid. As a result, the registration of CDCA was phased out in several countries. In the Netherlands, having a relatively small population and relatively high costs for keeping a drug on the market, this soon resulted in CDCA becoming hardly available in the pharmacy. Many of the pharmacists took the decision to replace the prescription for CDCA for UDCA acid. For CTX-patients, this replacement can worsen symptoms as it has been shown that Ursodeoxycholic acid is an ineffective inhibitor of bile acid synthesis [20]. It took interventions from clinical specialists towards the pharmacies to get them to go after a form of CDCA that was still available elsewhere. From 2009 until 2017, Xenbilox (CDCA) was available in the Netherlands, imported from Germany.

In 2017, CDCA was reintroduced in Europe as an orphan medicine for the treatment of CTX (CDCA-Leadiant), with an outrageous increase in price (500 fold), although the reintroduction was not accompanied with significant pharmaceutical enhancement. This medicine was rejected for reimbursement by all Dutch health insurances due to its high price. To ensure treatment for the patients in the

Netherlands, a magistral CDCA formula by a local Amsterdam UMC pharmacy was developed [21], which is reimbursed. Pharmacy compounded medicines can provide a good alternative for the treatment of patients with rare diseases.

References

1. Van Bogaert L, Scherer H, Epstein E. Une forme cérébrale de la cholestérinose généralisée. Paris: Masson et Cie; 1937.
2. Cali JJ, Hsieh CL, Francke U, Russell DW. Mutations in the bile acid biosynthetic enzyme sterol 27-hydroxylase underlie cerebrotendinous xanthomatosis. J Biol Chem. 1991;266(12):7779–83.
3. Cali JJ, Russell DW. Characterization of human sterol 27-hydroxylase. A mitochondrial cytochrome P-450 that catalyzes multiple oxidation reaction in bile acid synthesis. J Biol Chem. 1991;266(12):7774–8.
4. Björkhem I, Hansson M. Cerebrotendinous xanthomatosis: an inborn error in bile acid synthesis with defined mutations but still a challenge. Biochem Biophys Res Commun. 2010;396(1):46–9.
5. Panzenboeck U, Andersson U, Hansson M, Sattler W, Meaney S, Björkhem I. On the mechanism of cerebral accumulation of cholestanol in patients with cerebrotendinous xanthomatosis. J Lipid Res. 2007;48(5):1167–74.
6. Salen G, Meriwether TW, Nicolau G. Chenodeoxycholic acid inhibits increased cholesterol and cholestanol synthesis in patients with cerebrotendinous xanthomatosis. Biochem Med. 1975;14(1):57–74.
7. Verrips A. Cerebrotendinous xanthomatosis. Some clinical, radiological, genetic and pathophysiological aspects. Thesis, Nijmegen, The Netherlands, 2000.
8. Haas D, Gan-Schreier H, Langhans CD, et al. Differential diagnosis in patients with suspected bile acid synthesis defects. World J Gastroenterol. 2012;18(10):1067–76.
9. Chiang JYL. Regulation of bile acid synthesis: pathways, nuclear receptors, and mechanisms. J Hepatol. 2004;40(3):539–51.
10. Chiang JYL. Negative feedback regulation of bile acid metabolism: impact on liver metabolism and diseases. Hepatology. 2015;62(4):1315–7.
11. Crosignani A, Zuin M, Allocca M, Del Puppo M. Oxysterols in bile acid metabolism. Clin Chim Acta. 2011;412(23–24):2037–45.
12. Fuchs M. Bile acid regulation of hepatic physiology: III. Regulation of bile acid synthesis: past progress and future challenges. Am J Physiol Gastrointest Liver Physiol. 2003;284(4):551–7.
13. Koopman BJ, Wolthers BG, van der Molen JC, Nagel GT, Waterreus RJ, Oosterhuis HJ. Capillary gas chromatographic determinations of urinary bile acids and bile alcohols in CTX patients proving the ineffectivity of ursodeoxycholic acid treatment. Clin Chim Acta. 1984;142(1):103–11.
14. Verrips A, Nijeholt GJ, Barkhof F, et al. Spinal xanthomatosis: a variant of cerebrotendinous xanthomatosis. Brain. 1999;122(Pt 8):1589–95.
15. Stelten BML, Bonnot O, Huidekoper HH, van Spronsen FJ, van Hasselt PM, Kluijtmans LAJ, Wevers RA, Verrips A. Autism spectrum disorder in cerebrotendinous xanthomatosis. J Inherit Metab Dis. 2018;41(4):641–6. Corrigendum: J Inherit Metab Dis 2021; 44(6): 1507.
16. Stelten BML, van de Warrenburg BPC, Wevers RA, Verrips A. Movement disorders in cerebrotendinous xanthomatosis. Parkinsonism Relat Disord. 2019;58:12–6.
17. Stelten BML, Raal FJ, Marais AD, Riksen NP, Roeters van Lennep JE, Duell PD, van der Graaf M, Kluijtmans LAJ, Wevers RA, Verrips A. Cerebrotendinous xanthomatosis without neurological involvement. J Intern Med. 2021;290(5):1039–47.

18. Stelten BML, Huidekoper HH, van de Warrenburg BPC, et al. Long-term treatment effect in cerebrotendinous xanthomatosis depends on age at treatment start. Neurology. 2019;92(2):e83–95.
19. Stelten BML, Lycklama À, Nijeholt GJ, et al. Long-term MRI findings in patients with cerebrotendinous xanthomatosis treated with chenodeoxycholic acid. Neurology. 2002;99(13):559–66.
20. Batta AK, Salen G, Tint GS. Hydrophilic 7 beta-hydroxy bile acids, lovastatin, and cholestyramine are ineffective in the treatment of cerebrotendinous xanthomatosis. Metabolism. 2004;53(5):556–62.
21. Polak Y, Jacobs BAW, Kemper EM. Pharmacy compounded medicines for patients with rare diseases: lessons learned from chenodeoxycholic acid and cholic acid. Front Pharmacol. 2021;12:758210.

4 Landscape of Cerebrotendinous Xanthomatosis (CTX) Clinical Practice and Research in Brazil

Paulo Ribeiro Nóbrega, Helena Fussiger, and Jonas Alex Morales Saute

Cerebrotendinous xanthomatosis (CTX) is a rare autosomal recessive inherited metabolic lipid storage disorder related to bile acid biosynthesis pathways, caused by bi-allelic pathogenic variants in *CYP27A1* [14]. It was initially described in 1937 by Van Bogaert [20], and in 1968, the storage of cholesterol and cholestanol in tissues was demonstrated [13], enabling its biochemical diagnosis. Reports of CTX treatment with off-label use of chenodeoxycholic acid began in the 1970s [3], with the description of efficacy on neurological manifestations with long-term treatment more extensively described in 1984 by Berginer et al. [2]. More recently, in the 2010s, gene panel sequencing or exome sequencing by massive parallel sequencing (MPS) became available in clinical practice with repercussions for CTX diagnosis [4]. As we will see later, the availability of diagnostic technologies for CTX has had

P. R. Nóbrega
Division of Neurology, Department of Clinical Medicine, Universidade Federal do Ceará, Fortaleza, Brazil

Neurogenetics Unit, Department of Neurology, School of Medicine of Universidade de São Paulo, São Paulo, Brazil

H. Fussiger
Graduate Program in Medicine: Medical Sciences, Universidade Federal do Rio Grande do Sul, Porto Alegre, Brazil

J. A. M. Saute (✉)
Graduate Program in Medicine: Medical Sciences, Universidade Federal do Rio Grande do Sul, Porto Alegre, Brazil

Medical Genetics Service, Hospital de Clínicas de Porto Alegre, Porto Alegre, Brazil

Neurology Service, Hospital de Clínicas de Porto Alegre, Porto Alegre, Brazil

Department of Internal Medicine, Universidade Federal do Rio Grande do Sul, Porto Alegre, Brazil
e-mail: jsaute@hcpa.edu.br

A. Federico et al. (eds.), *Cerebrotendinous Xanthomatosis*, https://doi.org/10.1007/978-3-031-92526-9_4

a significant impact on patient access to diagnosis, as well as on the development of research projects focused on this condition carried out in Brazil.

On August 2 and 28, 2023, the CTX International Scientific Meeting took place in Jerusalem, Israel. During the Experience & Disease Spectrum for International CTX Patient Cohorts session, the study "Landscape of cerebrotendinous xanthomatosis clinical practice and research in Brazil" was presented. To construct this panorama, a search was conducted on MEDLINE/PubMed using the following terms: (Cerebrotendinous Xanthomatoses OR Xanthomatoses, Cerebrotendinous OR Cerebrotendinous Xanthomatosis OR Cerebral Cholesterinosis OR Cerebral Cholesterinoses OR Van Bogaert-Scherer-Epstein Disease OR Bogaert-Scherer-Epstein Disease, Van OR Disease, Van Bogaert-Scherer-Epstein OR Van Bogaert Scherer Epstein Disease) combined with the Boolean operator AND for the specific country, Brazil, and all countries in South America. The search was repeated in April 2024, yielding the same results. In total, 13 studies were found in Brazil, with the first one published in 2004. Additionally, through manual search, we found an additional reference from 1983, which seems to be the first report of the condition in the country, detailed below. The second country with the highest number of studies on CTX in South America was Chile, with 7, followed by Argentina with 4, Colombia with 3, and Suriname with 2. No studies were found in the other countries in the region (Fig. 4.1).

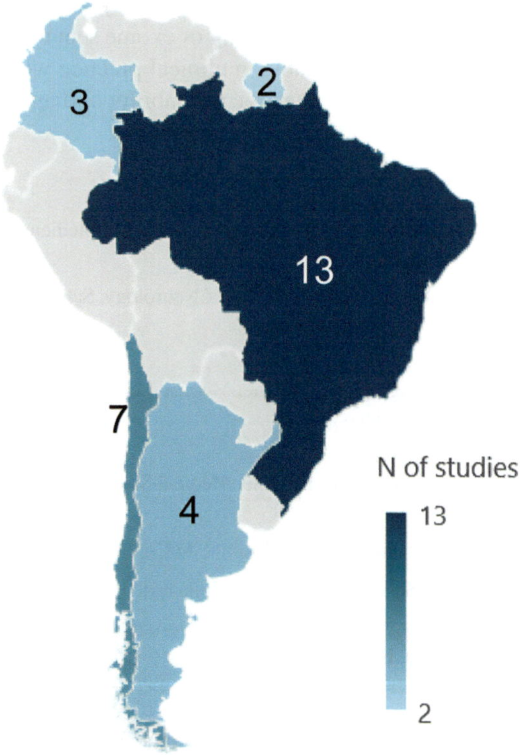

Fig. 4.1 Number of studies related to CTX found in MEDLINE search (April, 2024) among South American countries

CTX in Brazil

The first description of CTX in Brazil appears to have been made in 1983 by Canelas et al., who reported the case of two siblings born to a consanguineous couple, presenting with dementia, cataracts, and multiple xanthomas. In one of the cases, marked pyramidal findings were observed. Diagnostic confirmation was achieved by detecting significantly elevated levels of cholestanol in blood, bile, and tendon xanthomas [5]. There was a 20-year gap until the next report in 2004, which described the clinical history of two siblings with CTX from the Southern region of Brazil diagnosed through molecular analysis of *CYP27A1* [12]. These were likely the first CTX cases with identification of the causal genetic variant in Brazil, specifically the variant c.1183C > T/(p.Arg395Cys) in homozygosity. Other authors reported lipid peaks in cerebral Magnetic Resonance Spectroscopy of three patients with biochemical diagnosis of CTX [8], a single case of a patient with early-onset epilepsy as the main neurological manifestation also with biochemical diagnosis through cholestanol levels [16]. In 2014, a group of Brazilian authors participated in the validation of quantification of plasma ketosterol bile acid precursors by isotope dilution liquid chromatography-electrospray ionization-tandem mass spectrometry [7]. One of the cases whose samples were utilized in this validation was further detailed in 2015, highlighting spastic paraparesis as the primary neurological phenotype [19]. Additionally, two other variants in *CYP27A1*, namely, c.1435C > G/(p.Arg479Gly) and c.1435C > T/(p.Arg479Cys), were identified in compound heterozygosity. From this report onward, except for an educational article on neuroimaging aspects of a CTX case, all other cases reported in original articles were initially investigated through genetic testing rather than biochemical methods [4, 9–11].

Three main explanations may have driven this shift toward molecular testing as a first-tier diagnostic approach for CTX. The first is the unavailability of plasma cholestanol measurement by local Brazilian laboratories. In the case reported by Saute et al. [19], patient samples had to be sent to a reference laboratory in Oregon, USA, for confirmation, a scenario similar to other cases reported in the literature, highlighting the barrier to accessing biochemical diagnosis for this condition. The second explanation is that, starting in 2014, there was a greater local availability of massive parallel sequencing (MPS) analyses. This allowed for the sequencing of the *CYP27A1* gene through gene panel sequencing or even whole exome sequencing at Brazilian facilities. The third explanation is a local founder effect in Rio Grande do Sul (the southernmost state in Brazil) related to the findings described in the article by Burguez et al. in [4], detailed below.

Detecting CTX in Massive Parallel Sequencing and Hereditary Spastic Paraplegia as a Major Disease Phenotype

The case report by Saute et al. described a male patient presenting with spastic paraparesis starting at 28 years of age, with the sole neurological finding being pyramidal signs [19]. This was accompanied by Achilles tendon xanthomas present since adolescence, with no abnormalities found on spinal MRI. In reviewing this article, emphasis was given to the form of CTX most comprehensively described by Verrips et al. [21], known as spinal xanthomatosis, where, in addition to pyramidal and cataract findings, abnormalities in white matter on MRI were observed, with the presence of xanthomas being rare. The case described by Saute et al. and the spinal xanthomatosis phenotype described by Verrips led the Brazilian research group to consider the likely existence of CTX cases among patients with hereditary spastic paraplegias (HSP), both pure and complicated forms, that did not present with xanthomas or other manifestations clearly suggestive of CTX. In such cases, the diagnostic suspicion of CTX would not be strong enough to request a targeted confirmatory test. Therefore, the diagnosis would only become possible through a broader investigation, using gene panels that include *CYP27A1* or exome sequencing. In this scenario, patients with suspected HSP would be considered an enriched population for disease detection.

In 2014–2015, Saute and colleagues began describing the clinical and genetic aspects of HSP in Rio Grande do Sul through MPS, designing a panel that included 12 genes related to the most common subtypes of this group of diseases worldwide and potentially treatable subtypes, such as SPG5 and remarkably CTX. In 2017, the initial results with this panel were published. Among 29 index cases suspected of HSP, one patient with CTX homozygous for the variant in *CYP27A1*:c.1421G > A/ (p.Arg474Gln) was identified, presenting with a phenotype of HSP complicated by ataxia, parkinsonism, and early-onset cataracts without prior suspicion of CTX [4]. Currently, the concept of HSP phenotype being one of the main clinical presentations of CTX is well established, with pyramidal findings being more frequent than cerebellar signs, with several case reports of spinal xanthomatosis described as pure forms of spastic paraplegias [14]. The updated results from the case series in Southern Brazil in early 2023, investigating 95 index cases of HSPs, described CTX as the third most common form of HSP in the state (in six families), being the second most common autosomal recessive form, tied with SPG11 and SPG76, and only less frequent than SPG7 [9].

Clinicogenetic Characterization of Cerebrotendinous Xanthomatosis in Brazil

In 2022 and 2023, driven by the initiation of a randomized controlled placebo trial evaluating the efficacy of chenodeoxycholic acid (CDCA) on biomarkers related to bile acid metabolism (NCT04270682) in CTX patients across three Brazilian centers, there was a multicenter effort to characterize the Brazilian cases, which was also accelerated by the CTX International Scientific Meeting. In the poster titled "Clinicogenetic Characterization of Cerebrotendinous Xanthomatosis in Brazil" [15] presented at that meeting, the authors reported data from 38 Brazilian patients from six centers across four out of five regions of Brazil (North, Middle west, South, and Southeast). Main demographic and clinical data are presented in Table 4.1, with the distributions of age at onset and age at onset of neurological symptoms depicted in Fig. 4.2a-b.

Table 4.1 Clinical and demographic characteristics of Brazilian CTX patients

Families/patients	26/38	
Female sex (%)	18/38 (47.4%)	
Ethnicity		
Caucasian	18 (47.4%)	
Hispanic/Latin American	12 (31.6%)	
Latin American/ admixture	6 (15.8%)	
Oriental	1 (2.6%)	
Pardo	1 (2.6%)	
Brazilian region		
North	6 (15.8%)	
Northeast	5 (13.2%)	
South	8 (21.1%)	
Southeast	19 (50%)	
Phenotype ($n = 37$)		
Classic	32 (86.5%)	
Spinal	4 (10.8%)	
Non-neurologic	1 (2.7%)	
	Mean (SD)	*Median (IQR)*
Age	32.6 (14.7)	32 (18)
Age at onset[a] ($N = 36$)	11.2 (9.6)	9.5 (13)
Disease duration[a] ($N = 35$)	22.7 (14)	19 (22)
Age at onset of neurological disease ($N = 22$)	23.9 (13)	25 (16)
Disease duration of neurological disease ($N = 21$)	15.9 (9.3)	14 (15)
Walking aid (%)	21/37 (56.7%)	
AWA[b] *(95%CI)*	36 (26.3–45.6)	
DDWA[b] *(95%CI)*	24 (10.8–37.2)	
NDDWA (95%CI)	9 (6.9–11)	
Wheelchair bound (%)	9/37 (24.3%)	
AWC[b] *(95%CI)*	50 (39.2–60.7)	
DDWC[b] *(95%CI)*	43 (30.8–55.2)	
NDDWA (95%CI)	27 (16.5–37.5)	

Adapted from [15]

AWA age at walking aid dependency, *AWC* age at wheelchair dependency, *DDWA* disease duration at walking aid dependency, *DDWC* disease duration at wheelchair dependency, *NDDWA* neurologic disease duration at walking aid dependency, *NDDWC* neurologic disease duration at wheelchair dependency *IQR* interquartile range, *SD* standard deviation; [a] variables without normal distribution; [b] median from Kaplan-Meyer survival analysis

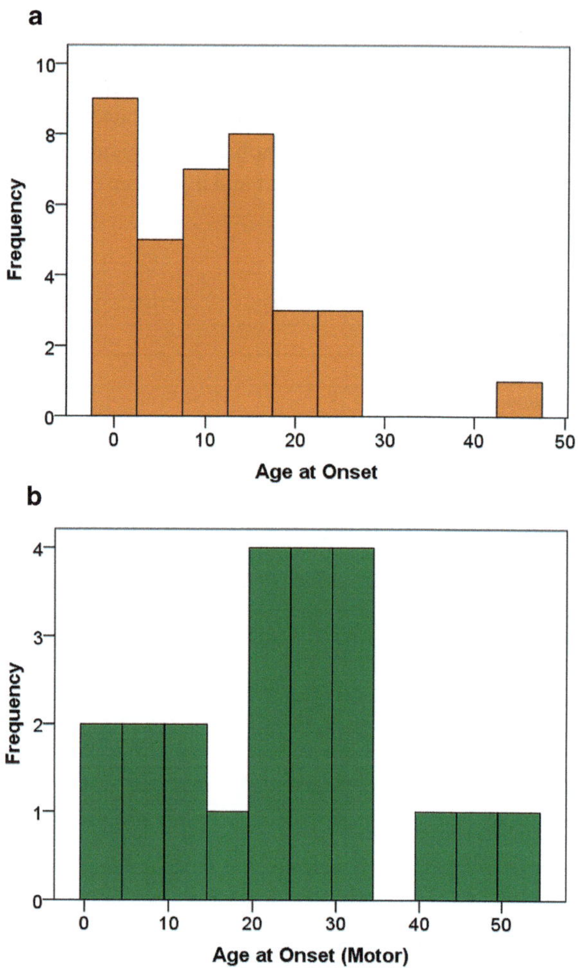

Fig. 4.2 Distribution of age at onset (**a**) and onset age of neurological symptoms (**b**) in CTX Patients from Brazil. Adapted from [15]

Genetic Characterization of the Brazilian Cohort

Genetic diagnosis was obtained in 37 out of 38 CTX probands (in one case, the diagnosis was solely based on cholestanol levels). Cholestanol levels were measured in 21/38 cases (55.2%), and they were elevated in all. The mean (standard deviation, SD) cholestanol level for cases in which values were reported was 1.15 (0.27) mg/dL. Thirteen variants in the *CYP27A1* (NM_000784.4) were identified, including three variants that had not been previously described (three likely pathogenic and one variant of uncertain significance, Fig. 4.3). The most frequent variants in Brazil were c.1183C > T/(p.Arg395Cys) found in 19 alleles from 12 families, being more common in the Northeast (5 out of 10 alleles, 50%) and Southeast (13 out of 26 alleles, 46.4%) regions; and c.1421G > A/(p.Arg474Gln), present in 9 alleles from 6 families, being more frequent in the South (4 out of 10 alleles, 40%)

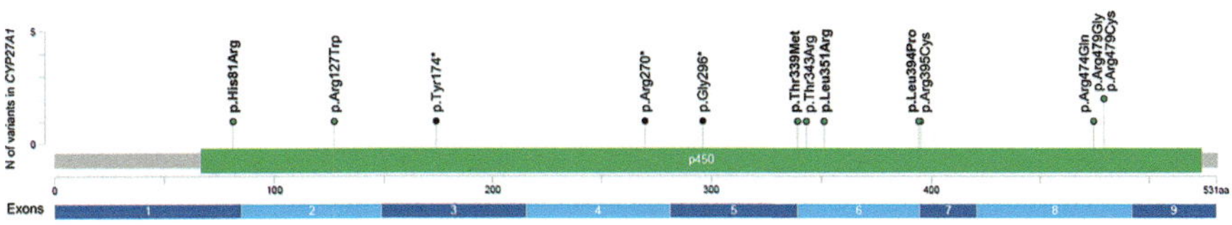

Fig. 4.3 Schematic representation of variants found in *CYP27A1* in CTX Patients from Brazil. Missense variants are represented with green dots and nonsense variants with black dots. Novel variants are depicted in bold. Adapted from [15].

Table 4.2 Variants in *CYP27A1 (NM_000784.4) in* CTX patients from Brazil

Nucleotide change	Classification	Alleles	Families	Brazilian region
c.1183C > T (p.Arg395Cys)	Pathogenic	19	12	5 NE, 1 S, 13 SE
c.1421G > A (p.Arg474Gln)	Pathogenic	9	6	1 NE, 4 S, 4 SE
c.1028C > G (p.Thr343Arg)	Pathogenic	5	4	1 S, 4 SE
c.1181 T > C (p.Leu394Pro)	**Likely pathogenic—PM2 sup, PM3, PP3 mod, PM1, PP4**	**3**	**2**	**2 NE, 1 SE**
c.1435C > G (p.Arg479Gly)	Pathogenic	3	2	1 S, 4 SE
c.245A > G (p.His81Arg)	**VUS—PM2 sup, PM3 sup, PP4**	**2**	**1**	**1 SE**
c.379C > T (p.Arg127Trp)	Pathogenic	2	1	1 N
c.1052 T > G (p.Leu351Arg)	**Likely pathogenic—PP3 strong, PM2 sup, PM3 sup, PP4**	**2**	**1**	**1 SE**
c.1016C > T (p.Thr339Met)	**Likely pathogenic—PP3 strong, PM2 sup, PP4**	**1**	**1**	**1 NE**
c.522 T > A (p.Tyr174*)	Pathogenic	1	1	1 S
c.808C > T (p.Arg270*)	Pathogenic	1	1	1 S
c.886C > T (p.Gly296*)	Pathogenic	1	1	1 NE
c.1435C > T (p.Arg479Cys)	Pathogenic	1	1	1 S

N North, *NE* Northeast, *SE* southeast, *S* South, *VUS* variant of uncertain significance. Novel variants are depicted in bold with 2015 American College of Medical Genetics [18] criteria provided. Adapted from [15]

and Southeast (4 out of 26 alleles, 15.4%, Table 4.2) regions. Only three variants were of the loss-of-function type, all of them being nonsense variants. All other variants were missense. The age of onset and phenotype of cases with loss-of-function variants were similar to those of others, but due to the small sample size, it was not possible to conduct statistical tests for genotype/phenotype correlations.

Clinical and Neuroimaging Findings

The most frequent initial symptom of CTX was cataract (27%), followed by xanthomas (24%), chronic diarrhea (13.5%), and developmental delay (13.5%). The most common non-neurological symptoms during the disease were cataract (83.8%) and xanthomas (70.3%, Fig. 4.4a), with a median (interquartile range, IQR) age at cataract diagnosis ($N = 13$) of 17 [15] years and at xanthoma appearance ($N = 8$) of 13.5 [10] years. The most frequent neurological signs/symptoms were cognitive decline (80.5%), with a mean (SD) onset at 20.5 (7.4) years ($N = 7$), and psychiatric symptoms (75%). The most common motor findings were spastic paraparesis (56.7%), with a mean onset at 23.2 (6.8) years ($N = 11$), and ataxia (48.6%) with a mean onset at 26.1 (14.9) years ($N = 9$). Other neurological findings present in over 5% of cases are shown in Fig. 4.4b. The most frequent brain magnetic resonance imaging (MRI)

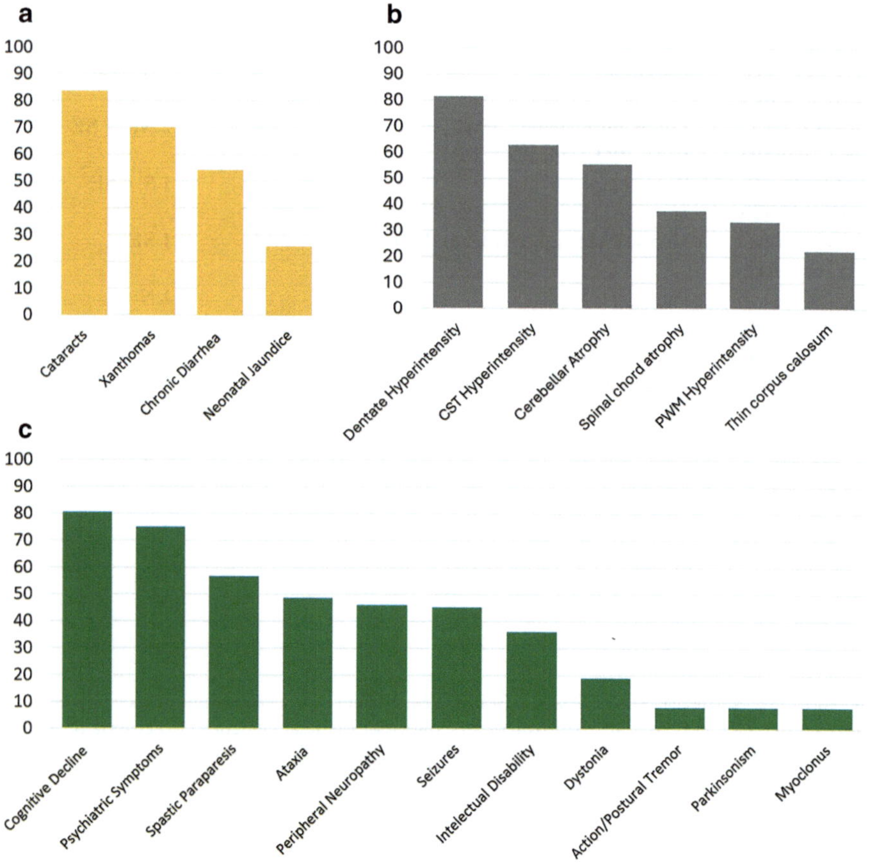

Fig. 4.4 Most frequent clinical and neuroimaging findings in CTX Patients from Brazil. (**a**) Most frequent systemic, (**b**) neurological, and (**c**) magnetic resonance imaging findings. Adapted from [15]. CST, corticospinal tract; PWM periventricular white matter

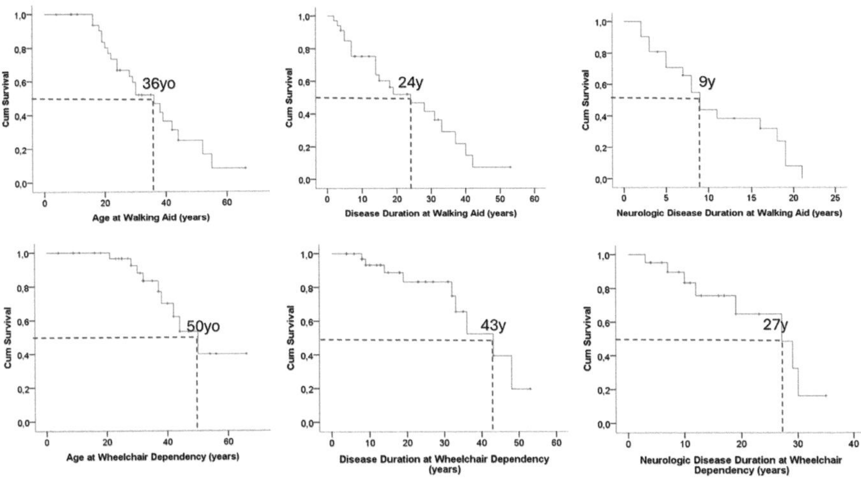

Fig. 4.5 Progression to major motor handicap in CTX patients from Brazil. Adapted from [15]

findings ($N = 27$) were hyperintensity in T2/FLAIR of dentate nuclei at the cerebellum (81.5%) and corticospinal tract (62.7%); and in spinal cord MRI ($N = 16$) spinal cord atrophy (37.5%), with only 1 out of 16 cases showing T2/FLAIR hyperintensity on the posterior funiculi, as detailed in Fig. 4.4c.

Regarding the progression of neurological impairment, the frequency of walking aids and wheelchair necessity, as well as the medians of age, disease duration, and neurological involvement duration when initiating the use of walking aids and wheelchairs, were presented in Table 4.1 and Fig. 4.5a-f. While the median disease duration until the need for walking aids and wheelchair was 24 and 43 years, respectively, the median for the need for walking aids dropped to 9 years when considering only the duration of the neurological symptoms. These results are important for understanding the clinical course of the disease and highlight that there is a significant interval between symptom onset and the onset of neurological symptoms, and that the reduction in mobility capacity and loss of functional independence will be associated with the neurological onset of the disease. In another perspective, the results draw attention to the detection of the disease while there is still no neurological picture, presenting an opportunity window for treatment, which seems to be effective in improving or reducing the progression of neurological symptoms when initiated earlier [19].

Pharmacological Treatment

In Brazil, the authorization for the use of medications is granted by the National Health Surveillance Agency (ANVISA), and treatment with CDCA does not have registration with ANVISA. Access to medications without ANVISA registration in Brazilian territory is very unusual and can individually occur through obtaining the medication from other countries through direct patient purchase, but for high-cost medications, this process is practically unfeasible. The Unified Health System of Brazil (SUS) was established in 1990 to fulfill the constitutional understanding that health is a right for all, and providing it is a duty of the Brazilian state. Article 196 of the Brazilian Federal Constitution, which considers health as a right of all and a duty of the state, serves as the starting point for the judicialization of access to high-cost treatments like CDCA [6]. The absence of registration with ANVISA becomes a significant barrier to obtaining such treatments, even through judicial means. This results in highly unequal access to such treatments in Brazilian territory and does not allow for collective purchase of the medication and negotiation of its price.

CDCA in Brazil

In the Brazilian case series, only 16 out of 38 (42.1%) patients received treatment with CDCA, of which three discontinued treatment—one due to poor adherence, one due to persistent transaminase elevation that resolved upon treatment discontinuation, and one due to unknown reasons. However, the treatment coverage in practice was much lower, as only six patients were on CDCA for more than 1 year, and none of these cases reported symptom improvement, with stabilization or deterioration of the condition observed. Most patients receiving more recent treatment were enrolled in clinical trials with undisclosed results (NCT04270682). Seventeen out of 34 patients (50%) for whom information was available were on statins, with four of them concurrently taking CDCA and statins. The effect of statins in improving symptoms or prognosis of CTX is still controversial [17]. None of the patients was on cholic acid.

The absence of registration with ANVISA is not the only significant barrier to CDCA treatment in Brazil, both within the context of SUS and private insurances. Brazil is a middle-income country, and even in high-income countries like the Netherlands, there was a discontinuation of CDCA supply for CTX patients after it was approved by the European Medicines Agency as an orphan drug and obtained market authorization in 2017. This discontinuation was due to a drastic price increase that rendered health insurance companies unable to reimburse this drug, which subsequently affected the availability of CDCA for CTX patients [3]. In Brazil, the decision regarding reimbursement and adoption of novel therapies within SUS is based on scientific criteria, including evidence of efficacy, effectiveness, economic evaluation, and budget impact analysis. These evaluations are conducted by the National Committee for Health Technology Incorporation (Conitec), an organization established in 2011 and modeled after international agencies such as the National Institute for Health and Care Excellence (NICE) in the United Kingdom and Canada's Drug and Health Technology Agency (CADTH). Therefore, approval by ANVISA does not automatically guarantee access to therapies within the SUS context; approval and incorporation of this technology by Conitec are also necessary.

The price history of CDCA is noteworthy. In the case of the Netherlands, CDCA was initially commercialized for the treatment of gallstones under the brand name

Chenofalk®, priced at €0.28 per capsule, costing €308 per patient per treatment year at that time. Subsequently, after CDCA was developed as Xenbilox® by Sigma-Tau, this company acquired the rights for Chenofalk® and later for Chenix®, a Belgian firm. Through establishing a monopoly position, Sigma-Tau gradually increased the price to approximately €29 per capsule. In 2015, CDCA was removed from the Dutch market for gallstone treatment [1]. Following this, Sigma-Tau rebranded as Leadiant and registered CDCA as an orphan drug for CTX treatment in 2017, significantly increasing the price to approximately €150,000 per patient per year in the Dutch market, representing a price surge of 500 times. The utilization of orphan drug regulations to escalate prices and obtain 10 years of market exclusivity is likely to pose challenges to CDCA incorporation into SUS, unless a substantial deal with a marked price reduction is proposed. Low- and middle-income countries like Brazil should also explore the option of local production by national laboratories of generic or biosimilar CDCA to address the affordability issue for effective CTX treatment.

Conclusion

While reports of CTX are relatively few compared to the North American and European populations, the recently described Brazilian case series stands as one of the largest global series. It underscores the need to expand access to biochemical and genetic diagnostic methods for CTX in Brazilian territory, as well as to seek sustainable ways for patient treatment, ensuring that maximum benefit can be achieved at the appropriate time.

Acknowledgments We would like to express our gratitude to the other authors and centers that participated in the collaborative study of CTX in Brazil and who were co-authors of the poster presented at the CTX International Scientific Meeting [15] and in a manuscript that is currently under submission, listed as follows: Karina Carvalho Donis, Wladimir Bocca Vieira de Rezende Pinto, Luciana Negrão Almeida Morais, Fernando Kok, Emília Katiane Embiruçu de Araújo Leão, Pedro Lucas Grangeiro de Sá Barreto Lima, Fernando Freua, Pedro Braga-Neto, Antonette Souto El Husny, and Paulo Victor Sgobbi de Souza. We also extend our thanks to Brazilian patients and families affected by CTX. The English language revision was conducted with the assistance of an artificial intelligence language model developed by OpenAI.

References

1. Bayoumy AB, de Boer NKH, Ansari AR, Crouwel F, Mulder CJJ. Unrealized potential of drug repositioning in Europe during COVID-19 and beyond: a physician's perspective. J Pharm Policy Pract. 2020 Jul 17;13:45. https://doi.org/10.1186/s40545-020-00249-9.
2. Berginer VM, Salen G, Shefer S. Long-term treatment of cerebrotendinous xanthomatosis with chenodeoxycholic acid. N Engl J Med. 1984 Dec 27;311(26):1649–52. https://doi.org/10.1056/NEJM198412273112601.
3. Bouwhuis N, Jacobs BAW, Kemper EM. Product development and quality of pharmacy compounded chenodeoxycholic acid capsules for Dutch cerebrotendinous xanthomatosis patients. Front Pharmacol. 2023 Oct 17;14:1264997. https://doi.org/10.3389/fphar.2023.1264997.

4. Burguez D, Polese-Bonatto M, Scudeiro LAJ, Björkhem I, Schöls L, Jardim LB, Matte U, Saraiva-Pereira ML, Siebert M, Saute JAM. Clinical and molecular characterization of hereditary spastic paraplegias: a next-generation sequencing panel approach. J Neurol Sci. 2017 Dec 15;383:18–25. https://doi.org/10.1016/j.jns.2017.10.010.
5. Canelas HM, Quintão EC, Scaff M, Vasconcelos KS, Brotto MW. Cerebrotendinous xanthomatosis: clinical and laboratory study of 2 cases. Acta Neurol Scand. 1983 May;67(5):305–11. https://doi.org/10.1111/j.1600-0404.1983.tb04580.x.
6. D'Ippolito PIMC, Gadelha CAG. O tratamento de doenças raras no Brasil: a judicialização e o Complexo Econômico-Industrial da Saúde. Saúde debate. 2020 Jun 19;43(spe4):219–31.
7. DeBarber AE, Luo J, Giugliani R, Souza CF, Chiang JP, Merkens LS, Pappu AS, Steiner RD. A useful multi-analyte blood test for cerebrotendinous xanthomatosis. Clin Biochem. 2014 Jun;47(9):860–3. https://doi.org/10.1016/j.clinbiochem.2014.04.017.
8. Embiruçu EK, Otaduy MC, Taneja AK, Leite CC, Kok F, Lucato LT. MR spectroscopy detects lipid peaks in cerebrotendinous xanthomatosis. AJNR Am J Neuroradiol. 2010 Aug;31(7):1347–9. https://doi.org/10.3174/ajnr.A1885.
9. Fussiger H, Pereira BLDS, Padilha JPD, Donis KC, Rare-Genomes Project Consortium, Siebert M, Brusius-Facchin AC, Baldo G, Saute JAM. Copy number variations in SPAST and ATL1 are rare among Brazilians. Clin Genet. 2023 May;103(5):580–4. https://doi.org/10.1111/cge.14280.
10. Jacinto-Scudeiro LA, Dariva Machado G, Ayres A, Burguêz D, Polese-Bonato M, González-Salazar C, Siebert M, Cavalcante França M, Jr Olchik MR, Morales Saute JA. Are cognitive changes in hereditary spastic paraplegias restricted to complicated forms? Front Neurol. 2019a May 24;10:508. https://doi.org/10.3389/fneur.2019.00508.
11. Jacinto-Scudeiro LA, Machado GD, Ayres A, Burguêz D, Polese-Bonatto M, González-Salazar C, Siebert M, França Junior MC, Olchik MR, Saute JAM. Prevalence of oropharyngeal dysphagia in hereditary spastic paraplegias. Arq Neuropsiquiatr. 2019b Dec;77(12):843–7. https://doi.org/10.1590/0004-282X20190180.
12. Lange MC, Zétola VF, Teive HA, Scola RH, Trentin AP, Zavala JA, Pereira ER, Raskin S, Werneck LC, Sistermans EA. Cerebrotendinous xanthomatosis: report of two Brazilian brothers. Arq Neuropsiquiatr. 2004 Dec;62(4):1085–9. https://doi.org/10.1590/s0004-282x2004000600028.
13. Menkes JH, Schimschock JR, Swanson PD. Cerebrotendinous xanthomatosis. The storage of cholestanol within the nervous system. Arch Neurol. 1968 Jul;19(1):47–53. https://doi.org/10.1001/archneur.1968.00480010065004.
14. Nóbrega PR, Bernardes AM, Ribeiro RM, Vasconcelos SC, Araújo DABS, Gama VCV, Fussiger H, Santos CF, Dias DA, Pessoa ALS, Pinto WBVR, Saute JAM, de Souza PVS, Braga-Neto P. Cerebrotendinous Xanthomatosis: a practice review of pathophysiology, diagnosis, and treatment. Front Neurol. 2022 Dec 23;13:1049850. https://doi.org/10.3389/fneur.2022.1049850.
15. Nóbrega PR, Donis KC, Pinto WBVR, Morais LNA, Kok F, Leão EKEA, Camargos ST, Fussiger H, Lima PLGSB, Freua F, Braga-Neto P, El Husny AS, Sgobbi de Souza PV, Saute JA. Clinicogenetic characterization of Cerebrotendinous Xanthomatosis in Brazil. In: CTX international scientific meeting. Jerusalem; 2023.
16. Pedroso JL, Pinto WB, Souza PV, Santos LT, Abud IC, Avelino MA, Barsottini OG. Early-onset epilepsy as the main neurological manifestation of cerebrotendinous xanthomatosis. Epilepsy Behav. 2012 Jul;24(3):380–1. https://doi.org/10.1016/j.yebeh.2012.04.121.
17. Ribeiro RM, Vasconcelos SC, Lima PLGSB, et al. Pathophysiology and treatment of lipid abnormalities in Cerebrotendinous Xanthomatosis: An Integrative Review. Brain Sci. 2023;13(7):979. https://doi.org/10.3390/brainsci13070979.
18. Richards S, Aziz N, Bale S, Bick D, Das S, Gastier-Foster J, Grody WW, Hegde M, Lyon E, Spector E, Voelkerding K, Rehm HL. ACMG laboratory quality assurance committee. Standards and guidelines for the interpretation of sequence variants: a joint consensus recommendation of the American College of Medical Genetics and Genomics and the Association for Molecular Pathology. Genet Med. 2015 May;17(5):405–24. https://doi.org/10.1038/gim.2015.30.

19. Saute JA, Giugliani R, Merkens LS, Chiang JP, DeBarber AE, de Souza CF. Look carefully to the heels! A potentially treatable cause of spastic paraplegia. J Inherit Metab Dis. 2015;38(2):363–4. https://doi.org/10.1007/s10545-014-9745-0. Epub 2014 Aug 12. PMID: 25112387.
20. Stelten BML, Huidekoper HH, van de Warrenburg BPC, Brilstra EH, Hollak CEM, Haak HR, Kluijtmans LAJ, Wevers RA, Verrips A. Long-term treatment effect in cerebrotendinous xanthomatosis depends on age at treatment start. Neurology. 2019 Jan 8;92(2):e83–95. https://doi.org/10.1212/WNL.0000000000006731.
21. Van Bogaert L, Scherer HJ, Froehlich A, Epstein E. Une deuxieme observation de cholesterinose tendineuse avec symptomes cerebraux. Ann Med. 1937;42:69–101.
22. Verrips A, Nijeholt GJ, Barkhof F, Van Engelen BG, Wesseling P, Luyten JA, Wevers RA, Stam J, Wokke JH, van den Heuvel LP, Keyser A, Gabreëls FJ. Spinal xanthomatosis: a variant of cerebrotendinous xanthomatosis. Brain. 1999 Aug;122(Pt 8):1589–95. https://doi.org/10.1093/brain/122.8.1589.

Cerebrotendinous Xanthomatosis (CTX) in France

5

Fanny Mochel

Introduction

Given the overall estimated prevalence of cerebrotendinous xanthomatosis (CTX), from 1/50,000 (East and South Asia) to 1/150,000 (Europe, America, and Africa) [2], the number of patients reported so far in France is rather low. Indeed, in 2022, the national platform for rare diseases in France (Banque Nationale de Données Maladies Rares) has registered only 21 French patients with CTX. This may be explained by the variety of medical specialists who take care of CTX patients in France, several of them who do not belong to reference centers for inherited metabolic diseases. This includes isolated cases seen by endocrinologists—especially patients with predominantly tendon xanthomas and no overt neurological diseases [6]—but also psychiatrists. Overall, it is likely that there are no less than 50 patients with CTX in France.

Our national reference center for inherited metabolic diseases in La Pitié-Salpêtrière hospital (director: Prof. Fanny Mochel) focuses primarily on adult neurometabolic diseases. As a result, we follow most of French adult patients with CTX. In 2016, we reported the natural history study of 14 patients for whom reliable retrospective data were available [3]. In 2018, we reported therapeutic outcomes of 13 patients treated with chenodeoxycholic acid (CDCA) with standardized neurological and neuroimaging measures [1]. Our center also participated to the international expert opinion study on diagnosis and treatment of CTX, together with Dutch, Italian, Israeli, Turkish, and Northern American centers [7].

F. Mochel (✉)
Reference Center for Adult Neurometabolic Diseases and Leukodystrophies, Department of Medical Genetics of APHP, Sorbonne University, Paris Brain Institute (ICM), La Pitié-Salpêtrière University Hospital, Paris, France
e-mail: fanny.mochel@icm-institute.org

A. Federico et al. (eds.), *Cerebrotendinous Xanthomatosis*,
https://doi.org/10.1007/978-3-031-92526-9_5

Natural History of French Patients with CTX

We enrolled nine female and four male patients with CTX in a natural retrospective history study [3]. The higher proportion of women has already been described in CTX. Our main observations were that almost all patients were diagnosed in adulthood—mean and median age at diagnosis were 30.4 ± 14.9 years and 24.5 years (range: 14–55), respectively—whereas all patients had symptom onset as children. Likewise, the mean and median disease duration at the time of diagnosis were 26.2 ± 11.6 years and 21.5 years (range: 13.5–54.5), respectively. This finding has two major implications. First is the need for pediatricians to search for CTX in any child with chronic diarrhea, or liver dysfunction, or cataract. Second is the relevance of newborn screening programs. Indeed, as the development of symptoms can be halted or prevented by supplementation with CDCA, early treatment is essential. Nevertheless, it is unknown yet whether attenuated phenotypes [6] will be detected by NBS, but if they are, it does raise a concern about the common principle of treating all CTX patients detected by NBS [4].

Another important finding of our natural history study was the phenotypic spectrum that we observed, as well as the sequence of these symptoms. Of course, this is biased by our primary expertise in neurometabolic disorders and, therefore, predominant referral of patients with neurological symptoms. Accordingly, clinical tendon xanthomas were rare, and none of our patients had a history of infantile liver dysfunction. Instead, infantile chronic diarrhea was very common, followed by cataract and school difficulties between 5 and 15 years of age (Fig. 5.1). It took another 5–15 years for patients to develop motor (pyramidal, cerebellar, and/or neuropathic) and/or psychiatric symptoms (Fig. 5.1), emphasizing the need for an early diagnosis of CTX during childhood or adolescence. No patient had developed cardiovascular symptoms, but osteopenia was documented in a third of them. All patients had T2- or FLAIR-weighted hyperintensities of the dentate nuclei and increased plasma cholestanol at the time of diagnosis. We did not measure bile acids concentrations in our cohort.

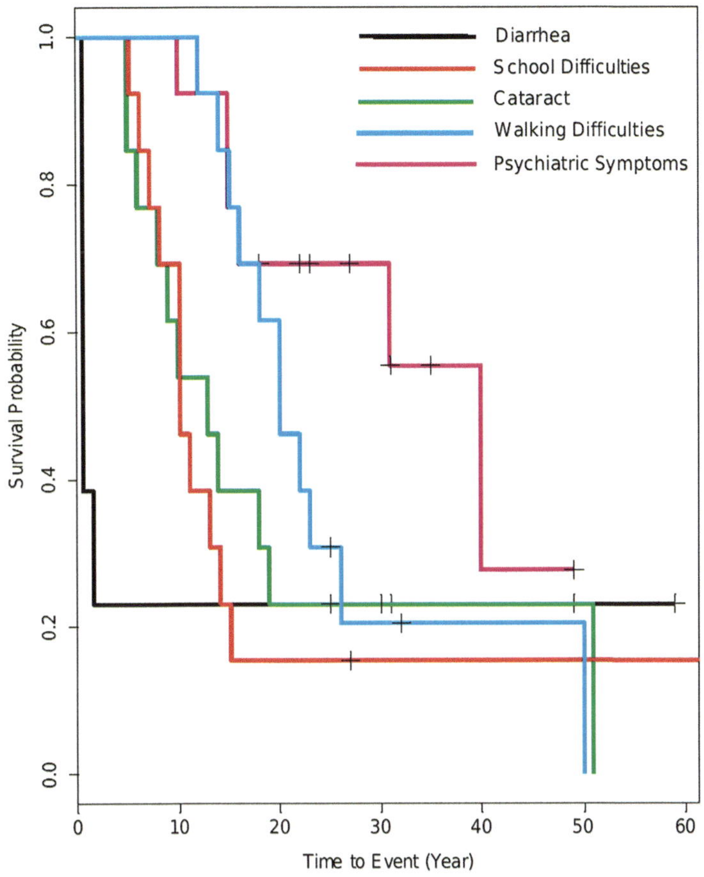

Fig. 5.1 Kaplan–Meier analyses indicate the natural history of 13 patients with CTX for time to diarrhea, cataract, school difficulties, walking difficulty, and psychiatric symptoms

French Experience with CDCA in CTX

All patients followed in our reference center for inherited metabolic diseases have had long-term access to CDCA, initially under compassionate use, then early access programs up until CDCA was commercialized in France. In our report of retrospective neurological and neuroimaging outcomes of patients treated with CDCA for 2–9 years, we enrolled 11 women and 3 men with CTX [1]. Our main observation was that CDCA was well tolerated in all patients, without liver toxicity, and led to disease stabilization or improvement in most patients. The few patients who kept deteriorating under CDCA had the longest treatment delay (>25 years after neurological symptom onset), as reported in other cohorts [5, 8].

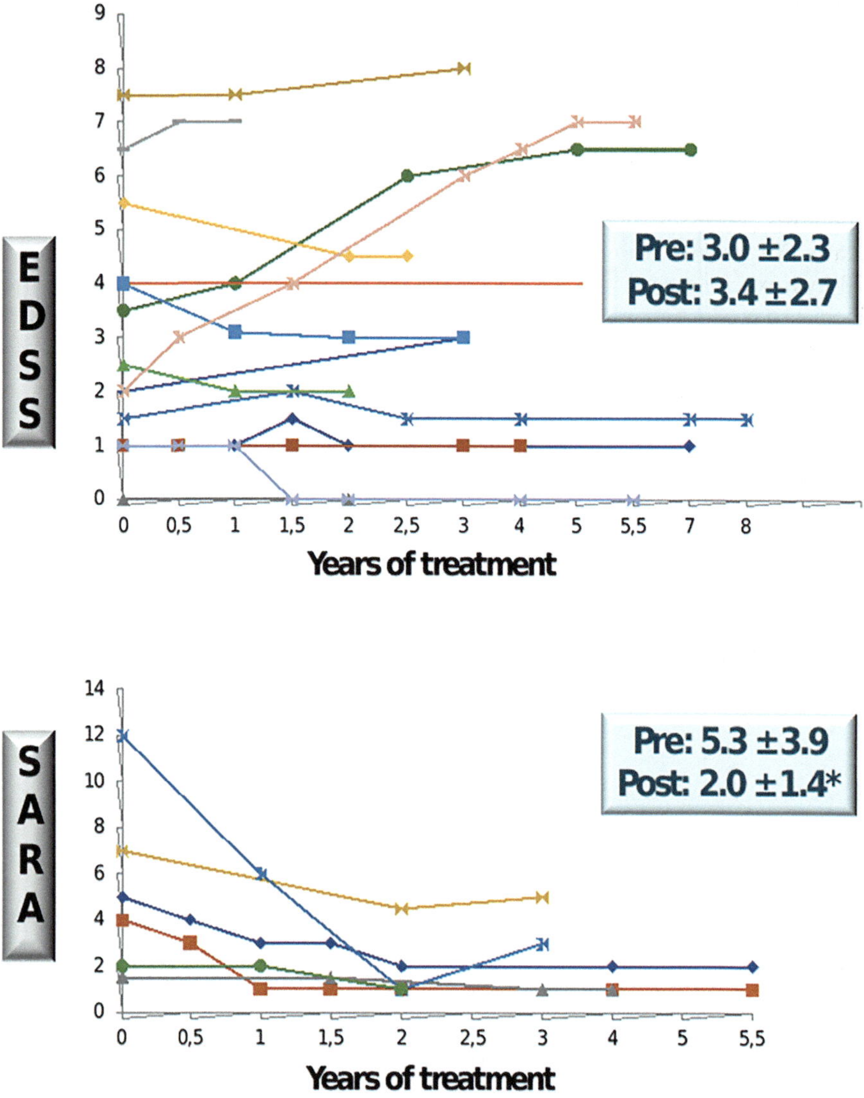

Fig. 5.2 Evolution of the Expanded Disability Status Scale (EDSS, $n = 14$) and Scale for the Assessment and Rating of Ataxia (SARA, $n = 6$) in patients before (pre) and on (post) CTX treated with CDCA. *Significant change

Despite the retrospective nature of our data, we were able to demonstrate that CDCA led to significant improvement of standardized neurological scores (Fig. 5.2), such as the Expanded Disability Status Scale (EDSS) and the Scale for the Assessment and Rating of Ataxia (SARA), as well as nerve conduction parameters. This is remarkable as very few neurodegenerative disorders can benefit from treatments that can reverse neurological dysfunctions.

We completed our cohort study with neuroimaging analyses that comprised both volumetric analyses and measures of white matter trophicity using diffusion tensor imaging (DTI). Although we had a small sample size, we observed no overt volume loss in CTX patients treated with CDCA. Instead, we found an improvement in a fraction of anisotropy and radial diffusivity with CDCA in regions of interest in CTX, i.e., the pontocerebellar tracts and the internal capsules [1].

Conclusion

Our French experience in CTX is very much in line with what has been reported in other countries. The natural history study emphasizes that most patients exhibit symptoms as children. The treated cohort study highlighted that neurological dysfunction can be halted, and even reversed, by metabolic intervention such as CDCA supplementation if treatment onset is early enough. Both studies support the development of newborn screening programs. The observation that not all adult patients with CTX develop neurological dysfunction calls for the identification of sensitive biomarkers to detect brain disease activity before the onset of neuropsychiatric manifestations.

References

1. Amador MDM, et al. Treatment with chenodeoxycholic acid in cerebrotendinous xanthomatosis: clinical, neurophysiological, and quantitative brain structural outcomes. J Inherit Metab Dis. 2018;41(5):799–807. https://doi.org/10.1007/s10545-018-0162-7.
2. Appadurai V, et al. Apparent underdiagnosis of cerebrotendinous xanthomatosis revealed by analysis of ~60,000 human exomes. Mol Genet Metab. 2015;116(4):298–304. https://doi.org/10.1016/j.ymgme.2015.10.010.
3. Degos B, et al. Natural history of cerebrotendinous xanthomatosis: a paediatric disease diagnosed in adulthood. Orphanet J Rare Dis. 2016;11:41. https://doi.org/10.1186/s13023-016-0419-x.
4. Hollak CEM. Expanding the clinical spectrum of cerebrotendinous xanthomatosis: implications for newborn screening, follow-up and treatment. J Intern Med. 2021;290(5):942–3. https://doi.org/10.1111/joim.13276.
5. Stelten BML, et al. Long-term treatment effect in cerebrotendinous xanthomatosis depends on age at treatment start. Neurology. 2019;92(2):e83–95. https://doi.org/10.1212/WNL.0000000000006731.
6. Stelten BML, et al. Cerebrotendinous xanthomatosis without neurological involvement. J Intern Med. 2021;290(5):1039–47. https://doi.org/10.1111/joim.13277.
7. Stelten BML, et al. Expert opinion on diagnosing, treating and managing patients with cerebrotendinous xanthomatosis (CTX): a modified Delphi study. Orphanet J Rare Dis. 2021;16(1):353. https://doi.org/10.1186/s13023-021-01980-5.
8. Yahalom G, et al. Neurological outcome in cerebrotendinous xanthomatosis treated with chenodeoxycholic acid: early versus late diagnosis. Clin Neuropharmacol. 2013;36(3):78–83. https://doi.org/10.1097/WNF.0b013e318288076a.

Cerebrotendinous Xanthomatosis (CTX) in Japan

6

Shingo Koyama and Yoshiki Sekijima

Introduction

Cerebrotendinous xanthomatosis (CTX: OMIM#213700) is a rare autosomal-recessive lipid storage disorder caused by pathogenic variants in the *CYP27A1* gene, which encodes the key enzyme in bile acid synthesis, sterol 27-hydroxylase (CYP27A1, EC 1.14.15.15) [1]. To date, over 100 pathogenic variants, including missense, nonsense, splice-site, and insertion/deletion variants, have been reported worldwide [2]. Decreased activity of sterol 27-hydroxylase leads to impaired bile acid synthesis, resulting in reduced production of bile acids, especially chenodeoxycholic acid (CDCA), in addition to elevated serum cholestanol and urine bile alcohols. Clinical presentation is characterized variably by neonatal jaundice or cholestasis, refractory diarrhea, juvenile cataracts, tendon xanthomas, osteoporosis, coronary heart disease, and progressive neuropsychiatric disturbances including intellectual disability or dementia, psychiatric symptoms, pyramidal and cerebellar signs, progressive myelopathy, peripheral neuropathy, extrapyramidal manifestations, and seizures though symptoms vary tremendously between patients [3–10]. The broad and diverse clinical symptoms likely contribute to a substantial diagnostic delay [3–5, 9, 10]. Replacement treatment with CDCA in the early stage of the disease has been reported to improve or even prevent clinical symptoms of CTX [11, 12]; however, there is a crucial "point of no return," after which treatment initiation can no longer reverse signs and symptoms or halt the progression of the

S. Koyama (✉)
Department of Neurology, National Hospital Organization Yamagata National Hospital, Yamagata, Japan
e-mail: skoyama@med.id.yamagata-u.ac.jp

Y. Sekijima
Department of Medicine (Neurology & Rheumatology), Shinshu University School of Medicine, Matsumoto, Japan

A. Federico et al. (eds.), *Cerebrotendinous Xanthomatosis*,
https://doi.org/10.1007/978-3-031-92526-9_6

disease [13]. CTX patients have been reported worldwide, but prevalence of the disease is considered to be underestimated [14, 15]. Although several large series of CTX patients have been reported from the Netherlands [3], Italy [5], and the United States [8], only one nationwide survey has been conducted in Spain, in which 25 CTX patients were reported, and the minimum estimated prevalence was one in 1,800,000 individuals [4]. A genetic epidemiological study based on the Exome Aggregation Consortium (ExAC) cohort estimated the incidence of CTX. Among East Asians, including Japanese population, the estimated incidence is 1:64,247–1:64,712 [16]. Surprisingly, based on this estimation, the number of Japanese patients is calculated to be between 1961 and 1975. However, CTX is likely to be underdiagnosed, and the precise epidemiology of CTX is largely unknown. Therefore, we conducted a nationwide survey on CTX in Japan [9]. In this chapter, we will focus on the results of our survey and discuss the issues on CTX that should be resolved in Japan.

Nationwide Survey on CTX in Japan

To elucidate the frequency, clinical characteristics, and molecular genetics of Japanese CTX patients, we conducted the first nationwide survey on CTX. Detailed information on CTX patients was analyzed based on the questionnaires. In the primary survey, we contacted 2541 departments of neurology, cardiology, and pediatrics across Japan to investigate the number of patients with suspected or confirmed CTX who had visited affiliated hospitals between September 2012 and August 2015, and 1032 (40.6%) returned completed. In the secondary survey, we collected clinical data, including symptoms, *CYP27A1* genotype, cholestanol/cholesterol levels, radiological findings, physiological findings, and treatment response. A diagnosis of CTX was made if the patient fulfilled the criteria of definite or probable CTX described in Table 6.1.

Diagnosis of CTX and Definition of Clinical Phenotype

We established original criteria in this study that included clinical symptoms, biochemical findings, genetic testing, and differential diagnosis (Table 6.1). At least one CTX clinical symptom and elevated serum cholestanol are necessary for diagnosing possible CTX. Excluding other conditions with elevated cholestanol is necessary for diagnosing probable CTX. A definite diagnosis of CTX is confirmed by the presence of biallelic pathogenic variants in the *CYP27A1* gene. In our study, CTX was categorized into three phenotypes: the classical form, spinal form, and non-neurological form. Classical form CTX patients exhibited neurological symptoms attributed to the brain (cerebrum, cerebellum, and/or brainstem). In the present study, we defined spinal form as CTX patients whose neurological symptoms were limited to the spinal cord. The non-neurological form CTX patients were without

Table 6.1 Diagnostic criteria for cerebrotendinous xanthomatosis used in this study

A. Symptoms
1. Tendon xanthoma
2. Progressive neurological dysfunctions[a] or intellectual disability
3. Juvenile cataract
4. Juvenile coronary artery disease
5. Chronic unexplained diarrhea
6. Juvenile osteoporosis
7. Prolonged neonatal cholestasis
B. Biochemical finding
Elevated serum cholestanol level (>4.5 μg/mL)
C. Genetic testing
Pathogenic variants in the *CYP27A1* gene (homozygosity or compound heterozygosity)
D. Differential diagnosis
Increased serum cholestanol level due to following diseases should be excluded
Familial hypercholesterolemia
Sitosterolemia
Obstructive biliary tract diseases
Hypothyroidism
<Diagnostic category>
Definite: At least one of symptom in A and B + C + D
Probable: At least one of symptom in A and B + D
Possible: At least one of symptom in A and B

Reprinted by permission of the publisher [10]

[a]Representative progressive neurological dysfunctions include cognitive dysfunction, cerebellar symptoms, pyramidal symptoms, extrapyramidal symptoms, seizure, peripheral neuropathy, and sensory disturbance attributed to spinal cord

any apparent neurological symptoms. In the non-neurological form CTX, patients without genetic testing were excluded from the study because it is difficult to distinguish this phenotype from sitosterolemia without genetic testing.

Demographic, Clinical, and Radiological Features of Japanese CTX Patients

In our survey, 40 patients (20 male and 20 female) met the criteria of definite (18 subjects) or probable (22 subjects) and were included in the analysis. Thirty-four patients were registered from the department of neurology, three patients from the department of metabolism/endocrinology, and one patient each from the departments of cardiology, orthopedics, and dermatology. No patients were reported from the department of pediatrics. The age of onset ranged from 0 to 50 years (mean ± standard deviation [SD]: 24.5 ± 13.6 years, Fig. 6.1a) and the age at diagnosis ranged from 5 to 71 years (mean ± SD: 41.0 ± 11.6 years, Fig. 6.1b). The duration of illness from onset of signs or symptoms to diagnosis ranged from 0 to 57 years (mean ± SD:

16.5 ± 13.5 years) and displayed a bimodal distribution (Fig. 6.1c). The duration of illness from onset to diagnosis was significantly longer in patients who developed CTX before the age of 15 (mean ± SD: 27.1 ± 16.8 years) compared to those whose onset was 15 years or older (mean ± SD: 12.4 ± 9.6 years, $P = 0.008$), suggesting a notable diagnostic delay, particularly among pediatric patients.

At the time of the survey, the most common symptom was tendon xanthoma ($n = 38$, 95.0%), followed by intellectual disability/cognitive impairment ($n = 28$, 70.0%), spastic paraplegia ($n = 26$, 65.0%), juvenile cataract ($n = 24$, 60.0%), cerebellar ataxia ($n = 17$, 42.5%), sensory disturbance attributed to spinal cord/disturbance of posterior column ($n = 13$, 32.5%), coronary artery disease ($n = 8$, 20.0%), chronic unexplained diarrhea ($n = 8$, 20.0%), parkinsonism/dystonia ($n = 8$, 20.0%), peripheral neuropathy ($n = 5$, 12.5%), epilepsy ($n = 4$, 10.0%), and juvenile osteoporosis/pathologic fracture ($n = 4$, 10.0%) (Fig. 6.2). In our survey, the majority of cases showed xanthomas in Japan. However, it is noteworthy that the presence of xanthomas is a characteristic feature of the disease, but it is not mandatory for CTX diagnosis [17]. Although the high frequency of xanthomas could be due to the potential underdiagnosis of pediatric patients who have not yet developed xanthomas, CTX patients without xanthomas may be overlooked in Japan.

All subjects underwent brain MRI, and abnormal hyperintense signals on T2-weighted and/or fluid-attenuated inversion recovery (FLAIR) images were observed in 85.0% of patients. Primary sites of abnormal intensity were the dentate nucleus of the cerebellum ($n = 25$, 62.5%), cerebral white matter ($n = 17$, 42.5%), corticospinal tract ($n = 13$, 32.5%), cerebellar white matter ($n = 8$, 20.0%), substantia nigra ($n = 4$, 10.0%), corpus striatum ($n = 2$, 5.0%), globus pallidus ($n = 2$, 5.0%), and thalamus ($n = 2$, 5.0%). Atrophy of the cerebrum was observed in 40.0% ($n = 16$), cerebellum in 45.0% ($n = 18$), and brainstem in 22.5% ($n = 9$) of patients. Spinal cord MRI of 21 patients revealed abnormal hyperintense signals on T2-weighted images in eight patients. Abnormal intensity was mainly located in the cervical cord ($n = 8$), followed by the thoracic cord ($n = 4$) and lumbar cord ($n = 2$), in the dorsal and/or lateral column. These abnormal findings are consistent with previously reported MRI characteristics of CTX patients [18–20].

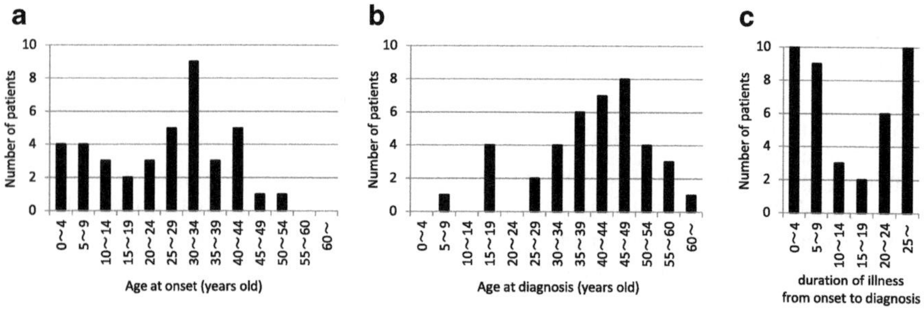

Fig. 6.1 Distribution of age at onset (**a**), age at diagnosis (**b**), and duration of illness from onset to diagnosis (**c**) among Japanese cerebrotendinous xanthomatosis patients

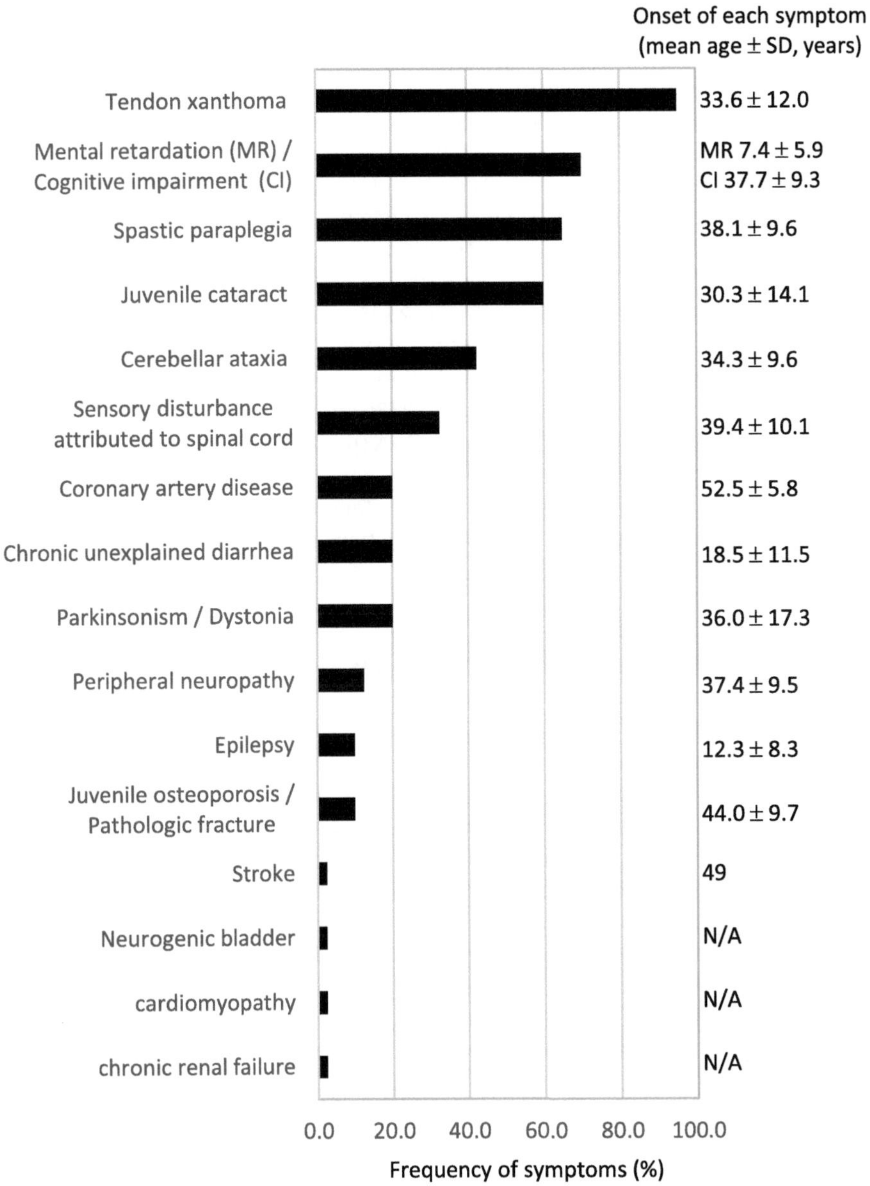

Fig. 6.2 Frequency of symptoms and onset of each symptom among Japanese cerebrotendinous xanthomatosis patients. N/A indicates data on age of onset was not available

CYP27A1 Genotype in Japanese CTX Patients

Genetic analysis of the *CYP27A1* gene, performed on 19 patients, revealed 10 different variants in our survey. The most common variant in Japanese CTX patients was c.1214G>A (p.R405Q, 31.6%), followed by c.1421G>A (p.R474Q, 26.3%), c.435G>T (p.G145=, 13.2%), c.1420C>T (p.R474W, 7.9%), c.1176_1117delGA (5.3%), c.254A>G (p.Q85R, 2.6%), c.673C>T (p.R225C, 2.6%), c.1004C>T (p.A335V, 2.6%), c.1238T>A (p.V413D, 2.6%), and c.1342_1343insCACC (2.6%). A clustering of *CYP27A1* variants in particular ethnic groups has been reported: c.1016C>T (p.T339M), c.1183C>T (p.R395C), and c.1263+1G>A in the Netherlands [21], c.646G>C (p.A216P), c.1183C>T (p.R395C), c.1184+1G>A, c.1263+1G>A, and a 1.9 kb deletion including exons 7–9 in Italy [22], c.1183C>T (p.R395C) in northwestern Spain, and c.1213C>T (p.R405W) in southern Spain [4]. The present survey revealed that c.1214G>A (p.R405Q), c.1421G>A (p.R474Q), and c.435G>T (p.G145=) were the three most common variants in Japanese CTX, accounting for >70% of variant alleles. This finding seems consistent with the allele frequency of these variants in six global populations reported in the ExAC database (Table 6.2).

Comparison Between Clinical Subtypes

There were 30 patients with the classical form, six with the spinal form, and four with the non-neurological form. In addition to the classical and spinal forms, we have introduced the non-neurological form of CTX as a third clinical subtype in this study. This form has also been described by investigators in the Netherlands [23]. Although patients with the non-neurological form may later develop neurological symptoms, two genetically confirmed CTX patients in their 50s showed no evidence of neurological symptoms even after more than 20 years since first symptom onset. One developed tendon xanthoma at age 27 and was diagnosed with CTX at age 48. At the time of investigation at age 50, the symptoms were tendon xanthoma and cataracts. The other had tendon xanthoma at age 30 and was diagnosed with CTX at age 45. There were no symptoms other than tendon xanthoma at the time of investigation at age 50. After the diagnosis, they received combination therapy of CDCA and HMG-CoA inhibitor. Therefore, we regarded the non-neurological form as a distinct clinical phenotype of CTX. The spinal form patients tended to develop the symptoms of disease later in life (mean ± SD age: 32.8 ± 5.5 years) as compared with those exhibiting the classical form (mean ± SD age: 22.5 ± 14.5 years) or the non-neurological form (mean ± SD age: 27.3 ± 11.6 years), although the differences were not statistically significant. The spinal form patients also showed significantly lower serum cholestanol levels as compared with the classical form (Table 6.3), in contrast to a previous report [4]. A possible reason for this discrepancy may lie in the definition of the spinal form CTX: spinal form patients in the present study

Table 6.2 Allele frequencies of *CYP27A1* variants according to Exome Aggregation Consortium database (version 0.3)

Variant	AFR	AMR	EAS	FIN	NFE	SAS
p.G145=	0.00000	0.00000	0.00040	0.00000	0.00000	0.00000
p.A216P	0.00000	0.00000	0.00000	0.00000	0.00004	0.00000
p.T339M	0.00000	0.00000	0.00010	0.00000	0.00002	0.00007
p.R395C	0.00010	0.00020	0.00000	0.00030	0.00020	0.00006
p.R405W	0.00000	0.00009	0.00000	0.00000	0.00000	0.00006
p.R405Q	0.00010	0.00009	0.00050	0.00000	0.00004	0.00000
p.R474W	0.00000	0.00000	0.00000	0.00000	0.00002	0.00000
p.R474Q	0.00000	0.00000	0.00010	0.00000	0.00002	0.00000
c.1184+1G>A	0.00000	0.00000	0.00000	0.00000	0.00006	0.00070
c.1263+1G>A	0.00000	0.00009	0.00010	0.00000	0.00007	0.00000

Reprinted by permission of the publisher [11]
AFR African, *AMR* Admixed American, *EAS* East Asian, *FIN* Finnish, *NFE* Non-Finnish European, *SAS* South Asian

Table 6.3 Demographic and characteristics of the patient population separated by clinical phenotype of cerebrotendinous xanthomatosis

Clinical phenotypes	Classical form	Spinal form	Non-neurological form
Sex	M 17, F 13	M 2, F 4	M 1, F 3
Age at onset (years old)	22.5 ± 14.5	32.8 ± 5.5	27.3 ± 11.6
Age at diagnosis (years old)	39.3 ± 10.4	50.8 ± 12.3	38.5 ± 15.1
Age at survey (years old)	45.6 ± 13.3	58.0 ± 13.2	41.3 ± 14.4
Serum cholestanol level (μg/ml)*	24.0 ± 9.5	11.9 ± 9.6	12.3 ± 12.3
Tendon xanthoma	96.7%	83.3%	100%
Diarrhea	26.7%	0%	0%
Cataract	66.7%	50.0%	25.0%
Osteoporosis	13.3%	0%	0%
Coronary artery disease	16.7%	33.3%	25.0%
Modified Rankin Scale**	3.1 ± 1.2	2.8 ± 1.8	0.5 ± 0.6
CYP27A1 genotype	p.R474Q 40.9%, p.R474W 13.6% p.R405Q 22.7%, p.G145 = 9.1% c.1176_1117delGA 9.1% p.A335V 4.5%, p.V413D 4.5% c.1342_1343insCACC 4.5%	p.R405Q 87.5% p.Q85R 12.5%	p.G145 = 37.5% p.R405Q 25.0% p.R225C 12.5% p.R474Q 12.5%

Reprinted by permission of the publisher [10]
M male, *F* female
*Classical form vs Spinal form: $P = 0.03$
**Classical form vs Non-neurological form: $P = 0.003$, Spinal form vs Non-neurological form: $P = 0.03$

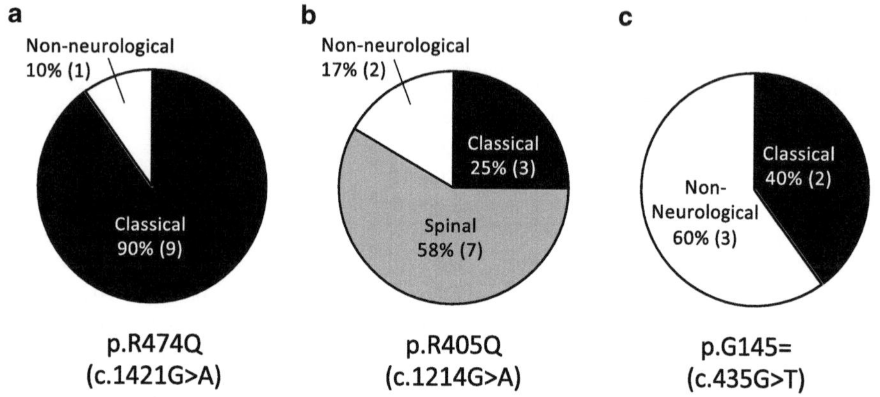

Fig. 6.3 Genotype–phenotype correlation among Japanese cerebrotendinous xanthomatosis patients. The percentage of alleles (number of alleles) associated with each clinical phenotype is shown. (**a**) p.R474Q (c.1421G>A). (**b**) p.R405Q (c.1214G>A). (**c**) p.G145 = (c.435G>T).

possessed no neurological symptoms other than myelopathy, while those described by Pilo-de-la-Fuente showed various neurological symptoms other than myelopathy [4]. The classical form patients were more likely to have general symptoms, including diarrhea, cataract, and osteoporosis, compared to other subtypes. As expected, subjects with the non-neurological form showed significantly lower modified Rankin Scale, as compared with the other clinical phenotypes (vs. classical form: $P = 0.003$, vs. spinal form: $P = 0.03$, Table 6.3). Whereas earlier reports indicated no correlation between any given variant and any specific symptom, onset age, or severity [3, 4], this survey revealed possible associations between c.1421G>A (p.R474Q) and classical form CTX, c.1241G>A (p.R405Q) and spinal form CTX, and c.435G>T and non-neurological form CTX (Table 6.3 and Fig. 6.3), despite considerable phenotypic variation among patients with the same genotype. However, due to the small number of cases, further investigations are necessary to clarity potentially more precise genotype-phenotype correlation of CTX.

Treatment Response

Fifteen patients received CDCA monotherapy, two received 3-hydroxy-3-methylglutaryl coenzyme A reductase (HMGR) inhibitor monotherapy, 18 received combination therapy of CDCA and HMGR inhibitor, and three underwent low-density lipoprotein (LDL) apheresis: all three patients received CDCA and two received additional HMGR inhibitor (Table 6.4). No patients received cholic acid in our survey. All treatment modalities reduced serum

Table 6.4 Efficacy of treatments for cerebrotendinous xanthomatosis

Treatment	Number of patients	Details of each treatment	Serum cholestanol before treatment (μg/ml)	Serum cholestanol after treatment (μg/ml)	*P* value	Change in clinical symptoms	Adverse effects
CDCA	15	Dosage of CDCA: 250–750 mg/day (mean ± SD: 442.5 ± 155.2)	23.2 ± 10.1	5.2 ± 3.3	0.0005	Improved 6 (tremor 2, ataxia 1, cognitive dysfunction 1, psychiatric symptom 1, tendon xanthoma 1) Unchanged 9	Liver injury 3
HMGR inhibitor	2	Dosage of HMGR inhibitor: Atorvastatin 10 mg/day Lovastatin 2.5 mg/day	13.3 ± 10.8	8.2 ± 0.1	0.6	Unchanged 2	None
CDCA + HMGR inhibitor	18	Dosage of CDCA: 125–900 mg/day (mean ± SD: 438.2 ± 169.6) Dosage of HMGR inhibitor: Atorvastatin 10–20 mg/day Lovastatin 2.5–5 mg/day Pitavastatin 2–4 mg/day Pravastatin 5–10 mg/day Simvastatin 10 mg/day	21.6 ± 11.7	8.8 ± 11.3	0.009	Improved 6 (gait disturbance 3, spasticity 1, cognitive dysfunction 2) Unchanged/unknown 11 Deteriorated 1	Liver injury 1 (due to CDCA)
LDL-apheresis + CDCA + (HMGR inhibitor)	3	Apheresis was performed 9–70 times. Dosage of CDCA: 250–500 mg/day (mean ± SD: 416.7 ± 144.3) Dosage of HMGR inhibitor: (HMGR inhibitor was administered in two patients) Lovastatin 2.5–5 mg/day	23.7 ± 7.1	6.3 ± 1.0	0.049	Improved 2 (gait disturbance 2, spasticity 1, weakness 1, cognitive dysfunction 1) Unchanged 1	None

Reprinted by permission of the publisher [10]

cholestanol level, among which CDCA monotherapy, combination CDCA and HMGR inhibitor, and combination LDL apheresis and CDCA/HMGR inhibitor decreased cholestanol significantly. However, the effect of statin monotherapy was modest. The percent decrease of cholestanol by combination therapy (59.3%) was not superior to that by CDCA monotherapy (77.6%), and so the efficacy of HMGR inhibitor add-on therapy to CDCA remains unproven; CDCA remains standard of care treatment worldwide. Symptomatic improvement was observed in six patients in the CDCA group, six in the combination of CDCA and statins group, and two in the LDL apheresis-performed group. The clinical symptoms in the HMGR inhibitor group remained unchanged. Four patients had liver injury apparently associated with CDCA.

Issues on CTX Diagnosis and Treatment in Japan

In this study, we established an elevated cholestanol level as an essential requirement, serving as a diagnostic biological marker because, apart from specific research facilities, clinically available biochemical tests for CTX for commercial use are limited to serum cholestanol in Japan. This enables the diagnosis of probable CTX even without genetic testing, making it possible to include it as a subject of our survey. However, CTX patients with normal or close to normal cholestanol may be overlooked in Japan [24]. It is desirable that biomarkers other than cholestanol, such as 7α-hydroxy-4-cholesten-3-one, 27-hydroxycholesterol, and urine bile alcohols, be available for diagnosis and monitoring treatment adherence and effectiveness [25, 26].

CTX is a treatable metabolic disorder; however, once significant neurological symptoms are established, clinical deterioration can occur despite normalization of cholestanol levels after treatment with CDCA [4, 13, 21, 27, 28]. After the landmark study published in 1984, in which the long-term safety and efficacy of oral CDCA were demonstrated, it became a standard first-line treatment for CTX [11]. However, CDCA is approved only for the treatment of gallstones and is not approved for CTX in Japan: it has to be used off-label. Clinical trials of CDCA for CTX have been completed in Japan, and we are currently preparing to apply for PMDA approval. Recently, cholic acid was approved for inborn errors of bile acid metabolism, including CTX in Japan.

Our nationwide survey revealed an average 16.5-year diagnostic delay, consistent with retrospective cohort studies on CTX that have shown a significant diagnostic delay of 15–25 years [3–5]. The early diagnosis of CTX presents a significant challenge in Japan, and it may indeed be considered a worldwide issue. Our survey revealed a notable diagnostic delay, particularly among pediatric patients. Juvenile cataracts are arguably an important cue for early diagnosis of CTX. A screening for CTX among 170 patients with idiopathic bilateral cataracts diagnosed between the ages of 2 and 21 years identified 3 cases [29]. There is no CTX patient advocacy organization in Japan. We need additional awareness-raising activities for CTX and collaboration, particularly with pediatrics and ophthalmology societies, for early diagnosis. As one of the initiatives for awareness-raising activities, we have launched the clinical practice guidelines and genetic testing registration website for CTX in Japanese (http://www.ctx-guideline.jp/guideline/). Through this initiative, 22 genetically confirmed cases of CTX have been identified from 2017 to the present. In the future, CTX should be considered for universal newborn screening as effective newborn dried bloodspot screening for CTX is available [30–32]; however, it is currently not included in Japan.

References

1. Cali JJ, Hsieh CL, Francke U, Russell DW. Mutations in the bile acid biosynthetic enzyme sterol 27-hydroxylase underlie cerebrotendinous xanthomatosis. J Biol Chem. 1991;266:7779–83.
2. Salen G, Steiner RD. Epidemiology, diagnosis, and treatment of cerebrotendinous xanthomatosis (CTX). J Inherit Metab Dis. 2017;40:771–81.
3. Verrips A, Hoefsloot LH, Steenbergen GC, Theelen JP, Wevers RA, Gabreëls FJ, van Engelen BG, van den Heuvel LP. Clinical and molecular genetic characteristics of patients with cerebrotendinous xanthomatosis. Brain. 2000;123:908–19.
4. Pilo-de-la-Fuente B, Jimenez-Escrig A, Lorenzo JR, Pardo J, Arias M, Ares-Luque A, Duarte J, Muñiz-Pérez S, Sobrido MJ. Cerebrotendinous xanthomatosis in Spain: clinical, prognostic, and genetic survey. Eur J Neurol. 2011;18:1203–11.
5. Mignarri A, Gallus GN, Dotti MT, Federico A. A suspicion index for early diagnosis and treatment of cerebrotendinous xanthomatosis. J Inherit Metab Dis. 2014;37:421–9.
6. Nie S, Chen G, Cao X, Zhang Y. Cerebrotendinous xanthomatosis: a comprehensive review of pathogenesis, clinical manifestations, diagnosis, and management. Orphanet J Rare Dis. 2014;9:179.
7. Wong JC, Walsh K, Hayden D, Eichler FS. Natural history of neurological abnormalities in cerebrotendinous xanthomatosis. J Inherit Metab Dis. 2018;41:647–56.
8. Duell PB, Salen G, Eichler FS, DeBarber AE, Connor SL, Casaday L, Jayadev S, Kisanuki Y, Lekprasert P, Malloy MJ, Ramdhani RA, Ziajka PE, Quinn JF, Su KG, Geller AS, Diffenderfer MR, Schaefer EJ. Diagnosis, treatment, and clinical outcomes in 43 cases with cerebrotendinous xanthomatosis. J Clin Lipidol. 2018;12:1169–78.
9. Sekijima Y, Koyama S, Yoshinaga T, Koinuma M, Inaba Y. Nationwide survey on cerebrotendinous xanthomatosis in Japan. J Hum Genet. 2018;63:271–80.
10. Koyama S, Sekijima Y, Ogura M, Hori M, Matsuki K, Miida T, Harada-Shiba M. Cerebrotendinous xanthomatosis: molecular pathogenesis, clinical spectrum, diagnosis, and disease-modifying treatments. J Atheroscler Thromb. 2021;28:905–25.
11. Berginer VM, Salen G, Shefer S. Long-term treatment of cerebrotendinous xanthomatosis with chenodeoxycholic acid. N Engl J Med. 1984;311:1649–52.
12. van Heijst AF, Verrips A, Wevers RA, Cruysberg JR, Renier WO, Tolboom JJ. Treatment and follow-up of children with cerebrotendinous xanthomatosis. Eur J Pediatr. 1998;157:313–6.
13. Yahalom G, Tsabari R, Molshatzki N, Ephraty L, Cohen H, Hassin-Baer S. Neurological outcome in cerebrotendinous xanthomatosis treated with chenodeoxycholic acid: early versus late diagnosis. Clin Neuropharmacol. 2013;36:78–83.

14. Lorincz MT, Rainier S, Thomas D, Fink JK. Cerebrotendinous xanthomatosis: possible higher prevalence than previously recognized. Arch Neurol. 2005;62:1459–63.
15. Pramparo T, Steiner RD, Rodems S, Jenkinson C. Allelic prevalence and geographic distribution of cerebrotendinous xanthomatosis. Orphanet J Rare Dis. 2023;18:13.
16. Appadurai V, DeBarber A, Chiang PW, Patel SB, Steiner RD, Tyler C, Bonnen PE. Apparent underdiagnosis of Cerebrotendinous Xanthomatosis revealed by analysis of ~60,000 human exomes. Mol Genet Metab. 2015;116:298–304.
17. Verrips A, van Engelen BG, Wevers RA, van Geel BM, Cruysberg JR, van den Heuvel LP, Keyser A, Gabreëls FJ. Presence of diarrhea and absence of tendon xanthomas in patients with cerebrotendinous xanthomatosis. Arch Neurol. 2000;57:520–4.
18. De Stefano N, Dotti MT, Mortilla M, Federico A. Magnetic resonance imaging and spectroscopic changes in brains of patients with cerebrotendinous xanthomatosis. Brain. 2001;124:121–31.
19. Barkhof F, Verrips A, Wesseling P, van Der Knaap MS, van Engelen BG, Gabreëls FJ, Keyser A, Wevers RA, Valk J. Cerebrotendinous xanthomatosis: the spectrum of imaging findings and the correlation with neuropathologic findings. Radiology. 2000;217:869–76.
20. Verrips A, Nijeholt GJ, Barkhof F, Van Engelen BG, Wesseling P, Luyten JA, Wevers RA, Stam J, Wokke JH, van den Heuvel LP, Keyser A, Gabreëls FJ. Spinal xanthomatosis: a variant of cerebrotendinous xanthomatosis. Brain. 1999;122:1589–95.
21. Stelten BML, Huidekoper HH, van de Warrenburg BPC, Brilstra EH, Hollak CEM, Haak HR, Kluijtmans LAJ, Wevers RA, Verrips A. Long-term treatment effect in cerebrotendinous xanthomatosis depends on age at treatment start. Neurology. 2019;92:e83–95.
22. Gallus GN, Dotti MT, Federico A. Clinical and molecular diagnosis of cerebrotendinous xanthomatosis with a review of the mutations in the CYP27A1 gene. Neurol Sci. 2006;27:143–9.
23. Stelten BML, Raal FJ, Marais AD, Riksen NP, Roeters van Lennep JE, Duell PB, van der Graaf M, Kluijtmans LAJ, Wevers RA, Verrips A. Cerebrotendinous xanthomatosis without neurological involvement. J Intern Med. 2021;290:1039–47.
24. Guenzel AJ, DeBarber A, Raymond K, Dhamija R. Familial variability of cerebrotendinous xanthomatosis lacking typical biochemical findings. JIMD Rep. 2021;59:3–9.
25. DeBarber AE, Connor WE, Pappu AS, Merkens LS, Steiner RD. ESI-MS/MS quantification of 7alpha-hydroxy-4-cholesten-3-one facilitates rapid, convenient diagnostic testing for cerebrotendinous xanthomatosis. Clin Chim Acta. 2010;41:43–8.
26. DeBarber AE, Luo J, Giugliani R, Souza CF, Chiang JP, Merkens LS, Pappu AS, Steiner RD. A useful multi-analyte blood test for cerebrotendinous xanthomatosis. Clin Biochem. 2014;47:860–3.
27. Dotti MT, Lütjohann D, von Bergmann K, Federico A. Normalisation of serum cholestanol concentration in a patient with cerebrotendinous xanthomatosis by combined treatment with chenodeoxycholic acid, simvastatin and LDL apheresis. Neurol Sci. 2004;25:185–91.
28. Koyama S, Okabe Y, Suzuki Y, Igari R, Sato H, Iseki C, Tanji K, Suzuki K, Ohta Y. Differing clinical features between Japanese siblings with cerebrotendinous xanthomatosis with a novel compound heterozygous CYP27A1 mutation: a case report. BMC Neurol. 2022;22:193.
29. Freedman SF, Brennand C, Chiang J, DeBarber A, Del Monte MA, Duell PB, Fiorito J, Marshall R. Prevalence of cerebrotendinous xanthomatosis among patients diagnosed with acquired juvenile-onset idiopathic bilateral cataracts. JAMA Ophthalmol. 2019;137:1312–6.
30. Vaz FM, Bootsma AH, Kulik W, Verrips A, Wevers RA, Schielen PC, DeBarber AE, Huidekoper HH. A newborn screening method for cerebrotendinous xanthomatosis using bile alcohol glucuronides and metabolite ratios. J Lipid Res. 2017;58:1002–7.

31. DeBarber AE, Kalfon L, Fedida A, Fleisher Sheffer V, Ben Haroush S, Chasnyk N, Shuster Biton E, Mandel H, Jeffries K, Shinwell ES, Falik-Zaccai TC. Newborn screening for cerebrotendinous xanthomatosis is the solution for early identification and treatment. J Lipid Res. 2018;59:2214–22.
32. Hong X, Daiker J, Sadilek M, DeBarber AE, Chiang J, Duan J, Bootsma AH, Huidekoper HH, Vaz FM, Gelb MH. Toward newborn screening of cerebrotendinous xanthomatosis: results of a biomarker research study using 32,000 newborn dried blood spots. Genet Med. 2020;22:1606–12.

Cerebrotendinous Xanthomatosis (CTX): Remaining Challenges and the Need for International Collaboration

7

Hidde H. Huidekoper

Unresolved Issues Within the Field of CTX

In the last decades, much progress has been made in understanding the clinical spectrum of CTX with the delineation of three phenotypic subtypes. The vast majority of patients will exhibit 'classical CTX' in which they develop a broad spectrum of progressive neuropsychiatric symptoms in addition to characteristic somatic features like cataracts, intractable diarrhea, and tendon xanthomas [1, 2]. Patients with 'spinal CTX' will develop predominantly pyramidal signs with a more attenuated clinical course, often without clear somatic symptoms [3]. More recently, a 'non-neurological CTX' phenotype has been described in which patients only develop somatic symptoms at a later age without neurological involvement [4]. The exact distribution between these phenotypes remains unclear; (inter)national cohort studies, as conducted in Japan [5], are needed to establish this.

Although our knowledge on the clinical spectrum of CTX has greatly improved, many aspects of this complex and heterogeneous disorder still need to be resolved. Many pathogenic *CYP27A1* variants have now been described, but no clear genotype—phenotype, either clinical or biochemical, associations have been established to date [1, 2, 6]. This is exemplified by CTX patients within the same family who were demonstrated to have a very different disease course, which could not be attributed to a difference in treatment or lifestyle circumstances [7, 8]. Adding to this complexity is the fact that we have not yet identified accurate prognostic biomarkers that can be used for the assessment of disease severity and disease monitoring. This makes it difficult to predict the course of disease in newly diagnosed CTX patients.

H. H. Huidekoper (✉)
Department of Pediatrics, Center for Lysosomal and Metabolic Diseases, Erasmus MC University Medical Center, Rotterdam, The Netherlands
e-mail: h.huidekoper@erasmusmc.nl

A. Federico et al. (eds.), *Cerebrotendinous Xanthomatosis*,
https://doi.org/10.1007/978-3-031-92526-9_7

This is very relevant in view of the possible inclusion of CTX in newborn screening programs in the near future. It has been clearly demonstrated that CTX is a treatable condition in which symptoms can be prevented if treatment with chenodeoxycholic acid is started at an early age [9–11]. As now several newborn screening methods for CTX have been validated [12, 13], CTX is a very good candidate for inclusion in newborn screening according to the screening criteria of Wilson and Jungner [14]. Currently, efforts are being made to get CTX nominated for the Recommend Uniform Screening Panel (RUSP) in the USA, whereas in the Netherlands and Israel, steps are already being taken to implement newborn screening for CTX. As no symptoms are expected to develop when treatment is started shortly after confirmation of the diagnosis after a positive newborn screening test panelists in a recent Delphi study agreed this is the best treatment option. Starting treatment upon symptom onset was considered to be the second best option [15]. Chenodexocholic acid (CDCA) has been approved as an orphan drug treatment for CTX in Europe and is available as CDCA Leadiant (Leadiant GmbH, Germany). In the USA market authorization of CDCA for CTX was recently obtained based on the recently reported results of the RESTORE trial [16]. However, chenodeoxycholic acid has been used off-label for the treatment of CTX for many decades and the designation of CDCA Leadiant as an orphan drug for CTX has led to a 500-fold price increase in comparison to the original CDCA formulation used off-label without making any significant pharmaceutical enhancements [17]. This jeopardized the continuation of treatment of patients with CTX in the Netherlands as CDCA Leadiant was not eligible for reimbursement and resulted in the production of pharmacy compounded CDCA capsules to ensure treatment of Dutch CTX patients [18]. In addition, large fines were given by Dutch, Israeli, Italian, and Spanish authorities for competition regulation because of this unwarranted excessive price increase [19–21]. Because of the now significant price of CDCA for the treatment of CTX, and because of the large clinical variability in which patients may develop symptoms only at a later age and may never develop neuropsychiatric symptoms, it has been suggested that a watchful waiting policy should be adapted with implementation of newborn screening for CTX and treatment should only be initiated beyond symptom onset [22]. It is therefore likely that countries may adapt different implementation strategies for CTX newborn screening, and it would be very valuable to compare outcomes in patients with different treatment strategies.

Need for an International CTX Patient Registry

In order to address the issues raised setting up an international patient registry for CTX will allow us to collect standardized outcome data from countries with different strategies for diagnosing (i.e. implementation of newborn screening; diagnostic capabilities) and treating (i.e. availability of CDCA; cholic acid (CA) versus CDCA; use of statins as adjuvant therapy) patients with CTX. This will help us to further establish and refine the standard of care for the diagnosis and treatment of CTX and to develop criteria for starting treatment in CTX patients identified through newborn screening in countries that wish to adapt a watchful waiting policy. In addition, an international registry will help us to further delineate the clinical spectrum in CTX, may help us to establish genotype–phenotype associations, and will help to identify and prioritize unmet medical needs in patients.

There are many examples of international patient registries within the field of inborn errors of metabolism, including the European registry and network for Intoxication type Metabolic Diseases (E-IMD; https://www.e-imd.org/), the European network and registry for Homocystinurias and methylation Defects (E-HOD; https://www.e-hod.org/), the Unified European Registry for Inherited Metabolic Disorders (U-IMD; https://u-imd.org/), the International Niemann-Pick Disease Registry (INPDR; https://inpdr.org/) and the Galactosemia Patient Registry (https://www.galactosemianetwork.org/registry), as well as many other examples in other rare disease fields. These registries have proven to be of great value in establishing the natural history, clinical spectrum, and outcomes on current treatments in rare disorders.

During the 2023 CTX International Scientific Meeting in Jerusalem, setting up an international CTX patient registry was discussed with a panel of experts and patient representatives during a workshop meeting. All attendees received a survey prior to the meeting in which they could give their input on what outcome parameters would be most valuable to include with respect to clinical symptoms and signs, biochemical markers, neuroimaging, other medical investigations, and patient reported outcome and experience measures. The survey was used to fuel the discussions and the collected input will be used to design the outline for the registry. It was agreed that the registry should be set up independent from pharmaceutical companies, as to promote the unbiased collection of data, and should have an international steering committee as a governing body to oversee registry participation, adherence to the registry protocol, requests for data analysis and publications and presentations derived from registry data.

The next steps will be to draft an outline for the registry in collaboration with a core working group, write a registry protocol including a description of the informed consent procedure in order to obtain institutional review board (IRB) approval in participating countries, identify possible sources of funding, and identify a data capture platform on which the registry can be hosted.

Development of a CTX Clinical Severity Score

In addition to discussing setting up an international CTX patient registry during the 2023 CTX International Scientific Meeting, it was also proposed to start the development of a CTX clinical severity score. Because of the large clinical heterogeneity in CTX patients, descriptions in literature vary greatly, which makes it difficult to compare patients. Developing a clinical severity score based on clearly defined clinical outcome parameters will help to standardize phenotypic descriptions in CTX patients and will provide us with a tool for assessing the efficacy of current and future therapeutic interventions. The value of such a clinical severity score has been well established in Niemann-Pick type C disease [23]. A Delphi consensus procedure should be adapted for developing the CTX clinical severity score, as this method has been used successfully for the development of various clinical assessment tools [24].

Concluding Remarks

International collaboration in the field of CTX, as well as in other ultra rare disorders, where health care professionals work together with patient advocacy groups to mitigate unresolved issues, close knowledge gaps, and identify unmet medical needs, is essential to improve prospects for patients. We are confident that setting up an international CTX patient registry and developing a CTX clinical severity score will greatly contribute towards this aim. Therefore, this should be the focus of the international scientific CTX community in the upcoming years.

References

1. Salen G, Steiner RD. Epidemiology, diagnosis, and treatment of cerebrotendinous xanthomatosis (CTX). J Inherit Metab Dis. 2017;40(6):771–81.
2. Nie S, Chen G, Cao X, Zhang Y. Cerebrotendinous xanthomatosis: a comprehensive review of pathogenesis, clinical manifestations, diagnosis, and management. Orphanet J Rare Dis. 2014;9:179.
3. Verrips A, Nijeholt GJ, Barkhof F, Van Engelen BG, Wesseling P, Luyten JA, et al. Spinal xanthomatosis: a variant of cerebrotendinous xanthomatosis. Brain. 1999;122(Pt 8):1589–95.
4. Stelten BML, Raal FJ, Marais AD, Riksen NP, Roeters van Lennep JE, Duell PB, et al. Cerebrotendinous xanthomatosis without neurological involvement. J Intern Med. 2021;290(5):1039–47.
5. Sekijima Y, Koyama S, Yoshinaga T, Koinuma M, Inaba Y. Nationwide survey on cerebrotendinous xanthomatosis in Japan. J Hum Genet. 2018;63(3):271–80.
6. Verrips A, Hoefsloot LH, Steenbergen GC, Theelen JP, Wevers RA, Gabreels FJ, et al. Clinical and molecular genetic characteristics of patients with cerebrotendinous xanthomatosis. Brain. 2000;123(Pt 5):908–19.
7. Zádori D, Szpisjak L, Madar L, Varga VE, Csányi B, Bencsik K, et al. Different phenotypes in identical twins with cerebrotendinous xanthomatosis: case series. Neurol Sci. 2017;38(3):481–3.
8. Guenzel AJ, DeBarber A, Raymond K, Dhamija R. Familial variability of cerebrotendinous xanthomatosis lacking typical biochemical findings. JIMD Rep. 2021;59(1):3–9.
9. Stelten BML, Huidekoper HH, van de Warrenburg BPC, Brilstra EH, Hollak CEM, Haak HR, et al. Long-term treatment effect in cerebrotendinous xanthomatosis depends on age at treatment start. Neurology. 2019;92(2):e83–95.
10. Degrassi I, Amoruso C, Giordano G, Del Puppo M, Mignarri A, Dotti MT, et al. Case report: early treatment with chenodeoxycholic acid in cerebrotendinous xanthomatosis presenting as neonatal cholestasis. Front Pediatr. 2020;8:382.
11. Berginer VM, Gross B, Morad K, Kfir N, Morkos S, Aaref S, et al. Chronic diarrhea and juvenile cataracts: think cerebrotendinous xanthomatosis and treat. Pediatrics. 2009;123(1):143–7.
12. Vaz FM, Jamal Y, Barto R, Gelb MH, DeBarber AE, Wevers RA, et al. Newborn screening for Cerebrotendinous Xanthomatosis: a retrospective biomarker study using both flow-injection and UPLC-MS/MS analysis in 20,000 newborns. Clin Chim Acta. 2023;539:170–4.

13. Hong X, Daiker J, Sadilek M, DeBarber AE, Chiang J, Duan J, et al. Toward newborn screening of cerebrotendinous xanthomatosis: results of a biomarker research study using 32,000 newborn dried blood spots. Genet Med. 2020;22(10):1606–12.
14. Wilson JMG, Jungner G. Principles and practice of screening for disease. Geneva: World Health Organization; 1968. Contract No.: 34.
15. Stelten BML, Dotti MT, Verrips A, Elibol B, Falik-Zaccai TC, Hanman K, et al. Expert opinion on diagnosing, treating and managing patients with cerebrotendinous xanthomatosis (CTX): a modified Delphi study. Orphanet J Rare Dis. 2021;16(1):353.
16. Kisanuki YY, Nobrega PR, Himes R, Jayadev S, Bernat JA, Prakash V, et al. RESTORE Study Group Collaborators. Efficacy, safety, and tolerability of chenodeoxycholic acid (CDCA) in adult patients with cerebrotendinous xanthomatosis (RESTORE): a randomized withdrawal, double-blind, placebo-controlled, crossover phase 3 study. Genet Med. 2025;25:101449.
17. Polak Y, Jacobs BAW, Kemper EM. Pharmacy compounded medicines for patients with rare diseases: lessons learned from chenodeoxycholic acid and cholic acid. Front Pharmacol. 2021;12:758210.
18. Bouwhuis N, Jacobs BAW, Kemper EM. Product development and quality of pharmacy compounded chenodeoxycholic acid capsules for Dutch cerebrotendinous xanthomatosis patients. Front Pharmacol. 2023;14:1264997.
19. After Netherlands and Israel, now Italy: Leadiant fined for excessive price. Pharmaceutical Accountability Foundation; 2022. Available from: https://www.pharmaceuticalaccountability.org/2022/06/02/after-netherlands-and-israel-now-italy-leadiant-fined-for-excessive-price/.
20. ACM imposes fine on drug manufacturer Leadiant for CDCA's excessive price. Netherlands Authority for Consumers and Markets; 2021. Available from: https://www.acm.nl/en/publications/acm-imposes-fine-drug-manufacturer-leadiant-cdcas-excessive-price.
21. The CNMC fines the pharmaceutical company Leadiant 10.25 million for selling its orphan drug for the treatment of a rare disease at an excessive price. Comisión Nacional de los Mercados y la Competencia; 2022. Available from: https://www.cnmc.es/sites/default/files/editor_contenidos/Notas%20de%20prensa/2022/20221114_NP_S_0028_20_LEADIANT_COM_en_GB.pdf.
22. Hollak CEM. Expanding the clinical spectrum of cerebrotendinous xanthomatosis: implications for newborn screening, follow-up and treatment. J Intern Med. 2021;290(5):942–3.
23. Evans W, Patterson M, Platt F, Guldberg C, Mathieson T, Pacey J. International consensus on clinical severity scale use in evaluating Niemann-Pick disease Type C in paediatric and adult patients: results from a Delphi Study. Orphanet J Rare Dis. 2021;16(1):482.
24. Nasa P, Jain R, Juneja D. Delphi methodology in healthcare research: how to decide its appropriateness. World J Methodol. 2021;11(4):116–29.

Part II

Genetic and Biochemical Aspects of Cerebrotendinous Xanthomatosis (CTX)

Genetics of Cerebrotendinous Xanthomatosis (CTX)

8

Jennifer Hanson and Penelope E. Bonnen

Introduction

Cerebrotendinous xanthomatosis (CTX) is an inborn error of metabolism the hallmark features of which include chronic diarrhea, juvenile-onset cataracts, tendinous xanthomas, and progressive neurological dysfunction (OMIM 213700). CTX is an autosomal recessive genetic condition caused by biallelic variants in *CYP27A1*, which codes for the sterol 27-hydroxylase enzyme that functions in bile acid synthesis. Bi-allelic pathogenic variants in this gene result in decreased cholic acid and especially chenodeoxycholic acid synthesis and consequently cause elevations of cholestanol, bile acid intermediates, and bile alcohols. Diagnosis can be made with clinical diagnostic testing of plasma cholestanol, bile acid intermediate and bile alcohol levels, urinary bile alcohol levels, and/or genetic testing of *CYP27A1*. Understanding of the genetics of CTX can help facilitate diagnosis. Here we discuss the medical genetics, population genetics, and genotype phenotype correlations of *CYP27A1*.

Medical Genetics of CTX

The gene that encodes the sterol 27-hydroxylase enzyme, *CYP27A1*, was cloned in 1991 [1], and shortly thereafter the first pathogenic variants that cause CTX were identified [2]. This first report of pathogenic variants in *CYP27A1* described two unrelated patients each of whom was presumed homozygous for a different variant. The reference sequence for *CYP27A1* has changed over time and so has the variant

J. Hanson · P. E. Bonnen (✉)
Department of Molecular and Human Genetics, Baylor College of Medicine, Houston, TX, USA
e-mail: pbonnen@bcm.edu

A. Federico et al. (eds.), *Cerebrotendinous Xanthomatosis*,
https://doi.org/10.1007/978-3-031-92526-9_8

nomenclature. The first two pathogenic variants reported in *CYP27A1* were: NM_000784.1:c.1456C>T;p.(Arg446Cys) now known as NM_000784.4:c.1435C>T;p.(Arg479Cys) and NM_000784.1 c.1204c>T; p.(Arg362Cys), which is now reported as NM_000784.4 c.1183C>T; p.(Arg395Cys). Expression of each of these missense variants in cultured cells showed reduced 27-hydroxylase protein levels and significantly diminished enzyme activity for p.(Arg479Cys) and no enzyme activity for p.(Arg395Cys) [2].

The gene structure of *CYP27A1* was subsequently delineated as being comprised of nine exons and eight introns [3], which we now appreciate span approximately 33Kb (hg38 2:218781749-218815293). The *CYP27A1* cDNA has 1596 nucleotides and the protein includes 532 amino acids (NM_000784.4(CYP27A1)). This same study reported additional pathogenic variants in *CYP27A1* which were the first frameshift and splice variants reported in CTX patients (NM_000784.4: c.819del;p.(Asp273GlufsTer13) and NM_000784.4: c.845-1G>A; splice) [3]. These two variants were demonstrated to be loss of function alleles through analysis of mRNA in patient fibroblasts; no stable sterol 27-hydroxylase mRNA was detected in patients' cells [3].

Since the cloning of *CYP27A1*, over 200 pathogenic variants have been identified in individuals with CTX; pathogenic variants are present in every exon of *CYP27A1*. ClinVar currently lists 151 loss of function (LOF) variants for *CYP27A1* (66 frameshift, 49 nonsense, 36 canonical splice site variants) as Pathogenic or Likely Pathogenic. ClinVar contains 25 missense variants in *CYP27A1* categorized as Pathogenic or Likely Pathogenic for CTX. However, we have identified 54 missense variants in the literature reported as causing CTX; some of these 54 missense variants are not listed in ClinVar at all, and others are in ClinVar listed as variants of uncertain significance (VUS). Under ACMG/AMP variant classification guidelines for clinical interpretation of variants, LOF can be presumed to be Likely Pathogenic even if that specific variant has not been reported in a prior patient as causing disease; missense variants are not presumed to be Likely Pathogenic without additional supporting evidence. As a result, there are many missense VUS and almost no LOF VUS for *CYP27A1*. The only frameshift and nonsense variants that are not presumed to be LOF variants in ClinVar are frameshift and nonsense variants that occur in the last 10 amino acids of the protein; because they occur in the very end of the protein, it is uncertain what effect they may have on protein function.

Population Genetics of CTX

Understanding the frequency that disease-causing variants have in a population can facilitate identification of patients as well as shed light on the incidence of disease. We queried one of the largest population genetic databases (gnomAD 4.0.0, $N = 807{,}000$, Jan 2024) for all pathogenic variants in *CYP27A1*. Analysis of these data across four global populations, African/African American $N = 37{,}545$, Admixed American $N = 30{,}019$, Asian $N = 67{,}994$, and European $N = 622{,}057$, shed light on the frequency of the variants that cause CTX across the world. A total 126 LOF variants in *CYP27A1* were identified in gnomAD; and of the 54 missense variants published in the literature as causing CTX, 43 were found in gnomAD. The allele frequency of all pathogenic variants combined was 0.0018 in African, Admixed American, and European populations (Fig. 8.1). The frequency of pathogenic variants in Asia was 0.0035 (Fig. 8.1).

CTX has been under-diagnosed likely due to the complex constellation of clinical features progressing over decades. Moreover, under-diagnosis leads to an incomplete ascertainment of variants that cause disease. In order to overcome these challenges, we reported the very first use of combining population genetics with bioinformatics to identify pathogenic variants and calculate incidence of a monogenic disorder [4]. We conducted a bioinformatics assessment of the variants that were reported in the literature to cause CTX and leveraged population genetics of those pathogenic variants and the variants present in a population-based database (ExAC, $N = 60{,}000$) that were predicted to be pathogenic based on the bioinformatic features of the variants present in CTX patients. We showed that most disease-causing variants had similar frequencies in global populations. Incidence of CTX was estimated to be 1 in 468,624 in African population, 1/148,914 in the American population, 1/70,000 in the Asian population, and 1/461,358 in Europeans [4]. This range of incidences underscored the point that CTX is underdiagnosed.

The power of the gnomAD 4.0 database with 800,000 individuals is greater, and we calculated incidence using just the *CYP27A1* LOF variants in the database plus

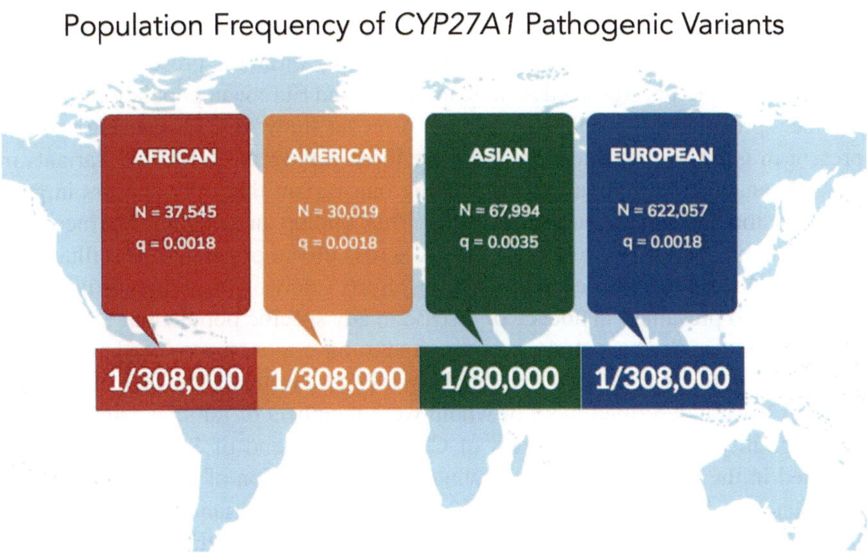

Fig. 8.1 Population based estimate of CTX incidence. The incidence of CTX was estimated in four global populations by applying Hardy Weinberg principle to heterozygote allele frequencies for pathogenic CTX variants in *CYP27A1*. N = the number of individuals in each population included in the allele frequency calculation. q is the sum of the allele frequencies of all pathogenic variants in a population. Incidence estimates are shown as $1/X$ number of individuals

the published pathogenic missense variants. A bioinformatics component was not included. Under this model, incidence for African, Admixed American, and European populations was the same: 1 in 308,000. The Asian population incidence was significantly higher at 1 in 80,000 (Fig. 8.1).

The incidence of CTX has been reported to be high in certain population isolates including various Jewish populations and Druze [3, 5–9]. There appear to be *CYP27A1* variants that have risen to high frequency in these groups resulting in more cases of CTX. The variant that appears in the Druze population is c.355delC; p.(Arg119GlyfsTer24) [8]. Druze is a religious faith practiced by approximately one million individuals, most of whom live in Syria, Lebanon, and Israel. This variant was identified in a Druze village in Israel. This variant is present in just 2 out of 152,000 chromosomes in gnomAD. Those two individuals were in the gnomAD Middle Eastern population, which is consistent with Druze originating and predominantly living in the Middle East. This variant serves as a classic example of a founder mutation in an isolated population.

There are a handful of variants that are found in high frequency in Sephardic Jews [3, 5–7, 9]. A high frequency of CTX was reported in Israel prior to the cloning of the gene [5]. As soon as *CYP27A1* was cloned, pathogenic variants were identified in Jewish individuals. The first of these was c.819del;p.(Asp273GlufsTer13), which was identified in Moroccan Sephardic Jews [3]. This variant is present in 1 allele out of 1,461,890 in gnomAD, making it very rare. In the same paper, c.845-1G>A was reported in a Moroccan Sephardic Jewish CTX patient. This variant is present in gnomAD in 41/1,614,078 alleles, which is also rare at a frequency of 0.000025. In contrast, a *CYP27A1* variant was identified in an Algerian Sephardic Jew with CTX, c.1016C>T;p.(Thr339Met) [9]. This variant is present in gnomAD in African American, Admixed American, Asian, and European populations making it wider spread across global populations. A recent study of CTX-causing variants present in gnomAD revealed that there are three pathogenic *CYP27A1* variants in the Ashkenazi Jewish population, including one variant that only appears in gnomAD in the Ashkenazi population [10]. This finding underscores the need for genetic or biochemical screening for CTX across global population and illustrates one of the limitations of focusing screening efforts solely on prior knowledge of the presence and presumed incidence of disease in any specific population.

The island of Sardinia, Italy, was reported to have a 'recurrent' variant when it was found in two purportedly unrelated families in Sardinia [11]. Two individuals with CTX were described, both of whom were members of families with reported consanguinity. No additional cases of CTX on the island of Sardinia have been reported in the medical literature leaving open the question of whether this island experiences a high prevalence of CTX. The pathogenic variant observed in these families, c.1435C>T;p.(Arg479Cys), is also present in the population database gnomAD predominantly in the European population as well as in African American, Admixed American, and Asian populations.

Genotype Phenotype Association in CTX

Clinical diagnostic criteria refer to cardinal features of CTX: cataracts, tendon xanthomas, cerebellar signs, pyramidal signs, peripheral neuropathy, and chronic diarrhea [12–14]. However, many studies report that CTX clinical presentation is highly variable across individuals, even within families [12, 15–18]. No genotype-phenotype studies were identified that were conducted using a robust sample size or sufficiently powered statistical analysis. There does not appear to be a sufficient number of samples with the same genotype for powerful statistical analysis. For example, Verrips et al. (2000) conducted a comparison across individuals who were homozygous for the same *CYP27A1* pathogenic variant; in 79 individuals who had a homozygous genotype, there were 23 different variants [15]. No genotype-phenotype association was identified and the authors reported that one does not exist for CTX; however, with 23 variants tested among 79 individuals, the study was statistically underpowered. This is a common problem in rare disease, and new methods are needed to study genotype-phenotype associations for rare monogenic disorders like CTX.

Summary

Since the cloning of *CYP27A1*, the gene responsible for CTX, over 200 pathogenic variants have been identified in individuals with CTX. Pathogenic variants are present in every exon of *CYP27A1*. Population genetic analyses show that CTX is present across global populations, including some previously underappreciated. The combined knowledge base across the medical and population genetics of CTX points to a need for greater genetic and biochemical screening efforts.

Addendum: Note that additional data on CTX Epidemiology is reported in a separate chapter in this book and in Pramparo et al. [19].

Acknowledgments PEB is supported by NIH NINDS RO1 NS08372.

References

1. Cali JJ, Russell DW. Characterization of human sterol 27-hydroxylase. A mitochondrial cytochrome P-450 that catalyzes multiple oxidation reaction in bile acid biosynthesis. J Biol Chem. 1991;266(12):7774–8.
2. Cali JJ, Hsieh CL, Francke U, Russell DW. Mutations in the bile acid biosynthetic enzyme sterol 27-hydroxylase underlie cerebrotendinous xanthomatosis. J Biol Chem. 1991;266(12):7779–83.
3. Leitersdorf E, Reshef A, Meiner V, Levitzki R, Schwartz SP, Dann EJ, et al. Frameshift and splice-junction mutations in the sterol 27-hydroxylase gene cause cerebrotendinous xanthomatosis in Jews or Moroccan origin. J Clin Invest. 1993;91(6):2488–96.

4. Appadurai V, DeBarber A, Chiang PW, Patel SB, Steiner RD, Tyler C, et al. Apparent underdiagnosis of Cerebrotendinous Xanthomatosis revealed by analysis of ~60,000 human exomes. Mol Genet Metab. 2015;116(4):298–304.
5. Berginer VM, Abeliovich D. Genetics of cerebrotendinous xanthomatosis (CTX): an autosomal recessive trait with high gene frequency in Sephardim of Moroccan origin. Am J Med Genet. 1981;10(2):151–7.
6. Meiner V, Marais DA, Reshef A, Bjorkhem I, Leitersdorf E. Premature termination codon at the sterol 27-hydroxylase gene causes cerebrotendinous xanthomatosis in an Afrikaner family. Hum Mol Genet. 1994;3(1):193–4.
7. Meiner V, Meiner Z, Reshef A, Bjorkhem I, Leitersdorf E. Cerebrotendinous xanthomatosis: molecular diagnosis enables presymptomatic detection of a treatable disease. Neurology. 1994;44(2):288–90.
8. Leitersdorf E, Safadi R, Meiner V, Reshef A, Bjorkhem I, Friedlander Y, et al. Cerebrotendinous xanthomatosis in the Israeli Druze: molecular genetics and phenotypic characteristics. Am J Hum Genet. 1994;55(5):907–15.
9. Reshef A, Meiner V, Berginer VM, Leitersdorf E. Molecular genetics of cerebrotendinous xanthomatosis in Jews of north African origin. J Lipid Res. 1994;35(3):478–83.
10. Hanson J, Bonnen PE. Cerebrotendinous Xanthomatosis occurs at high frequency in Ashkenazi Jews. Mol Genet Metab. 2025;144(3):109041.
11. Mandrile G, Gallus GN, Mura G, Di Sapio A, Sotgiu MA, Montella A, et al. Cerebrotendinous xanthomatosis: recurrence of the CYP27A1 mutation p.Arg479Cys in Sardinia. Neurol Sci. 2014;35(8):1303–5.
12. Mignarri A, Gallus GN, Dotti MT, Federico A. A suspicion index for early diagnosis and treatment of cerebrotendinous xanthomatosis. J Inherit Metab Dis. 2014;37(3):421–9.
13. Wong JC, Walsh K, Hayden D, Eichler FS. Natural history of neurological abnormalities in cerebrotendinous xanthomatosis. J Inherit Metab Dis. 2018;41(4):647–56.
14. Sekijima Y, Koyama S, Yoshinaga T, Koinuma M, Inaba Y. Nationwide survey on cerebrotendinous xanthomatosis in Japan. J Hum Genet. 2018;63(3):271–80.
15. Verrips A, Hoefsloot LH, Steenbergen GC, Theelen JP, Wevers RA, Gabreels FJ, et al. Clinical and molecular genetic characteristics of patients with cerebrotendinous xanthomatosis. Brain. 2000;123(Pt 5):908–19.
16. Zádori D, Szpisjak L, Madar L, Varga VE, Csányi B, Bencsik K, et al. Different phenotypes in identical twins with cerebrotendinous xanthomatosis: case series. Neurol Sci. 2017;38(3):481–3.
17. Federico A, Dotti MT. Cerebrotendinous xanthomatosis: clinical manifestations, diagnostic criteria, pathogenesis, and therapy. J Child Neurol. 2003;18(9):633–8.
18. Moghadasian MH. Cerebrotendinous xanthomatosis: clinical course, genotypes and metabolic backgrounds. Clin Invest Med. 2004;27(1):42–50.
19. Pramparo T, Steiner RD, Rodems S, Jenkinson C. Allelic prevalence and geographic distribution of cerebrotendinous xanthomatosis. Orphanet J Rare Dis. 2023;18(1):13.

General Overview of the Biochemistry Relevant to Cerebrotendinous Xanthomatosis (CTX) with a Focus on the Clinical Laboratory

9

Peter Clayton

Abbreviations

7α12αC4	7α,12α-dihydroxycholest-4-en-3-one
CA	Cholic acid, 3α,7α,12α-trihydroxy-5β-cholanoic acid
CDCA	Chenodeoxycholic acid, 3α,7α-dihydroxy-5β-cholanoic acid
CTX	Cerebrotendinous xanthomatosis
DBS	Dried blood spot(s)
GlcA-tetrol	5β-cholestane,3α,7α,12α,25tetrol-3-*O*-β-D-glucuronide
ROS	Reactive oxygen species
t-CDCA	Taurochenodeoxycholic acid
THCA	Trihydroxycholestanoic acid, 3α,7α,12α-trihydroxy-5β-cholestanoic acid
t-THCA	Taurotrihydroxycholestanoic acid

Chemical Nomenclature

Historically, the reaction catalysed by the enzyme deficiency in CTX was described as 27-hydroxylation (hence the gene name, *CYP27A1*). However, it is chemically more correct to refer to the product of the reaction as 26-hydroxycholesterol (or its full name 25R,26-hydroxycholesterol).

P. Clayton (✉)
University College London Great Ormond Street Institute of Child Health, London, UK
e-mail: peter.clayton@ucl.ac.uk

A. Federico et al. (eds.), *Cerebrotendinous Xanthomatosis*,
https://doi.org/10.1007/978-3-031-92526-9_9

Biochemical Pathways

The main routes for catabolism of cholesterol are shown in Fig. 9.1. From the point of view of testing for cerebrotendinous xanthomatosis (CTX) in a Chemical Pathology laboratory, the important pathways are the neutral pathway for conversion of cholesterol to bile acids commencing with cholesterol 7α-hydroxylase (encoded by *CYP7A1*) and pathways including C25 hydroxylation (enzyme encoded by C25H). The acidic pathway of bile acid synthesis that starts with a reaction catalysed by the enzyme deficient in CTX (*CYP27A1*) leads to acidic pathway intermediates, but these are not easily measured in a routine Chemical Pathology laboratory (see below).

In CTX, the neutral pathway for bile acid synthesis is disrupted at the level of C26 hydroxylation of intermediates such as 7α-hydroxy-cholest-4-en-3-one, 7α,12α-dihydroxy-cholest-4-en-3-one (7α12αC4) and 5β-cholestane-3α,7α,12α-triol (Fig. 9.2). 7α-Hydroxy-cholest-4-en-3-one can be converted to cholestanol [1, 2] which, with cholesterol, builds up in the brain, atheromatous plaques and xanthomata (Fig. 9.3). 5β-Cholestane-3α,7α,12α-triol can undergo C25 hydroxylation, leading to the build-up of 5β-cholestane-3α,7α,12α,25-tetrol as the glucuronide (GlcA-tetrol) in blood and urinary excretion of a range of 5β-cholestane-pentol glucuronides (including 22,25-,23,25- and 24,25-pentols). There is reduced synthesis of metabolites distal to the C26-hydroxylation block in the neutral pathway—the concentration of the taurine conjugate of 3α,7,12α-trihydroxy-5β-cholestanoic acid (t-THCA) in blood is reduced [3].

In CTX, the acidic pathway for bile acid synthesis is inhibited at its first step (Fig. 9.4); there is reduced production of 25R,26-hydroxycholesterol (27-hydroxycholesterol). The reduced level of this signalling molecule is thought to

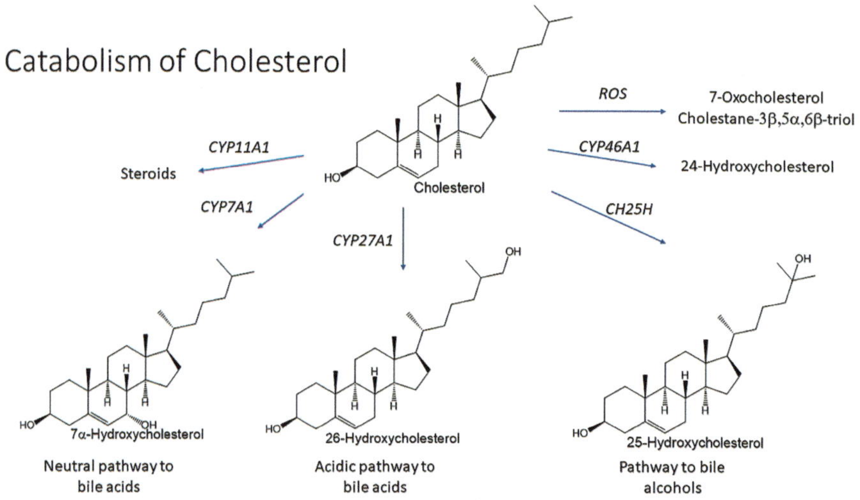

Fig. 9.1 Catabolism of cholesterol

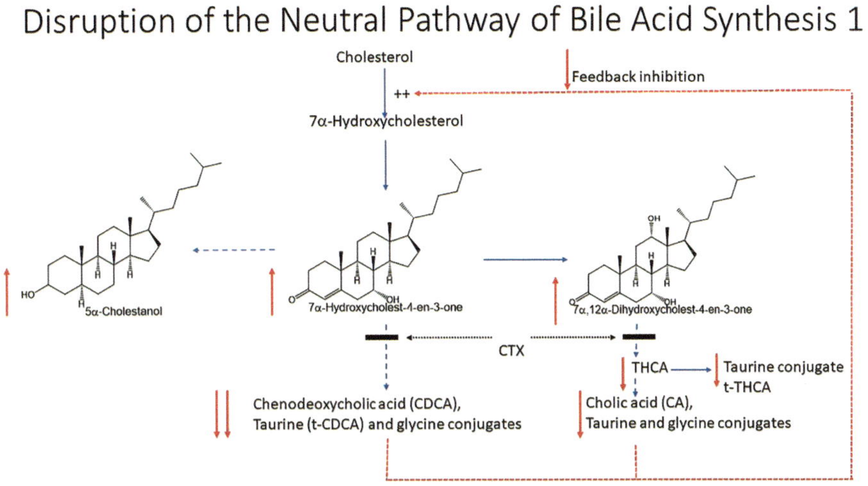

Fig. 9.2 Disruption of the neutral pathway of bile acid synthesis 1

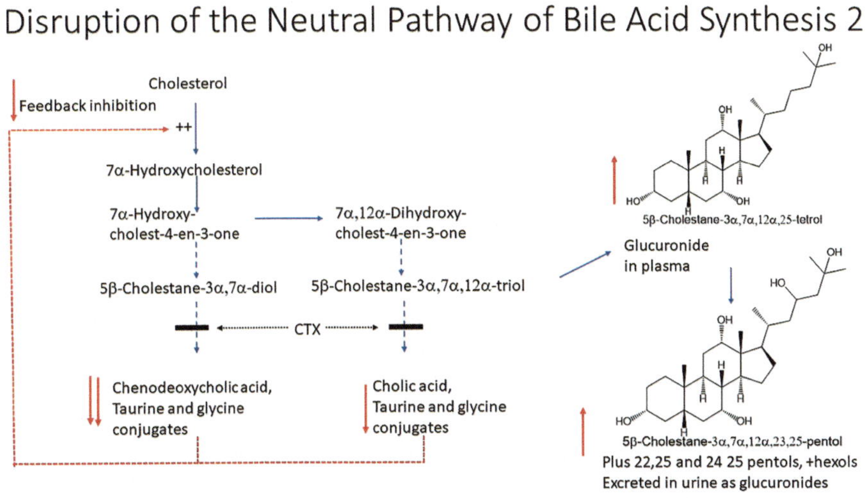

Fig. 9.3 Disruption of the neutral pathway of bile acid synthesis 2

play an important role in the increased rate of production of cholesterol and cholesterol precursors [such as lathosterol (Δ7-cholestenol, 5α-cholest-7-en-3β-ol)] from 3-hydroxy-3-methyl-glutaryl-CoA that was first described in an individual with CTX in 1977 [4]. The mechanisms by which reduced production of 27-hydroxycholesterol leads to increased cholesterol synthesis in CTX are becoming clearer from recent research.

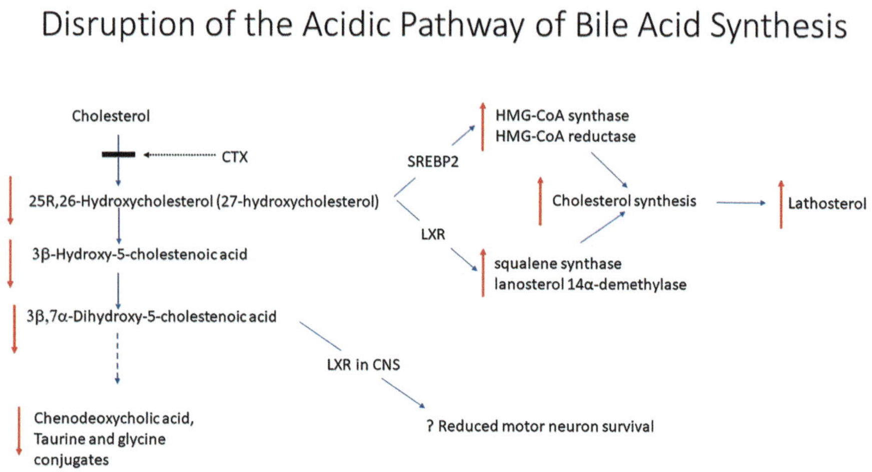

Fig. 9.4 Disruption of the acidic pathway of bile acid synthesis

(i) Low levels of oxysterols, such as 27-hydroxycholesterol, cause SREBP2 movement to the Golgi, proteolytic processing at two cleavage sites and nuclear localisation. SREBP2 is a potent activator of genes involved in cholesterol synthesis such as HMG-CoA synthase and HMG-CoA reductase [5, 6].
(ii) Reduced binding of 27-hydroxycholesterol to the liver X receptor (LXRα). LXRα negatively regulates two genes encoding enzymes in the cholesterol synthesis pathway, squalene synthase (*FDFT1*) and lanosterol 14α-demethylase (*CYP51A1*) [6, 7], so low levels of 27-hyroxycholesterol will activate these steps in the cholesterol synthesis pathway.

Plasma lathosterol is considered a useful marker of endogenous cholesterol synthesis and is increased in individuals with CTX [8, 9]. Plasma concentrations of 8(9)-cholestenol (5α-cholest-8(9)-en-3β-ol) and 8-dehydrocholesterol (cholesta-5,8-dien-3β-ol) can also be increased; the presence of Δ8 sterols in the plasma of individuals with CTX suggests partial inhibition of the Δ8–Δ7 isomerase.

Disruption of the acidic pathway for bile acid synthesis in CTX also leads to low levels of 3β,7α-dihydroxycholest–5–en–26–oic acid (3β,7α-diHCA) in the CSF [10]. This is important because 3β,7α-diHCA is a ligand for the liver X receptor which promotes motor neuron survival.

The combined disruption of the neutral and acidic pathways leads to reduced levels of bile acids such as taurine conjugated chenodeoxycholic acid (t-CDCA) in blood.

Table 9.1 Scenarios and presenting symptoms that might lead a clinician to request a biochemical diagnostic testing for CTX

Neonatal population screening	Ataxia
Neonatal cholestasis	Tremor
Infantile spasms	Psychiatric disorder (e.g. schizophrenia)
Developmental delay	Neuropathy
Protracted diarrhoea	Xanthomata
Cataracts	Premature atherosclerosis (e.g. ischemic heart disease)
Regression/dementia	Osteoporosis
Spastic paraparesis	
Expressive dysarthria/dysphasia	

Biochemical Diagnostic Testing for CTX

Table 9.1 lists the scenarios and presenting symptoms that might lead a clinician to request analysis of a biomarker for CTX. In the context of a patient with a particular presentation, it can be an advantage to have a test that can diagnose not only CTX but also other disorders with a similar presentation.

Neonatal Population-Based Screening

Early treatment of CTX can prevent most of the serious consequences of the disorder making it a good candidate for neonatal screening, but any test or combination of tests used for screening all newborns for a disorder should ideally have very close to 100% sensitivity and specificity and preferably use dried blood spots (DBS) which are routinely collected from newborns in developed countries. Biochemical tests can also be used to confirm a diagnosis of CTX made using DNA screening, especially when DNA screening identifies one or more variants of uncertain significance (VUS) or identifies only a single pathogenic variant in a patients with a high level of suspicion of disease.

In 2014, DeBarber et al. described a method for screening for CTX based on measurement of 7α,12α-dihydoxy-cholest-4-en-3-one (7α12αC4) in DBS [11]. In 2017, Vaz et al. described a method for screening for CTX using DBS from newborns, which involved measuring the ratio of cholestane 3α,7α,12α,25-tetrol glucuronide to taurochenodeoxycholic acid (GlcA-tetrol/t-CDCA) and also the ratio of taurotrihydroxycholestanoic acid to the tetrol (t-THCA/GlcA-tetrol) [3]. Hong et al. evaluated the screening methods on 32,000 newborn DBS. The measurement of 7α,12αC4 was abandoned because of isobaric interferences for the 7α,12αC4 derivatisation method used, but the measurements using the GlcA-tetrol alone or THCA/GlcA-tetrol achieved 100% sensitivity and specificity (a zero percent false positive rate) [12].

Monitoring Efficacy of Treatment of CTX

Treatment of CTX with chenodeoxycholic acid (CDCA) corrects many of the biochemical abnormalities such as the raised plasma cholestanol level and the raised urinary bile alcohol excretion. An expert panel recently recommended monitoring treatment of CTX with plasma cholestanol and neurological examination [13]. Cholestanol has been used as the primary blood biomarker for diagnosis and to monitor efficacy of therapy in CTX for >50 years, but this biomarker can also be elevated in some liver disease [14] and sitosterolemia [15] (and see following section). Methods for determination of cholestanol can often also detect the cholesterol precursors and raised lathosterol values rapidly normalise after initiation of chenodeoxycholic acid therapy [8]. DeBarber and Duell have pointed out that plasma cholestanol levels may take 3–6 months or even longer to normalise on treatment and have suggested that plasma 7α-hydroxy-choles-4-en-3-one and 7α,12α-dihydroxy-cholest-4-en-3-one may change more rapidly on treatment and thus may be superior for CDCA dose titration and monitoring of therapeutic efficacy in CTX; further studies are needed to verify this [16].

Neonatal Cholestasis

CTX can cause cholestatic liver disease of neonatal onset. Plasma cholestanol is not a good test in this scenario as other causes of cholestasis can give rise to raised plasma cholestanol. The DBS GlcA-tetrol/t-CDCA and t-THCA/GlcA-tetrol ratios proposed as newborn dried blood spot screening tests can distinguish CTX from other causes of neonatal/infantile cholestasis and can also detect peroxisomal disorders; however, there are other tests available through the chemical pathology laboratory that can diagnose not only CTX and peroxisomal disorders but also other treatable causes of neonatal/infantile cholestasis. Abnormal cholanoids (bile acids and bile alcohols) can be detected by a negative ion mass spectrometry scan of urine using either electrospray ionisation (ESI-MS) or fast atom bombardment ionisation (FAB-MS; also known as liquid secondary ionisation mass spectrometry) in highly specialised laboratories [17]. This can be achieved without chromatographic separation using a flow injection technique (Fig. 9.5). Peak identities can be confirmed by fragmentation of ions in a collision cell which produces specific daughter ions, e.g. m/z 74 for glycine conjugates, m/z 80 for taurine conjugates, m/z 97 for sulphates and m/z 85 for glucuronides. In CTX, the urinary cholanoid analysis shows massive excretion of cholestane pentol glucuronides (m/z 627 > 85) with lesser excretion of cholestane tetrol glucuronides (m/z 611 > 85) and cholestane hexol glucuronides (m/z 643 > 85). In normal infants and infants with cholestasis, there is a much lower level of excretion of bile alcohol glucuronides and the largest peak is attributable to 27-nor-5β-cholestane-3α,7α,12α,24,25-pentol (m/z 613 > 85).

The advantage of analysing a urinary cholanoid spectrum is that it can detect other disorders causing neonatal cholestasis (listed in Table 9.2), including two

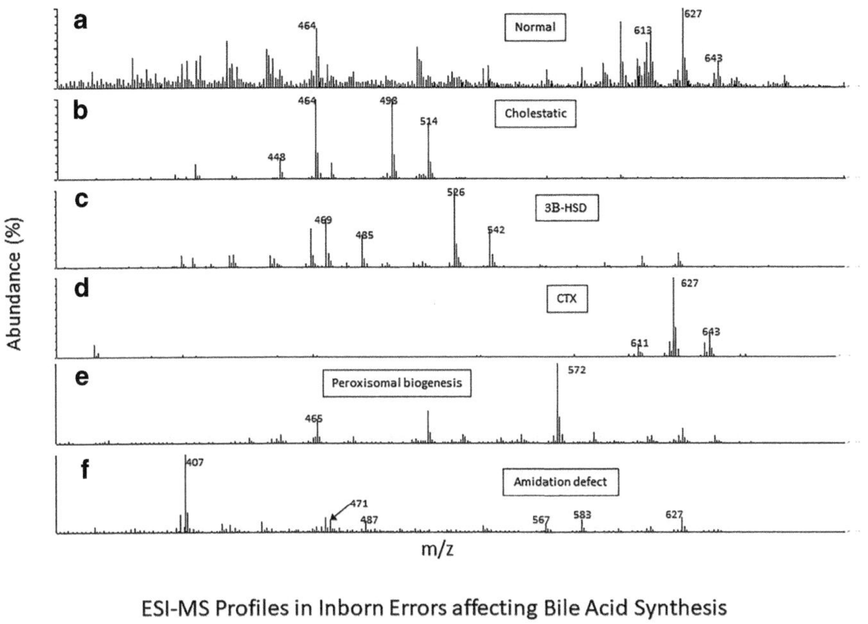

Fig. 9.5 ESI-MS profiles in inborn errors affecting bile acid synthesis

Table 9.2 Disorders causing neonatal cholestatic liver disease that can be diagnosed from a urine cholanoid spectrum

3β-Hydroxy-Δ^5-C_{27}-steroid dehydrogenase deficiency (*HSD3B7*)
Δ^4-3-Oxosteroid 5β-reductase deficiency (*SRD5B1/AKR1D1*)
α-Methyl-acyl-CoA racemase deficiency (*AMACR*)
Sterol 27-hydroxylase deficiency (Cerebrotendinous xanthomatosis; *CYP27A1*)
Peroxisome biogenesis disorders (*PEX* genes)
Zellweger/infantile Refsum's
Oxysterol 7α-hydroxylase deficiency (*CYP7B1*)
Bile acid CoA: amino acid N-acyl transferase deficiency (*BAAT*)
? Bile acid CoA ligase deficiency (*SLC27A5*)[a]
Acyl-CoA oxidase 2 deficiency (*ACOX2*)
Niemann Pick C disease (*NPC1* & *NPC2*)

[a]The urine bile acid spectrum can detect this enzyme defect, but it is not clear whether it causes neonatal cholestatic liver disease without other contributing factors

disorders for which bile acid treatment can reverse life-threatening liver disease—3β-hydroxy-Δ5-C27-steroid dehydrogenase deficiency and Δ4-3-oxosteroid 5β-reductase deficiency.

Cataracts

Bilateral juvenile cataracts are an early sign of CTX so an investigation that will make the diagnosis at the time of this presentation may enable treatment to commence before there have been any serious neurodevelopmental effects of the disease. Freedman et al., using plasma cholestanol and urine bile alcohol testing for CTX, showed that of 170 children diagnosed as having early-onset idiopathic bilateral cataracts, three patients (1.8%) had CTX [18]. Most laboratory methods for measurement of plasma cholestanol can detect other sterols/stanols so it is important that biomarkers of other causes of cataract are not missed. Table 9.3 lists sterols/stanols that can be diagnostic of other disorders. These disorders could, of course, be detected by DNA sequencing [19] with the usual caveat with regard to DNA testing that some gene variants detected will be VUS.

Table 9.3 Causes of cataracts that can be detected by analysis of sterols and stanols in plasma

Disorder	Gene	Enzyme	Sterol/stanol(s) detected
CTX	*CYP27A1*	Sterol 27-hydroxylase aka Sterol 26-hydroxylase	Cholestanol Lathosterol 8-Dehydrocholesterol Cholest-8(9)en-3β-ol
Conradi-Hunermann syndrome X-linked dominant chondrodysplasia punctata	*EBP*	Sterol Δ8–Δ7 isomerase	8-Dehydrocholesterol Cholest-8(9)en-3β-ol
Lathosterolosis	*SC5D*	Sterol-Δ5-desaturase	Lathosterol
Lanosterolosis	*CYP51A1*	Lanosterol C14-demethylase	Lanosterol 7-Dehydrocholesterol
Smith-Lemli-Opitz syndrome	*DHCR7*	7-Dehydrocholesterol reductase	7-Dehydrocholesterol 8-Dehydrocholesterol

Diarrhoea

Chronic diarrhoea is a common early symptom of CTX but CTX is not a cause of chronic diarrhoea that most paediatric gastroenterologists would have high on their list of differential diagnoses. The Clinical Pathology Laboratory should offer measurement of cholestanol and/or urinary cholanoid testing for CTX for unexplained chronic diarrhoea and disseminate the message that it is a cause to be considered and one that has specific effective treatment.

Neurodevelopmental Presentations

The neurological presentations of CTX are quite variable, but the earliest presentation can be developmental delay in a pre-school or school-aged child. This, in the author's view is a good reason why the Clinical Pathology Laboratory should include, in the work-up of a child with developmental delay, testing for CTX, such as the plasma sterol/stanol profile detecting cholestanol or the urinary cholanoid profile detecting the excretion of bile alcohol glucuronides characteristic of CTX.

Xanthomata and Atherosclerosis

CTX can present with xanthomata, the Achilles tendons being a typical site. It can also present with the consequences of atherosclerosis such as ischemic heart disease [20]. It is important to look at the plasma sterol and stanol profile in individuals with these presentations to detect the disorders that need different treatment to hypercholesterolemia including CTX and phytosterolemia (sitosterolemia) [21].

Conclusions

- It is 50 years since the pioneers of CTX research made the first important observations.
  - In 1968, Menkes et al. documented increased cholestanol in the CNS [22].
  - In 1971, Salen described the low concentration of chenodeoxycholic acid in bile and proposed use of blood cholestanol for identification of CTX [23].
  - In 1974, Setoguchi et al. reported the substantial production of bile alcohols in CTX [24].
- In these 50 years, we have come to understand a lot about the biochemical pathways in CTX that lead to these metabolite abnormalities.
- For neonatal screening of dried blood spots, the best method for detection of CTX appears to be the DBS ratios: GlcA-tetrol/t-CDCA and t-THCA/GlcA-tetrol.

- For biochemical diagnosis and for monitoring the efficacy of treatment of CTX, plasma cholestanol remains the choice of an expert panel, although additional urine bile alcohol testing can be helpful in that changes may occur more rapidly with bile alcohols and bile alcohol measurement can be useful to confirm a diagnosis of CTX.
- In the Clinical Pathology Laboratory, two analyses remain very useful in detecting CTX and disorders with similar presenting features:
  - Chromatography of plasma sterols and stanols, including cholestanol, e.g. by gas chromatography-mass spectrometry (GC-MS)
  - Urinary cholanoid (bile alcohol) profile by ESI-MS/MS

References

1. Salen G, Shefer S, Tint GS. Transformation of 4-cholesten-3-one and 7 alpha-hydroxy-4-cholesten-3-one into cholestanol and bile acids in cerebrotendinous xanthomatosis. Gastroenterology. 1984;87(2):276–83.
2. Buchmann MS, Björkhem I, Skrede S. Metabolism of the cholestanol precursor cholesta-4,6-dien-3-one in different tissues. Biochim Biophys Acta. 1987;922(2):111–7. https://doi.org/10.1016/0005-2760(87)90144-5.
3. Vaz FM, Bootsma AH, Kulik W, Verrips A, Wevers RA, Schielen PC, DeBarber AE, Huidekoper HH. A newborn screening method for cerebrotendinous xanthomatosis using bile alcohol glucuronides and metabolite ratios. J Lipid Res. 2017;58(5):1002–7. https://doi.org/10.1194/jlr.P075051. Epub 2017 Mar 17. PMID: 28314860; PMCID: PMC5408618.
4. Tint GS, Salen G. Evidence for the early reduction of the 24,25 double bond in the conversion of lanosterol to cholesterol in cerebrotendinous xanthomatosis. Metabolism. 1977;26(7):721–9. https://doi.org/10.1016/0026-0495(77)90059-2.
5. Madison BB. Srebp2: a master regulator of sterol and fatty acid synthesis. J Lipid Res. 2016;57(3):333–5. https://doi.org/10.1194/jlr.C066712. Epub 2016 Jan 21. PMID: 26798145; PMCID: PMC4766982.
6. Saito H, Tachiura W, Nishimura M, Shimizu M, Sato R, Yamauchi Y. Hydroxylation site-specific and production-dependent effects of endogenous oxysterols on cholesterol homeostasis: implications for SREBP-2 and LXR. J Biol Chem. 2023;299(1):102733. https://doi.org/10.1016/j.jbc.2022.102733. Epub 2022 Nov 22. PMID: 36423680; PMCID: PMC9792893.
7. Wang Y, Rogers PM, Su C, Varga G, Stayrook KR, Burris TP. Regulation of cholesterologenesis by the oxysterol receptor, LXRalpha. J Biol Chem. 2008;283:26332–9.
8. Wolthers BG, Walrecht HT, van der Molen JC, Nagel GT, Van Doormaal JJ, Wijnandts PN. Use of determinations of 7-lathosterol (5 alpha-cholest-7-en-3 beta-ol) and other cholesterol precursors in serum in the study and treatment of disturbances of sterol metabolism, particularly cerebrotendinous xanthomatosis. J Lipid Res. 1991;32(4):603–12.
9. Mignarri A, Magni A, Del Puppo M, Gallus GN, Björkhem I, Federico A, Dotti MT. Evaluation of cholesterol metabolism in cerebrotendinous xanthomatosis. J Inherit Metab Dis. 2016;39(1):75–83. https://doi.org/10.1007/s10545-015-9873-1. Epub 2015 Jul 8.
10. Theofilopoulos S, Griffiths WJ, Crick PJ, Yang S, Meljon A, Ogundare M, Kitambi SS, Lockhart A, Tuschl K, Clayton PT, Morris AA, Martinez A, Reddy MA, Martinuzzi A, Bassi MT, Honda A, Mizuochi T, Kimura A, Nittono H, De Michele G, Carbone R, Criscuolo C, Yau JL, Seckl JR, Schüle R, Schöls L, Sailer AW, Kuhle J, Fraidakis MJ, Gustafsson JÅ, Steffensen KR, Björkhem I, Ernfors P, Sjövall J, Arenas E, Wang Y. Cholestenoic acids regulate motor neuron survival via liver X receptors. J Clin Invest. 2014;124(11):4829–42. https://doi.org/10.1172/JCI68506. Epub 2014 Oct 1. PMID: 25271621; PMCID: PMC4347238.

11. DeBarber AE, Luo J, Star-Weinstock M, Purkayastha S, Geraghty MT, Chiang JP, Merkens LS, Pappu AS, Steiner RD. A blood test for cerebrotendinous xanthomatosis with potential for disease detection in newborns. J Lipid Res. 2014;55(1):146–54. https://doi.org/10.1194/jlr.P043273. Epub 2013 Nov 2. PMID: 24186955; PMCID: PMC3927472.
12. Hong X, Daiker J, Sadilek M, DeBarber AE, Chiang J, Duan J, Bootsma AH, Huidekoper HH, Vaz FM, Gelb MH. Toward newborn screening of cerebrotendinous xanthomatosis: results of a biomarker research study using 32,000 newborn dried blood spots. Genet Med. 2020;22(10):1606–12. https://doi.org/10.1038/s41436-020-0846-x. Epub 2020 Jun 10. PMID: 32523054; PMCID: PMC7529987.
13. Stelten BML, Dotti MT, Verrips A, Elibol B, Falik-Zaccai TC, Hanman K, Mignarri A, Sithole B, Steiner RD, Verma S, Yahalom G, Zubarioglu T, Mochel F, Federico A. Expert opinion on diagnosing, treating and managing patients with cerebrotendinous xanthomatosis (CTX): a modified Delphi study. Orphanet J Rare Dis. 2021;16(1):353. https://doi.org/10.1186/s13023-021-01980-5. PMID: 34362411; PMCID: PMC8349076.
14. Koopman BJ, van der Molen JC, Wolthers BG, de Jager AE, Waterreus RJ, Gips CH. Capillary gas chromatographic determination of cholestanol/cholesterol ratio in biological fluids. Its potential usefulness for the follow-up of some liver diseases and its lack of specificity in diagnosing CTX (cerebrotendinous xanthomatosis). Clin Chim Acta. 1984;137(3):305–15. https://doi.org/10.1016/0009-8981(84)90119-0.
15. Salen G, Kwiterovich PO Jr, Shefer S, Tint GS, Horak I, Shore V, Dayal B, Horak E. Increased plasma cholestanol and 5 alpha-saturated plant sterol derivatives in subjects with sitosterolemia and xanthomatosis. J Lipid Res. 1985;26(2):203–9.
16. DeBarber A, Duell PB. Update on cerebrotendinous xanthomatosis. Curr Opin Lipidol. 2021;32(2):123–31.
17. Clayton PT. Disorders of bile acid synthesis. J Inherit Metab Dis. 2011;34(3):593–604. https://doi.org/10.1007/s10545-010-9259-3. Epub 2011 Jan 13.
18. Freedman SF, Brennand C, Chiang J, DeBarber A, Del Monte MA, Duell PB, Fiorito J, Marshall R. Prevalence of cerebrotendinous xanthomatosis among patients diagnosed with acquired juvenile-onset idiopathic bilateral cataracts. JAMA Ophthalmol. 2019;137(11):1312–6. https://doi.org/10.1001/jamaophthalmol.2019.3639. PMID: 31536098; PMCID: PMC6753501.
19. Musleh M, Hall G, Lloyd IC, Gillespie RL, Waller S, Douzgou S, Clayton-Smith J, Kehdi E, Black GC, Ashworth J. Diagnosing the cause of bilateral paediatric cataracts: comparison of standard testing with a next-generation sequencing approach. Eye (Lond). 2016;30(9):1175–81. https://doi.org/10.1038/eye.2016.105. Epub 2016 Jun 17. PMID: 27315345; PMCID: PMC5023796.
20. Federico A, Gallus GN. Cerebrotendinous xanthomatosis. [Updated 2022 Mar 17]. In: Adam MP, Feldman J, Mirzaa GM, et al., editors. GeneReviews® [Internet]. Seattle: University of Washington; 1993–2024. Available from: https://www.ncbi.nlm.nih.gov/books/NBK1409/. 16 July 2003.
21. Liebeskind A, Peterson AL, Wilson D. Sitosterolemia. In: Feingold KR, Anawalt B, Blackman MR, Boyce A, Chrousos G, Corpas E, de Herder WW, Dhatariya K, Dungan K, Hofland J, Kalra S, Kaltsas G, Kapoor N, Koch C, Kopp P, Korbonits M, Kovacs CS, Kuohung W, Laferrère B, Levy M, McGee EA, McLachlan R, New M, Purnell J, Sahay R, Shah AS, Singer F, Sperling MA, Stratakis CA, Trence DL, Wilson DP, editors. Endotext [Internet]. South Dartmouth: MDText.com, Inc.; 2000. 10 Mar 2023.
22. Menkes JH, Schimschock JR, Swanson PD. Cerebrotendinous xanthomatosis. The storage of cholestanol within the nervous system. Arch Neurol. 1968;19(1):47–53. https://doi.org/10.1001/archneur.1968.00480010065004.
23. Salen G. Cholestanol deposition in cerebrotendinous xanthomatosis. A possible mechanism. Ann Intern Med. 1971;75(6):843–51. https://doi.org/10.7326/0003-4819-75-6-843.
24. Setoguchi T, Salen G, Tint GS, Mosbach EH. A biochemical abnormality in cerebrotendinous xanthomatosis. Impairment of bile acid biosynthesis associated with incomplete degradation of the cholesterol side chain. J Clin Invest. 1974;53(5):1393–401. https://doi.org/10.1172/JCI107688. PMID: 4825231; PMCID: PMC302628.

Atypical Cerebrotendinous Xanthomatosis (CTX) with Normal Cholestanol and Marked Elevations of Bile Acid Pathway Intermediates and Bile Alcohols

10

Maya Fowler, Jenefer DeKoning, and Andrea E. DeBarber

Abbreviations

23S-pentol	5β-cholestane-3α,7α,12α,23S,25-pentol
25-tetrol glucuronide	5β-cholestane-3α,7α,12α,25-tetrol-3-O-β-D-glucuronide
7α12αC4	7α,12α-dihydroxy-4-cholesten-3-one
7αC4	7α-hydroxy-4-cholesten-3-one
CDCA	Chenodeoxycholic acid
CTX	Cerebrotendinous xanthomatosis
LLOQ	Lower limit of quantification

Introduction

Cerebrotendinous xanthomatosis (CTX, OMIM 213700) is a rare autosomal recessive genetic disorder of bile acid synthesis associated with deficiency in the sterol 27-hydroxylase enzyme, encoded by *CYP27A1* [1, 2]. Disease progression in CTX can be effectively prevented by treatment with chenodeoxycholic acid (CDCA).

M. Fowler · J. DeKoning
University Shared Resources, Oregon Health & Science University (OHSU), Portland, OR, USA

A. E. DeBarber (✉)
School of Medicine, Oregon Health and Science University, Portland, OR, USA
e-mail: debarber@ohsu.edu

A. Federico et al. (eds.), *Cerebrotendinous Xanthomatosis*,
https://doi.org/10.1007/978-3-031-92526-9_10

The clinical presentation is quite heterogeneous for this disease, with variable symptoms, severity and progression, even for the same *CYP27A1* genotype within the same family [1, 2]. The mean age at diagnosis in a large series of 43 US cases was 32 years old [3]. Of the CTX patients, 53% suffered from chronic diarrhea in childhood, 74% had cognitive impairment, 70% had premature cataracts in childhood/adolescence, 77% developed tendon xanthomas by 25 years old, and 81% experienced neurologic disease beginning in the third or fourth decade of life (range 20–40 years of age) [3].

Data from population-based genetic studies suggests CTX patients as a group are likely under-diagnosed [4]. Those who are eventually diagnosed with CTX often remain undiagnosed for more than one to two decades after onset of initial symptoms, resulting in a significant burden of often irreversible neurologic disease [5]. Tools to mitigate under-diagnosis and late diagnosis include greater awareness of the disease among health care providers and access to genetic and (sensitive and specific) biochemical confirmatory testing.

It was first proposed >50 years ago by Salen that a biochemical diagnosis of CTX could be established through measurement of elevated cholestanol [6], which has been accepted as the primary biomarker for diagnosis of CTX for decades. A recent expert consensus study on diagnosing, treating and managing patients with CTX indicated genetic analyses and/or determination of circulating cholestanol levels should be used for diagnostic confirmation of CTX [7]. Expert panelists agreed that patients with CTX always have elevated circulating cholestanol at diagnosis and that measuring cholestanol is the diagnostic biomarker of choice. Conversely, identification of a normal cholestanol concentration has been considered definitive for exclusion of CTX.

Additional biomarkers or biochemical signatures for CTX have been identified as useful for diagnosis of CTX. For example, metabolic end-products of the sterol 27-hydroxylase enzyme (CYP27A1), such as CDCA, are deficient in CTX. In addition, elevated levels of cholesterol precursors consistent with an increased rate of cholesterol synthesis can be present in CTX [8, 9]. Activation of the cholesterol 7α-hydroxylase (CYP7A1) enzyme, which metabolizes cholesterol to 7α-hydroxycholesterol, is subject to diminished repression in CTX due to the lack of CDCA (see Fig. 10.1). This results in a high rate of bile acid pathway intermediate and bile alcohol synthesis and elevated levels in plasma and other tissues of the biomarkers shown in grey in Fig. 10.1, for example, 7α-hydroxy-4-cholesten-3-one (7αC4), 7α,12α-dihydroxy-4-cholesten-3-one (7α12αC4) [10, 11] and C27 bile alcohols [2]. Bile alcohols are highly elevated in CTX and are predominately present as their glucuronide conjugates [12, 13].

We have developed quantitative isotope-dilution liquid chromatography-tandem mass spectrometry (LC-MS/MS) assays for the bile acid pathway intermediates 7αC4 and 7α12αC4 and reported their typical concentration ranges in the blood of untreated CTX patients (see Fig. 10.2 and refer to [10, 11]). 7αC4 was proposed more than a decade ago by our group as a sensitive marker for diagnosis of CTX and for monitoring the efficacy of treatment with bile acids [10]. We have also developed a quantitative isotope-dilution LC-MS/MS assay for the predominant

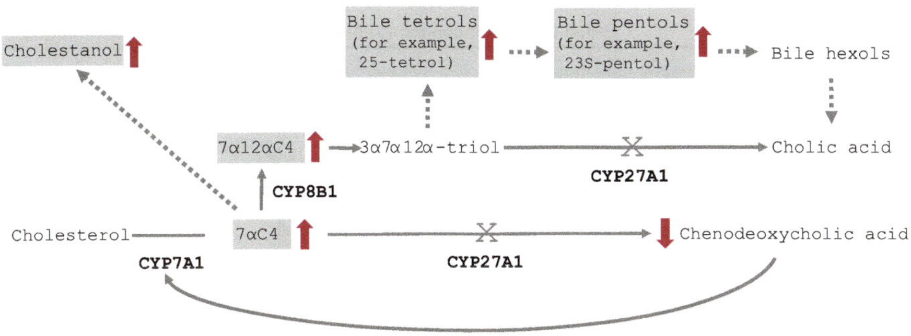

Fig. 10.1 "Classic" bile acid synthesis pathway in CTX. (Modified from Ref. [2]). Chenodeoxycholic acid (CDCA) normally acts as a ligand to activate FXR, providing an inhibitory cascade resulting in a loss of activation of CYP7A1 (and bile acid synthesis suppression). High expression of CYP7A1 is observed in CTX, that can be explained by deactivation of inhibitory pathway attributable to a reduced CDCA pool. This results in hyperactivation of the "classic" pathway of bile acid synthesis with increased production of 7α-hydroxy-cholesterol (not shown), its 7α-hydroxy-4-cholesten-3-one (7αC4) metabolite and increased production of derived metabolites including cholestanol, 7α,12α-dihydroxy-4-cholesten-3-one (7α12αC4), 5β-cholestan-3α,7α,12α-triol (3α7α12α-triol), 5β-cholestan-3α,7α,12α,25-tetrol (25-tetrol), 5β-cholestan-3α,7α,12α,23S,25-pentol (23S-pentol) and other bile alcohol isomers (tetrols, pentols and hexols), all predominantly present as their glucuronide conjugates. Note that some cholic acid is produced in untreated CTX through an atypical bile alcohol pathway. Pathway arrows may encompass multiple steps (with broken arrows additional major pathways present in CTX)

bile tetrol glucuronide present in bile and blood in CTX (5β-cholestane-3α,7α,12α,25-tetrol-3-O-β-D-glucuronide or 25-tetrol glucuronide [141516]), as well as the predominant bile pentol present in urine (5β-cholestane-3α,7α,12α,23S,25-pentol or 23S-pentol [17]), for which the assay requires cleavage of glucuronide conjugates prior to the measurement of total 23S-pentol. We have reported the typical concentration ranges of predominant bile alcohols in the blood and urine of untreated CTX patients (see Fig. 10.2 and refer to [141617]).

Recently, a number of atypical CTX cases with normal plasma cholestanol levels have been reported (at baseline prior to treatment with bile acids). We review here 16 cases of CTX with normal baseline cholestanol, many of which have been reported in the last few years [14, 18–28]. The highest normal concentration of plasma cholestanol was previously reported to range from 4.9 to 5.4 μg/ml (12.6 to 13.9 μmol/L) [29, 30]. In a large group of (normal) individuals analyzed by Schaefer et al (n = 333,379), the 99th percentile for plasma cholestanol was reported to be 5.4 μg/ml and this is the upper "normal" concentration value we have used for this review. For at least three cases of atypical CTX, full biochemical characterization was performed, including measurement of bile acid pathway intermediate and bile alcohol biomarkers, including after treatment with CDCA was initiated [14].

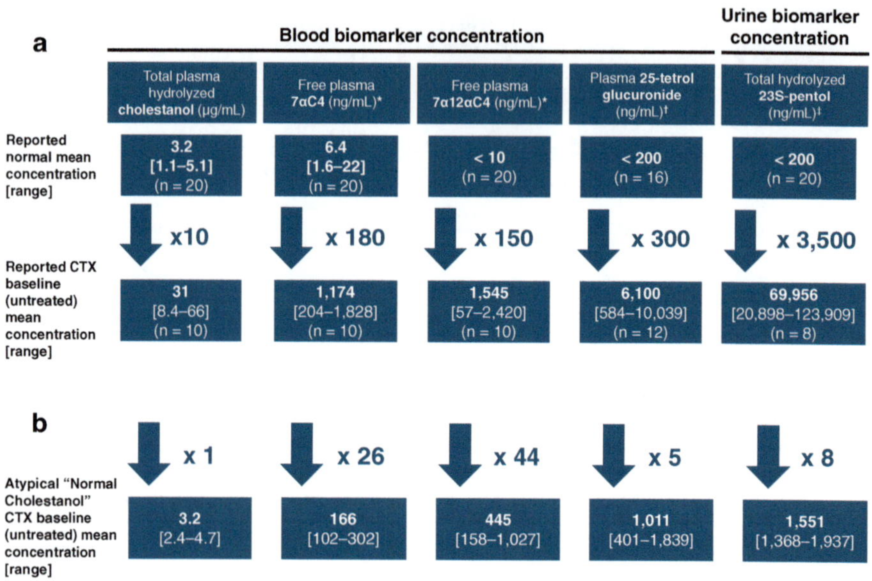

Fig. 10.2 Biomarker concentrations reported in patients with CTX. Panel (**a**): Highly elevated biomarker levels compared to normal mean concentration typically observed in CTX (with elevated cholestanol). Concentration mean and range is shown [14]. *In plasma; assay LLOQ is 10 ng/mL, †in dried blood; assay LLOQ is 200 ng/mL and ‡in urine; assay LLOQ is 200 ng/mL. Panel (**b**): Markedly elevated biomarker levels compared to normal mean concentration observed in atypical CTX (with normal cholestanol). *Averages of baseline mean concentrations from reported cases #1–3 [14]. 7αC4, 7α-hydroxy-4-cholesten-3-one; 7α12αC4, 7α,12α-dihydroxy-4-cholesten-3-one;25-tetrol glucuronide, 5β-cholestane-3α,7α,12α,25-tetrol-3-O-β-D-glucuronide; 23S-pentol, 5β-cholestane-3α,7α,12α,23S,25-pentol; CTX, cerebrotendinous xanthomatosis; LLOQ, lower limit of quantification

Results and Discussion

For the last 50 years, the standard for biochemical diagnosis of CTX has been the measurement of elevated levels of circulating cholestanol in plasma or serum. Identification of a normal circulating cholestanol concentration was believed to exclude a diagnosis of CTX. We review and provide a summary for 16 reported cases of clinically and/or genetically confirmed CTX with normal plasma cholestanol (designated as <5.4 μg/ml). Cases of CTX with normal or high normal circulating cholestanol may be more widespread than currently recognized, although their prevalence is currently unknown. CTX patients as a group are under-diagnosed, most likely due to the heterogeneous clinical presentation of CTX. Under-diagnosis may be exacerbated through the inability to confirm a biochemical diagnosis in CTX patients when using cholestanol as the primary diagnostic biomarker.

It is concerning that CTX cases may be missed when measurement of cholestanol is the only marker used for biochemical diagnosis of CTX. In reported case 1 (see Tables 10.1, 10.2, and 10.3 and refer to [14, 18]), the possibility of CTX was

Table 10.1 Clinical characteristics reported in atypical CTX patients with normal (or high normal) cholestanol

Clinical features	Age at diagnosis	Xanthomas	Cataracts	Cognitive impairment	Neurologic symptoms	Psychiatric symptoms	Additional symptoms
Case 1 [14, 18]	86 yr	+		+ (mild memory loss after stroke)			
Case 2 [14]	65 yr	+		+ (memory loss)	+		
Case 3 [14]	40 yr	+					
Case 4 [19]	57 yr	+			+		
Case 5 [19]	60 yr	+ (bilateral stiffness and swelling Achilles tendon)					
Case 6 [20]	11 yr	+		+ (pervasive developmental disorder)			Autism spectrum disorder
Case 7 [21]	65 yr	+		+ (memory impairment, dementia)	+	+	Epilepsy
Case 8 [22]	63 yr	+					Coronary atherosclerosis
Case 9 [23]	74 yr	+					Single stroke
Case 10 [24]	29 yr	+ (markedly thickened, occurred after neurological symptoms)	+ (small cortical)	+ (mild learning difficulties)	+		Epilepsy, diarrhea, neuroimaging features

(continued)

Table 10.1 (continued)

Clinical features	Age at diagnosis	Xanthomas	Cataracts	Cognitive impairment	Neurologic symptoms	Psychiatric symptoms	Additional symptoms
Case 11 [25]	35 yr	+					
Case 12 [26]	68 yr	+	+				
Case 13 [27]	17 yr		+	+	+		
Case 14 [27]	44 yr	+			+		
Case 15 [27]	31 yr	+	+	+	+		
Case 16 [28]	40 yr	+					

Table 10.2 Plasma and urine biomarker concentrations in atypical CTX patients with normal circulating cholestanol (at baseline prior to treatment and after CDCA therapy was initiated) [14]

	Blood biomarker concentration				Urine biomarker concentration	
CTX case ID	*Total Plasma hydrolyzed cholestanol (μg/mL)*	*Free plasma 7αC4 (ng/mL)*	*Free plasma 7α12α C4 (ng/mL)*	*Plasma 25-tetrol glucuronide (ng/mL)*	*Total hydrolyzed 23S-pentol (ng/mL)*	*23S-pentol/ creatinine (ng/mg)*
Case 1[a] Baseline (Case 1 [14])	**3.0: 2.4[b]**	**102: 116[b]**	**158: 219[b]**	**401: 495[b]**	**1368: 1478[b]**	**1505: 2514[b]**
Rx 1 month	*3.4*	*13.5*	*13.3*	*<200*	*272*	*338*
Rx 6 months	*2.9*	*11.3*	*<10*	*219.1*	*282*	*328*
Rx 8 months	*3.2*	*17.7*	*14.7*	*204.3*	*461*	*475*
Case 2 Baseline (Case 2 [14])	**4.7**	**302**	**1027**	**1839**	**1937**	**6943**
Rx 3 months	*3.5*	*<10*	*15*	*212*	*215*	*224*
Rx 6 months	*2.9*	*<10*	*<10*	*205*	*<200*	*<421*
Case 3 Baseline (Case 3 [14])	**2.8**	**139**	**308**	**580**	**1422**	**4309**
Rx 1.5 months	*2.6*	*43*	*113*	*425*	*1793*	*1207*

[a]Case previously reported [18] but not identified as CTX
[b]Samples taken 9 months apart prior to treatment

considered more than 30 years prior to diagnosis but was excluded on the basis of repeatedly normal plasma cholestanol concentrations (Table 10.2). In reported case 7 [21], the patient was not treated for CTX because of diagnostic delay, with a normal plasma cholestanol concentration despite neurological features suggestive of CTX, followed by progressive decline and death of the patient >2 years later. The post-mortem neuropathological findings documented a diagnosis of CTX, and the normal cholestanol concentration was later attributed to a possible technical error.

It may be that the concentration of cholestanol is low in some cases of CTX as a consequence of treatment with certain medications. For example, treatment with corticosteroids was proposed to have lowered the blood cholestanol concentration in case 10 (in this case the diagnosis of CTX was initially abandoned due to a normal cholestanol result, followed by marked neurological deterioration in the patient prior to treatment with CDCA 2 years later [24]). At least three atypical biochemical CTX patients reported with baseline normal cholestanol (prior to treatment with CDCA) were reported as being treated with ezetimibe (cases 3, 9 and 16), which may have lowered the plasma cholestanol concentration through inhibition of intestinal cholestanol absorption via the Niemann-Pick C1-like 1 (NPC1L1) sterol transporter. Although treatment with ezetimibe (with or without statins) may lower the plasma concentration of cholestanol in CTX [28] and could be a confounding factor

Table 10.3 *CYP27A1* variants reported in atypical CTX patients with normal (or high normal) circulating cholestanol

Patient ID	Baseline cholestanol[a] (μg/mL)	CYP27A1 molecular variant 1	Variant classification[b]	CYP27A1 molecular variant 2	Variant classification[b]
Case 1 [14, 18]	3.0, 2.4	c.785G>T (p.Arg262Leu)[c]	Uncertain significance[d]	c.1183C>T (p.Arg395Cys)	Pathogenic/ Likely pathogenic
Case 2 [14]	4.7	c.1184+1G>A (p.?)	Pathogenic	c.1537C>T (p.Arg513Cys)	Pathogenic/ Likely pathogenic
Case 3 [14]	2.8	c.753_754del (p.Tyr253fs or p.Tyr253CysfsTer34)	Pathogenic	c.1415G>C (p.Gly472Ala)	Pathogenic/ Likely pathogenic
Case 4 [19]	Not available; 2.9[e]	c.410G>A (p.Arg137Gln)	Pathogenic/ Likely pathogenic	c.1183C>T (p.Arg395Cys)	Pathogenic/ Likely pathogenic
Case 5 [19]	2.6	c.410G>A (p.Arg137Gln)	Pathogenic/ Likely pathogenic	c.1183C>T (p.Arg395Cys)	Pathogenic/ Likely pathogenic
Case 6 [20]	5.3	c.646G>C (p.Ala216Pro)[f]	Pathogenic/ Likely pathogenic	c.1183C>T (p.Arg395Cys)	Pathogenic/ Likely pathogenic
Case 7 [21]	2.7	c.1017G > C (p.Thr339=)	Pathogenic	c.1435C>T (p.Arg479Cys)	Pathogenic
Case 8 [22]	5.2	c.410G>A (p.Arg137Gln)	Pathogenic/ Likely pathogenic	c.410G>A (p.Arg137Gln)	Pathogenic/ Likely pathogenic
Case 9 [23]	3.1, 5.1	c.379C>T (p.Arg127Trp)	Pathogenic/ Likely pathogenic	c.1435C>G (p.Arg479Gly)	Pathogenic/ Likely pathogenic
Case 10 [24]	3.8	c.844+1G>A (p.?)	Pathogenic	c.844+1G>A (p.?)	Pathogenic
Case 11 [25]	3.9	c.254A>G (p.Gln85Arg)	Pathogenic/ Likely pathogenic	c.673C>T (p.Arg225Cys)	Benign[d, g]
Case 12 [26]	2.1	c.1016C>T (p.Thr339Met)	Pathogenic/ Likely pathogenic	c.844+4A>G (p.?)	Uncertain significance[d]
Case 13 [27]	4.4	c.1435C>T (p.Arg479Gly)	Pathogenic/ Likely pathogenic	c.1435C>T (p.Arg479Gly)	Pathogenic/ Likely pathogenic
Case 14 [27]	3.1	c.1538G >T (p.Arg513Leu)	Uncertain Significance[h]	c.1538G>T (p.Arg513Leu)	Uncertain Significance[h]

(continued)

Table 10.3 (continued)

Patient ID	Baseline cholestanol[a] (μg/mL)	CYP27A1 molecular variant 1	Variant classification[b]	CYP27A1 molecular variant 2	Variant classification[b]
Case 15 [27]	3.8	c.1476+2T>C (p.?)	Pathogenic	c.1476+2T>C (p.?)	Pathogenic
Case 16 [28]	9.4, 4.8[i]	c.1183C>T (p.Arg395Cys)	Pathogenic/ Likely pathogenic	c.1017+5G>C (p.?)	Uncertain signficance[d]

[a]Normal cholestanol designated as <5.4 μg/mL [30]
[b]ClinVar https://www.ncbi.nlm.nih.gov/clinvar/intro/; accessed 16October2024
[c]Correction of original paper from p.Arg262Gln to p.Arg262Leu based on data in ClinVar [14]
[d]Variants can now be considered likely pathogenic with the additional criteria that they are trans with a known pathogenic variant and that there is a specific clinical and/or biochemical phenotype present for the patient that correlates with the gene [14, 26, 28]
[e]Pretreatment result not available; result after 8 months of CDCA treatment [19]
[f]Reported in original reference [25] as c.646G>A (p.Ala261Pro) and updated in reference [14] as c.646G>A (p.Ala216Pro), however variant designated in ClinVar as c.646G>C (p.Ala216Pro)
[g]In addition to the CTX patient described [25] both variants have been described as causing a clinical phenotype in other patients. c.254AG was described in a spinal CTX patient [31]. c.673C, although was registered as a benign variant at the National Center for Biotechnology Information (https://www.ncbi.nlm.nih.gov/clinvar/variation/256798/) was described in one patient [32]
[h]Variant can now be considered likely pathogenic with a specific clinical and/or biochemical phenotype present for the patient that correlates with the gene [27, 32–34]
[i]Note that (second) cholestanol value obtained decreased on ezetimibe treatment (prior to diagnosis of CTX) [28]

for biochemical diagnosis of CTX using cholestanol as a biomarker, ezetimibe is not an accepted treatment for CTX and has not been demonstrated to normalize the production of 7αC4 and correct the aberrant bile acid pathway present in CTX. Medications that may potentially impact biochemical testing for CTX are listed in Table 10.4.

Since Guenzel, DeBarber and colleagues described two siblings in 2021 with genetically confirmed CTX but normal levels of serum cholestanol [19], to the best of our knowledge, an additional nine cases of atypical CTX with normal cholestanol have been reported. Prior to 2021, a handful of similar cases of CTX had been described, with normal cholestanol attributed in one case to a technical error [21] and in another case to treatment with corticosteroids [24]. A summary of the clinical characteristics of reported CTX cases without typical elevations observed in baseline plasma cholestanol is provided in Table 10.1. Of the 16 cases reviewed, 15 had evidence of xanthomas (94%), four had evidence of cataracts (25%), and nine had evidence of some cognitive impairment and/or neurological symptoms (56%; see Table 10.1). For the three atypical CTX patients where full biochemical characterization was performed, marked elevations of bile acid pathway intermediates and

Table 10.4 Potential impact of medications on biochemical testing for CTX

CTX case/ Reference	Medication(s)	Biomarker result	Potential impact on result	Comments
Case 10 [24]	Daily 100 mg Prednisone	Normal blood cholestanol	False negative	
Case 3 [14]	Daily 10 mg ezetimibe	Normal plasma cholestanol	False negative	
Case 9 [23]	Daily 10 mg ezetimibe and 40 mg atorvastatin	Normal plasma cholestanol	False negative	It is noted that analysis was after "15 days without hypolipidemic drug"; drug(s) not specified
Case 16 [28]	Daily 10 mg ezetimibe and 10 mg rosuvastatin	Normal blood cholestanol	False negative	
N/A [35]	Intravenous propofol anesthesia	Elevated urine bile alcohols	False positive	

bile alcohols in plasma and urine were observed (see mean concentrations for these patients in Fig. 10.2 and individual concentrations in Table 10.3). The plasma cholestanol concentrations and disease causing *CYP27A1* variants reported for all 16 CTX patients with atypical biochemical presentation are provided in Table 10.2.

It is unknown whether a diagnosis of CTX in a patient with a normal plasma cholestanol concentration has the same clinical implications and prognosis as a diagnosis of classical CTX with elevated cholestanol. The possibility of a milder "non-neurological" form of CTX has been suggested by Stelten et al. [36]. Of 19 patients with CTX described for the Stelten study [36], the majority (84%) presented with tendon xanthomas as the only or predominant feature. Although the study found some patients with the "non-neurological" form of CTX have a milder biochemical subtype with relatively normal cholestanol levels, the majority of patients showed increased plasma cholestanol levels. Overall, the study found no correlation between the "non-neurological" form of CTX, circulating cholestanol levels or *CYP27A1* genotype. In contrast, data from a different study [37] suggested that four patients with a milder clinical form of CTX may have lower serum cholestanol levels compared to typical levels for CTX.

More research is needed to confirm any correlations between *CYP27A1* genotype and biochemical or clinical phenotype in CTX. It may be possible that among patients with the atypical biochemical presentation reported, there may be sufficient partial sterol 27-hydroxylase (CYP27A1) enzyme activity to metabolize circulating cholestanol and prevent accumulation. In genetic diseases caused by enzyme deficiencies, the occurrence of hypomorphic genetic variants with some preservation of enzyme function is a common mechanism of variability in biochemical and clinical phenotypes between patients. For CTX, even for the same *CYP27A1* genotype within the same family, there can be a heterogeneous clinical presentation, suggesting factors in addition to the genotype must be contributory to the clinical phenotype. The possibility of a milder biochemical CTX presentation with partial enzyme activity could also have implications for CTX carriers heterozygous for a pathogenic variant. With 50% of normal CYP27A1 enzyme activity [38], CTX carriers heterozygous for a pathogenic variant are able to maintain normal levels of cholestanol in plasma, but when their bile acid synthesis pathway is stimulated (e.g., by treatment with cholestyramine), their levels of urinary bile alcohols may increase to levels comparable to those observed in the atypical patients described here [39].

The mechanism of pathophysiology in atypical CTX cases with normal circulating cholestanol is unknown. Accumulation of cholestanol in the central nervous system (CNS) in CTX was first described by Menkes, Schimschock and Swanson in 1968 [40] and has been proposed to contribute to neurological complications in CTX. Cholestanol cannot cross the blood-brain barrier, and cholestanol accumulation in the CNS is thought to be due to synthesis of cholestanol from plasma-derived 7αC4 that can cross the blood-brain barrier [41]. The marked elevation in 7αC4 observed in atypical CTX patients could lead to cholestanol accumulation in the brain, despite a normal concentration of cholestanol in plasma. A flux of only 2% of 7αC4 and other 7α-hydroxylated sterols from plasma into the brain is sufficient to explain cerebral accumulation of cholestanol in CTX [41]. Other factors may contribute to the pathophysiology of disease in atypical CTX cases with normal circulating cholestanol. For example, elevated levels of plasma bile alcohols may contribute to defective functioning of the blood-brain barrier as proposed by Salen and colleagues [42], who found increased amounts of albumin and apolipoprotein B in the cerebrospinal fluid of eight untreated patients with CTX. It is notable that treatment with a high dose of CDCA (1000 mg) daily suppressed plasma bile alcohol glucuronide concentrations in patients with CTX [12] and normalized the concentrations of sterols and apolipoproteins in cerebrospinal fluid, possibly due to restoration of selective permeability of the blood-brain barrier.

In the three atypical CTX cases for which full biochemical characterization was performed [14], the marked elevations of bile acid pathway intermediates and bile alcohols in plasma and urine samples decreased on treatment with oral CDCA (500–750 mg/day), the standard of care for treatment of CTX [1] (data from [14] is shown in Table 10.3). There was no discernable change or a slight downward trend in plasma cholestanol. Note that the urine total 23S-pentol concentration decreased on treatment with CDCA in all three cases when normalized to urine dilution using creatinine measurement. It is unknown what impact treatment with CDCA may have on clinical disease progression in CTX with atypical biochemical presentation with normal cholestanol and if the therapeutic benefits outweigh risks, particularly in the context of mild or absent neurological symptoms. Moreover, although decreased levels of biomarkers were reported in response to treatment with CDCA, the impact of treatment on clinical status or progression of disease in these patients could not be verified [14].

A clinical suspicion index for CTX was developed and demonstrated as a useful tool to decrease diagnostic delay by decades [5]. Early systemic signs such as neonatal cholestatic jaundice, diarrhea and cataract were considered strong indicators, together with neurological features such as intellectual impairment, psychiatric disturbances, ataxia, spastic paraparesis and dentate nuclei abnormalities at MRI. Tendon xanthomas were regarded as very strong indicators. An index score ≥100 warranted serum cholestanol assessment and elevated cholestanol or an index score ≥200 warranted *CYP27A1* gene analysis [5]. The cases described in this review document the existence of CTX patients with non-classical biochemical disease that would not be identified on the basis of measurement of plasma cholestanol alone. They highlight that measurement of cholestanol lacks sensitivity as the primary diagnostic tool for biochemical diagnosis of CTX, despite widespread acceptance of this diagnostic biomarker for decades. Clinicians need to be aware of the occurrence of atypical cases of CTX with normal concentrations of plasma cholestanol (and it should also be noted that treatment with ezetimibe may decrease baseline cholestanol in patients with CTX). The data presented here demonstrates that bile acid pathway intermediates and bile alcohols are sensitive biomarkers for atypical CTX with normal cholestanol, and that such testing is advised, along with *CYP27A1* gene analysis, in patients presenting with clinical symptoms despite normal or near normal cholestanol levels. These biomarkers may also be useful for monitoring the efficacy of bile acid treatment to repress aberrant bile acid synthesis in atypical CTX patients with normal cholestanol in the untreated state. Further studies are needed to verify the utility of using 7αC4 and 7α12αC4, and plasma and urine bile alcohols for monitoring of efficacy of treatment, as well as the impact of CDCA therapy on clinical outcomes in these patients.

Declaration of Interest (Conflict of Interest) Statement All authors are employees of Oregon Health & Science University, Portland, OR, an academic health center reference laboratory providing laboratory services to healthcare providers throughout the United States focusing on biochemical confirmation of genetic diseases of cholesterol synthesis, including CTX, and Andrea DeBarber serves as a volunteer Medical and Scientific Advisory Board member for the CTX Alliance and the United Leukodystrophy Foundation. Andrea DeBarber is a consultant for: Leadiant Biosciences, Travere Therapeutics and Mirum Pharmaceuticals. The OHSU Foundation and OSHU Departments have received gifts from Travere Therapeutics. These gifts, which have not been made specifically in connection with this research, have been reviewed by the OHSU integrity office.

References

1. Federico A, Gallus GN. Cerebrotendinous xanthomatosis. In: Adam MP, Feldman J, Mirzaa GM, Pagon RA, Wallace SE, Bean LJ, et al., editors. GeneReviews. Seattle: University of Washington; 2003. [Internet].
2. DeBarber AE, Duell PB. Update on cerebrotendinous xanthomatosis. Curr Opin Lipidol. 2021;32(2):123–31.
3. Duell PB, Salen G, Eichler FS, DeBarber AE, Connor SL, Casaday L, et al. Diagnosis, treatment, and clinical outcomes in 43 cases with cerebrotendinous xanthomatosis. J Clin Lipidol. 2018;12(5):1169–78.

4. Appadurai V, DeBarber A, Chiang PW, Patel SB, Steiner RD, Tyler C, et al. Apparent underdiagnosis of Cerebrotendinous Xanthomatosis revealed by analysis of ~60,000 human exomes. Mol Genet Metab. 2015;116(4):298–304.
5. Mignarri A, Gallus GN, Dotti MT, Federico A. A suspicion index for early diagnosis and treatment of cerebrotendinous xanthomatosis. J Inherit Metab Dis. 2014;37(3):421–9.
6. Salen G. Cholestanol deposition in cerebrotendinous xanthomatosis. A possible mechanism. Ann Intern Med. 1971;75(6):843–51.
7. Stelten BML, Dotti MT, Verrips A, Elibol B, Falik-Zaccai TC, Hanman K, et al. Expert opinion on diagnosing, treating and managing patients with cerebrotendinous xanthomatosis (CTX): a modified Delphi study. Orphanet J Rare Dis. 2021;16(1):353.
8. de Sain-van der Velden MGM, Verrips A, Prinsen BHCMT, de Barse M, Berger R, Visser G. Elevated cholesterol precursors other than cholestanol can also be a hallmark for CTX. J Inherit Metab Dis. 2008;31(Suppl 2):S387–93.
9. Mignarri A, Magni A, Del Puppo M, Gallus GN, Björkhem I, et al. Evaluation of cholesterol metabolism in cerebrotendinous xanthomatosis. J Inherit Metab Dis. 2016;36(1):75–83.
10. DeBarber AE, Connor WE, Pappu AS, Merkens LS, Steiner RD. ESI-MS/MS quantification of 7alpha-hydroxy-4-cholesten-3-one facilitates rapid, convenient diagnostic testing for cerebrotendinous xanthomatosis. Clin Chim Acta. 2010;411(1–2):43–8.
11. DeBarber AE, Luo J, Giugliani R, Souza CFM, Chiang JPW, Merkens LS, et al. A useful multi-analyte blood test for cerebrotendinous xanthomatosis. Clin Biochem. 2014;47(9):860–3.
12. Batta AK, Salen G, Shefer S, Tint GS, Batta M. Increased plasma bile alcohol glucuronides in patients with cerebrotendinous xanthomatosis: effect of chenodeoxycholic acid. J Lipid Res. 1987;28(8):1006–12.
13. Egestad B, Pettersson P, Skrede S, Sjövall J. Fast atom bombardment mass spectrometry in the diagnosis of cerebrotendinous xanthomatosis. Scand J Clin Lab Invest. 1985;45(5):443–6.
14. DeBarber AE, Schaefer EJ, Do J, Ray JW, Larson A, Redder S, et al. Genetically and clinically confirmed atypical cerebrotendinous xanthomatosis with normal cholestanol and marked elevations of bile acid precursors and bile alcohols. J Clin Lipidol. 2024;18(3):e465–76.
15. Kuramoto T, Suemura Y, Kihira K, Hiraoka T, Hoshita T. Determination of the glucurono-conjugated position in bile alcohol glucuronides present in a patient with cerebrotendinous xanthomatosis. Steroids. 1995;60(10):709–12.
16. DeBarber AE, Kalfon L, Fedida A, Fleisher Sheffer V, Ben Haroush S, Chasnyk N, et al. Newborn screening for cerebrotendinous xanthomatosis is the solution for early identification and treatment. J Lipid Res. 2018;59(11):2214–22.
17. Ganchuluun S, Jeffries KM, Duell PB, DeBarber AE. Quantification of urinary 5beta-cholestane-3alpha,7alpha,23S,25-pentol as a diagnostic test for cerebrotendinous xanthomatosis (CTX). Mol Genet Metab. 2019;127:219–320. Society Inborn Metabolic Diseases 41st Annual Meeting (April 6th–April 9th, 2019) Program and Abstracts; Poster # 57.
18. Vega GL, Illingworth DR, Grundy SM, Lindgren FT, Connor WE. Normocholesterolemic tendon xanthomatosis with overproduction of apolipoprotein B. Metabolism. 1983;32(2):118–25.
19. Guenzel AJ, DeBarber A, Raymond K, Dhamija R. Familial variability of cerebrotendinous xanthomatosis lacking typical biochemical findings. JIMD Rep. 2021;59(1):3–9.
20. Stelten BML, Bonnot O, Huidekoper HH, van Spronsen FJ, van Hasselt PM, Kluijtmans LAJ, et al. Autism spectrum disorder: an early and frequent feature in cerebrotendinous xanthomatosis. J Inherit Metab Dis. 2018;41(4):641–6.
21. Wallon D, Guyant-Maréchal L, Laquerrière A, Wevers RA, Martinaud O, Kluijtmans LAJ, et al. Clinical imaging and neuropathological correlations in an unusual case of cerebrotendinous xanthomatosis. Clin Neuropathol. 2010;29(6):361–4.
22. Tada H, Inaba S, Pozharitckaia D, Kawashiri M. Prominent tendon xanthomas and abdominal aortic aneurysm associated with cerebrotendinous xanthomatosis identified using whole exome sequencing. Intern Med. 2018;57(8):1119–22.
23. Bonnet JB, Couvert P, Di-Filippo M, Boissiere F, Cristol JP, Sutra T, et al. Tuberous xanthomatosis is not necessarily associated with increased plasma concentrations of cholestanol in cerebrotendinous xanthomatosis. J Intern Med. 2023;293(1):121–3.

24. Siman-Tov T, Meiner V, Gadoth N. Could steroids mask the diagnosis of cerebrotendinous xanthomatosis? J Neurol Sci. 2006;243(1–2):83–6.
25. Takahashi M, Okazaki H, Tada H, Ishibashi S. A case of cerebrotendinous xanthomatosis with massive xanthomas but without a considerable increase in serum cholestanol levels. J Clin Lipidol. 2023;17(6):834–8.
26. Alves RJ, Nunes VS, Junior NCDCB, Nakandakare ER, Quintão ECR. Rare genetic cerebrotendinous (CTX) cases without cholestanol elevation but with prominent cholesterol-rich tendon xanthomas. J Clin Lipidol. 2024:18(4):e631–e635.
27. Zubarioglu T, Kıykım E, Köse E, Eminoğlu FT, Kısa PT, Balcı MC, et al. Clinical, biochemical, and molecular insights into Cerebrotendinous Xanthomatosis: a nationwide study of 100 Turkish individuals. Mol Genet Metab. 2024;142(2):108493.
28. Guay SP, Paquette M, Poulin V, Levtova A, Baass A, Bernard S. The 20-year diagnostic odyssey of a milder form of cerebrotendinous xanthomatosis. JCEM Case Rep. 2024;2(2):luae004.
29. Stelten BML, Huidekoper HH, van de Warrenburg BPC, Brilstra EH, Hollak CEM, Haak HR, et al. Long-term treatment effect in cerebro-tendinous xanthomatosis depends on age at treatment start. Neurology. 2019;92(2):e83–95.
30. Schaefer EJ, Tsunoda F, Diffenderfer M, Polisecki E, Thai N, Asz-talos B. The measurement of lipids, lipoproteins, apolipoproteins, fatty acids, and sterols, and next generation sequencing for the diagnosis and treatment of lipid disorders. In: Endotext. South Dartmouth: MDText.com, Inc; 2000 [Internet].
31. Yanagihashi M, Kano O, Terashima T, Kawase Y, Hanashiro S, Sawada M, et al. Late-onset spinal form xanthomatosis without brain lesion: a case report. BMC Neurol. 2016;16:21.
32. Chen C, Zhang Y, Wu U, Sun YM, Cai YH, Wu JJ, et al. Clinical and molecular genetic features of cerebrotendinous xanthomatosis patients in Chinese families. Metab Brain Dis. 2017;32(5):1609–18.
33. Guan RY, Wu JJ, Ding ZT, Wang J, Sun YM. Clinical and genetic findings in a cohort of Chinese patients with autosomal recessive spinocerebellar ataxia. Clin Genet. 2020;97(3):532–5.
34. Jiang J, Chen G, Wu J, Luan X, Zhou H, Liu X, et al. c.1263+1GA Is a Latent Hotspot for CYP27A1 Mutations in Chinese Patients With Cerebrotendinous Xanthomatosis. Front Genet. 2020;11:682.
35. Claesen JLA, Koomen E, Schene IF, Jans JJM, Mast N, Pikuleve IA, et al. Misdiagnosis of CTX due to propofol: the interference of total intravenous propofol anaesthesia with bile acid profiling. J Inherit Metab Dis. 2020;43:843–51.
36. Stelten BML, Raal FJ, Marais AD, Riksen NP, Roeters van Lennep JE, Duell PB, et al. Cerebrotendinous xanthomatosis without neurological involvement. J Intern Med. 2021;290(5):1039–47.
37. Sekijima Y, Koyama S, Yoshinaga T, Koinuma M, Inaba Y. Nationwide survey on cerebrotendinous xanthomatosis in Japan. J Hum Genet. 2018;63(3):271–80.
38. Skrede S, Björkhem I, Kvittingen EA, East C, Grundy S, Skrede S. Reduced C27-steroid 26-hydroxylase activity in heterozygotes for cerebrotendinous xanthomatosis. Scand J Clin Lab Invest. 1998;48(5):425–9.
39. Koopman BJ, Waterreus RJ, Van den Brekel HW, Wolthers BG. Detection of carriers of cerebrotendinous xanthomatosis. Clin Chim Acta. 1986;158(2):179–85.
40. Menkes JH, Schimschock JR, Swanson PD. Cerebrotendinous xanthomatosis. The storage of cholestanol within the nervous system. Arch Neurol. 1968;19(1):47–53.
41. Björkhem I. Cerebrotendinous xanthomatosis. Curr Opin Lipidol. 2013;24(4):283–7.
42. Salen G, Berginer V, Shore V, Horak I, Horak E, Tint GS, et al. Increased concentrations of cholestanol and apolipoprotein B in the cerebrospinal fluid of patients with cerebrotendinous xanthomatosis. Effect of chenodeoxycholic acid. N Engl J Med. 1987;316(20):1233–8.

Part III

Biochemical Contributions to Pathology

Cholestanol Accumulation in the Brain and Eye in Cerebrotendinous Xanthomatosis (CTX)

11

Irina A. Pikuleva

Cerebrotendinous xanthomatosis (CTX) is a rare inherited metabolic disease due to deficiency in the enzymatic activity of cytochrome P450 27A1 or CYP27A1, a ubiquitous sterol 27-hydroxylase [1, 2]. CYP27A1 is a multifunctional enzyme, known to metabolize cholesterol in extrahepatic tissues, bile acid intermediates in the liver, and vitamin D_3 in the kidneys [3, 4]. Accordingly, CTX is manifested in the deposition of cholesterol and cholestanol (reduced form of cholesterol) in the brain and other tissues as well as reduced bile acid biosynthesis in the liver and hence deficient production of chenodeoxycholic acid (CDCA). Clinically, CTX is manifested in a broad range of symptoms, neurological and non-neurological [5], with the most serious neurologic symptoms (intellectual disability, dementia, cerebellar ataxia, and spinal cord paresis) believed to be caused at least in part by brain xanthomas [5].

In the brain, xanthomas are preferentially accumulated in the cerebellum [6]. The reason for this accumulation is not yet fully understood, although it is known that different pathways lead to cholestanol formation in the CTX-affected and healthy brain (Fig. 11.1). In CTX, 7α-hydroxy-4-cholesten-3-one (7HCO), a bile acid intermediate produced in the liver, cannot be metabolized by CYP27A1 [7, 8] and is therefore released in the systemic circulation [9]. 7HCO is then delivered to the brain [10–12] and is converted to cholesta-4,6-dien-3-one, 4-cholesten-3-one, 5α-cholestan-3-one, and finally to cholestanol [10, 13–17]. In contrast, in healthy brain, cholestanol is mainly synthesized from cholesterol, which is produced locally, likely via the 3β-hydroxy-Δ^5-dehydrogenation, to yield 4-cholesten-3-one and ultimately cholestanol [13] (Fig. 11.1). Much less is known about cholestanol elimination from the brain. Therefore, we decided to investigate this process and used wild

I. A. Pikuleva (✉)
Department of Ophthalmology and Visual Science, Case Western Reserve University, Cleveland, OH, USA
e-mail: iap8@case.edu

A. Federico et al. (eds.), *Cerebrotendinous Xanthomatosis*,
https://doi.org/10.1007/978-3-031-92526-9_11

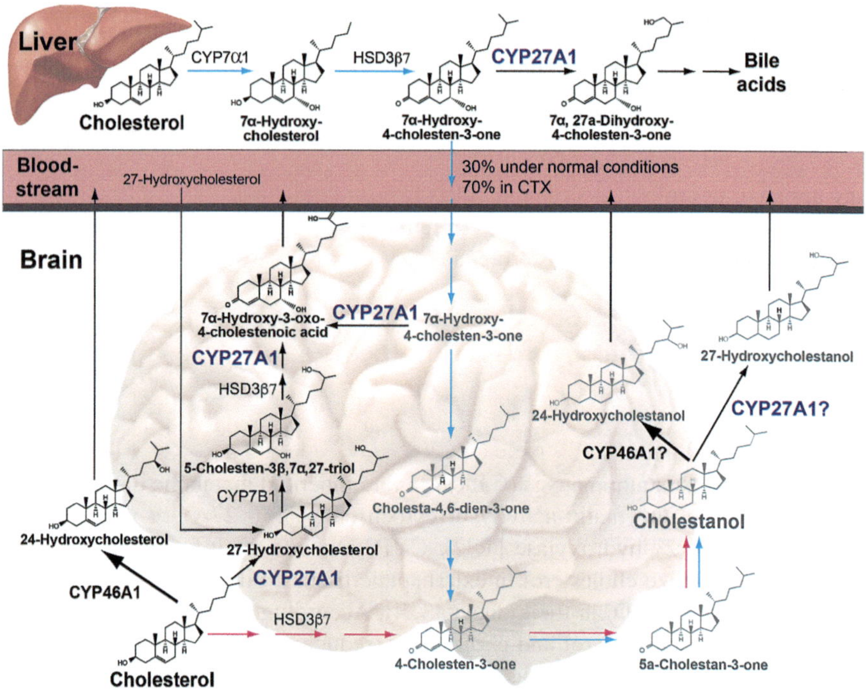

Fig. 11.1 Proposed pathways of cholestanol biosynthesis and elimination from the brain. The 7α-hydroxy-4-cholesten-3-one-dependent pathway is initiated in the liver and is indicated with cyan arrows; cholestanol precursors and metabolites in this pathway are shown in gray. The cholesterol-dependent pathway is initiated in the brain and is indicated with magenta arrows. In both pathways, the known enzymes are indicated; boldface arrows represent the major mechanism for cholesterol or cholestanol elimination from the brain. (Taken from Ref. [22] and modified)

type mice and those having a single (*Cyp27a1* or *Cyp46a1*) or double (both *Cyp27a1* and *Cyp46a1*) genetic abrogation. CYP46A1 was studied because this is the major cholesterol-metabolizing enzyme in the brain, accounting for elimination of 75–85% and 40–50% of cholesterol excess from human and mouse brains, respectively [18, 19].

Biochemical Abnormalities in the Plasma and Brain of *Cyp27a1*$^{-/-}$, *Cyp46a1*$^{-/-}$, and *Cyp27a1*$^{-/-}$*Cyp46a1*$^{-/-}$ Mice

Cyp27a1$^{-/-}$ mice do not develop xanthomas and CTX symptomatology, despite the fact they have increased levels of cholestanol in the systemic circulation CTX [20, 21]. Therefore, we first measured the cholestanol and 7HCO levels in mouse plasma, whole brain, and cerebellum to confirm that the *Cyp27a1*$^{-/-}$ genotype has the same biochemical abnormalities as those detected in CTX patients. Indeed, the levels of the plasma, whole brain, and cerebellar cholestanol were increased in *Cyp27a1*$^{-/-}$ mice as well as in *Cyp27a1*$^{-/-}$*Cyp46a1*$^{-/-}$ mice (Fig. 11.2), although were lower than observed in human disease. In addition, there was a much smaller increase in the cholestanol levels in the whole brain and cerebellum in *Cyp46a1*$^{-/-}$ mice [22]. This was likely due to lack of cholesterol metabolism by CYP46A1 in mouse brain and hence increased cholesterol availability for the production of cholestanol (Fig. 11.1). With respect to 7HCO, metabolite levels were increased up to 55-fold in the plasma of *Cyp27a1*$^{-/-}$ and *Cyp27a1*$^{-/-}$*Cyp46a1*$^{-/-}$ mice but decreased in these genotypes in the whole brain and cerebellum [22]. The latter was likely due to increased 7HCO utilization for the formation of cholestanol as this metabolite was no longer used to yield 7α-hydroxy-3-oxo-4-cholestenoic acid (Fig. 11.1). Thus, we documented that not only *Cyp27a1*$^{-/-}$ mice but also *Cyp27a1*$^{-/-}$*Cyp46a1*$^{-/-}$ mice had biochemical abnormalities characteristic for CTX and showed that CYP46A1 can also affect the cholestanol levels in the whole brain and cerebellum.

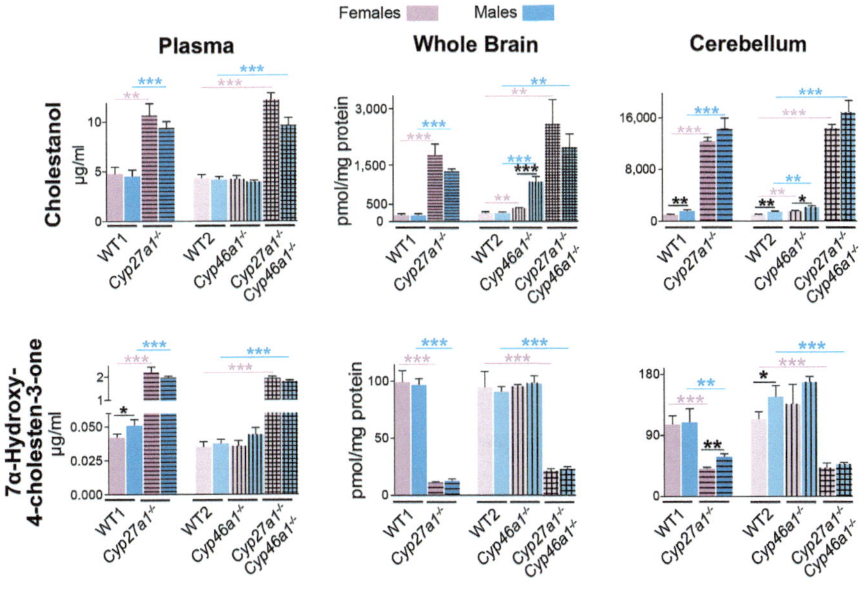

Fig. 11.2 Cholestanol and 7α-hydroxy-4-cholesten-3-one levels in mouse plasma and brain. The results are mean ± S.D. of the measurements in three to five mice per genotype and sex. Data were analyzed by two-way ANOVA followed by Bonferroni correction. Pink asterisks indicate significant changes between females of the knockout strains and females of the corresponding wild type (WT) strain. Blue asterisks indicate significant changes between males of the knockout strains and males of the corresponding WT strain. Black asterisks indicate significant changes between female and male mice of the same strain. *$P \leq 0.05$; **$P \leq 0.01$; ***$P \leq 0.001$. (Data were taken from Ref. [22])

Cholestanol Metabolism and Binding to CYP46A1 and CYP27A1 In Vitro

Cholestanol and cholesterol have very similar chemical structures, and cholestanol was previously found to undergo 24-hydroxylation in the incubations with CYP46A1-transfected HEK293 cells [23]. However, the product yield was very low, and the product was not characterized by mass spectrometry. CYP27A1 was already shown to metabolize cholestanol in the in vitro reconstituted system, but cholestanol was used in a 1:1, M/M, mixture with cholesterol, not alone [24]. Therefore, to ascertain whether cholestanol is indeed a substrate for CYP46A1 and CYP27A1 in vitro, we used purified recombinant CYP46A1 or CYP27A1 and cholestanol in the in vitro reconstituted system and ran the enzyme assays for different time (Figs. 11.3 and 11.4). Only one product peak was found during the gas chromatography separation of the incubations of CYP46A1 or CYP27A1 with

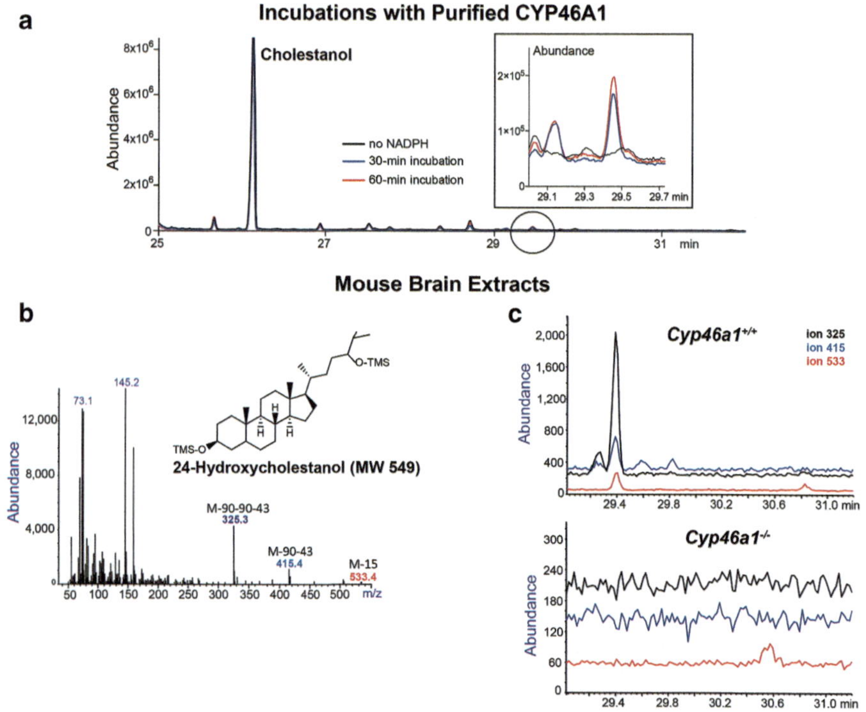

Fig. 11.3 Cholestanol is an endogenous substrate for CYP46A1 in mice. (**a**) Representative total ion chromatogram of sterol extract (after trimethylsilylation) from the in vitro incubations of cholestanol with purified recombinant CYP46A1. The peak at 29.46 min corresponding to the CYP46A1 product is circled and shown as an inset. (**b**) Mass spectrum of the peak at 29.46 min is consistent with the fragmentation pattern of 24-hydroxycholestanol. (**c**) Single ion monitoring chromatogram of the oxysterol fraction isolated from the whole brain of wild type (*Cyp46a1*$^{+/+}$) and *Cyp46a1*$^{-/-}$ mice. (Taken from Ref. [22] and modified)

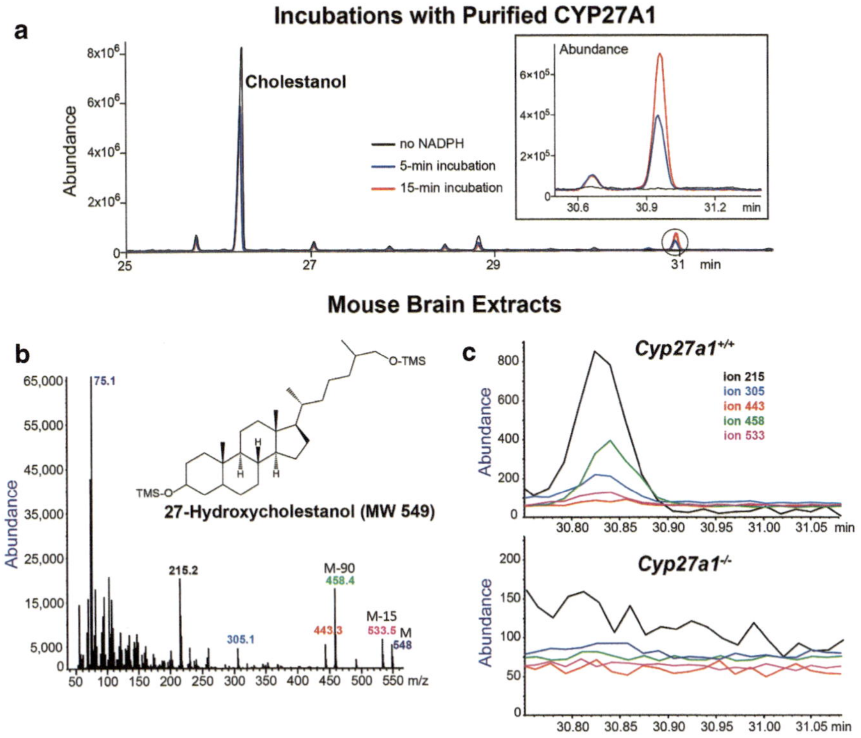

Fig. 11.4 Cholestanol is an endogenous substrate for CYP27A1 in mice. (**a**) Representative total ion chromatogram of sterol extract (after trimethylsilylation) from the in vitro incubations of cholestanol with purified recombinant CYP27A1. The peak at 30.96 min corresponding to the CYP27A1 product is circled and shown as an inset. (**b**) Mass spectrum of the peak at 30.96 min is consistent with the fragmentation pattern of 27-hydroxycholestanol. (**c**) Single ion monitoring chromatogram of the oxysterol fraction isolated from the whole brain of wild type (*Cyp27a1*$^{+/+}$) and *Cyp27a1*$^{-/-}$ mice. (Taken from Ref. [22])

cholestanol, and this peak was not seen in the control incubations lacking NADPH. The product peak showed the expected intensity increase with the incubation time (Figs. 11.3 and 11.4) and had a fragmentation pattern consistent with that of 24-hydroxycholestanol [the characteristic *m/z* values of 533, 415, and 325] or 27-hydroxycholestanol [the characteristic *m/z* values of 533, 458, 443, 305, and 215] (data are not shown) [22].

Then, we compared cholestanol and cholesterol as the substrates for CYP46A1 and CYP27A1 in the spectral binding assays and found that both sterols had the comparable apparent spectral K_d values (Table 11.1). These values were in the nanomolar range for CYP46A1, indicating tight sterol binding, and the low micromolar range for CYP27A1, indicating a less tight binding [22]. The apparent K_d values of cholestanol for CYP46A1 and CYP27A1 also suggested that we could estimate the cholestanol turnover numbers by the two enzymes from the data obtained in the in vitro enzyme assays (Figs. 11.3 and 11.4): 0.04 min^{-1} [0.11 min^{-1} for cholesterol

Table 11.1 Spectral binding of cholesterol and cholestanol to CYP27A1 and CYP46A1

P450	Ligand	K_d, μM
CYP27A1	Cholestanol	5.0 ± 0.6
	Cholesterol	6.3 ± 0.7
CYP46A1	Cholestanol	0.07 ± 0.03
	Cholesterol	0.05 ± 0.03

Taken from Ref. [22]
All results represent mean ± S.D. of three titrations of purified recombinant CYP27A1 or CYP46A1. The K_d values for CYP46A1 are much lower than the enzyme concentration in the assay; hence, they represent estimates only and reflect whether the substrate has low, intermediate, or high nanomolar affinity for CYP46A1

[25]] for CYP46A1 and 3.5 min^{-1} [3.0 min^{-1} for cholesterol [26]] for CYP27A1. Accordingly, the calculated values of catalytic efficiency of cholestanol hydroxylation (the cholesterol turnover number to K_d ratio, min^{-1}·μM^{-1}) were 0.57 for CYP46A1 and 0.70 for CYP27A1 or similar. For comparison, the numbers for the catalytic efficiency of cholesterol hydroxylation were 2.2 for CYP46A1 and 0.5 for CYP27A1, i.e., higher for CYP46A1, consistent with CYP46A1 being the major cholesterol-metabolizing enzyme in the brain [19]. Thus, under the optimal conditions of the in vitro assays, cholesterol was a better substrate for CYP46A1 than cholestanol, and cholestanol was metabolized by CYP46A1 and CYP27A1 with comparable catalytic efficiency.

Cholestanol Is an Endogenous Substrate for CYP46A1 and CYP27A1 in Mouse Brain

Since cholestanol was metabolized by CYP46A1 and CYP27A1 in vitro, mouse brains were analyzed for the presence of 24-hydroxycholestanol and 27-hydroxycholestanol. The ion peaks characteristic for 24-hydroxycholestanol and 27-hydroxycholestanol were indeed detected in the whole brain of wild type mice but not of *Cyp46a1*$^{-/-}$ and *Cyp27a1*$^{-/-}$ mice, respectively (Figs. 11.3 and 11.4), thus providing evidence that cholestanol is an endogenous substrate for both CYP46A1 and CYP27A1 [22]. Therefore, next, 24- and 27-hydroxycholestanols were quantified in mouse whole brain and cerebellum and compared with the enzyme expression.

In wild type mice, the content of 24-hydroxycholestanol was much lower in the cerebellum than in the whole brain, at least 20-fold, whereas 27-hydroxycholestanol was not detectable in the cerebellum and was only found in the whole brain (Fig. 11.5) [22]. Notably, the whole brain levels of 24-hydroxycholestanol were at least 4-times higher than that of 27-hydroxycholestanol, possibly a reflection of the 10-times higher expression of CYP46A1 than CYP27A1. Yet, neither 24-hydroxycholestanol nor 27-hydroxycholestanol was detected in animals with CYP46A1

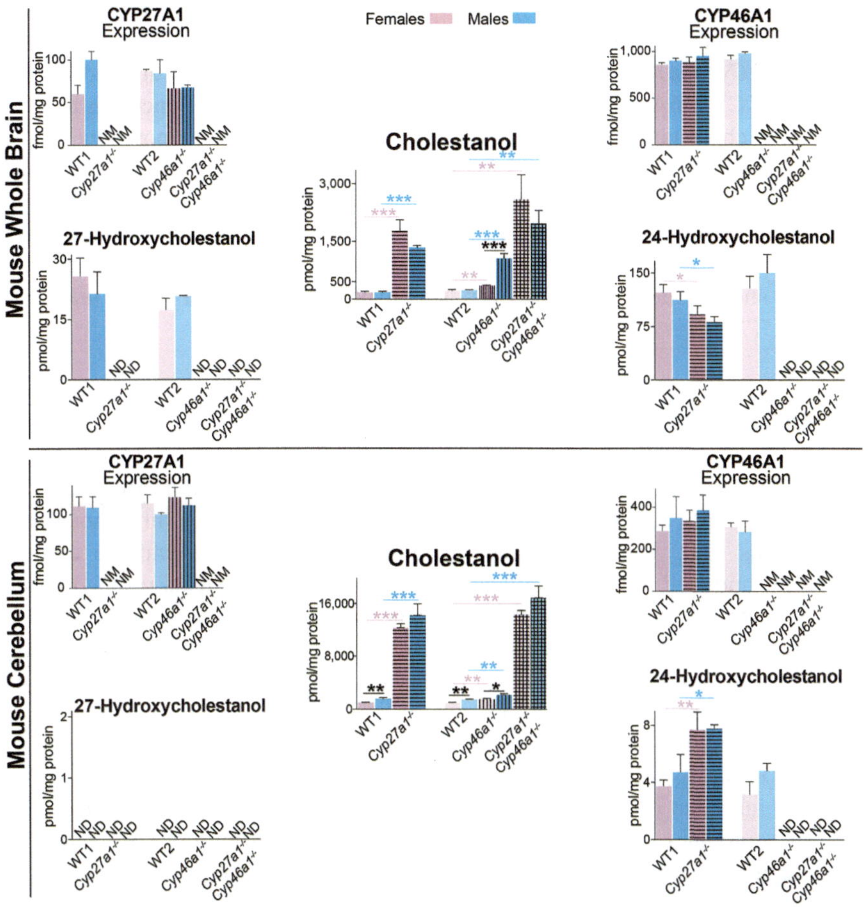

Fig. 11.5 Cholestanol is preferentially metabolized in mouse brain by CYP46A1 compared to CYP27A1. The levels of cholestanol, 24-hydroxycholestanol, and 27-hydroxycholestanol as well as protein expression of CYP46A1 and CYP27A1 in mouse brain and cerebellum. For sterol quantifications, the results are mean ± S.D. of the measurements in three to five mice per genotype and sex. For protein quantifications, the multiple reaction monitoring data from 3 to 4 transitions/peptide (3 peptides for CYP46A1 and 2 peptides for CYP27A1) were combined to determine the amount of each P450. Data represent mean ± S.D. of independent P450 measurements in three mice. Data were analyzed by two-way ANOVA followed by Bonferroni correction. Pink asterisks indicate significant changes between females of the knockout strains versus females of the corresponding wild type (WT) strain. Blue asterisks indicate significant changes between males of the knockout strains and males of the corresponding WT strain. Black asterisks indicate significant changes between female and male mice of the same strain. $^{*}P \leq 0.05$; $^{**}P \leq 0.01$; $^{***}P \leq 0.001$. (Data were taken from Ref. [22])

deficiencies (*Cyp46a1*$^{-/-}$ and *Cyp27a1*$^{-/-}$*Cyp46a1*$^{-/-}$ mice) nor was 27-hydroxycholestanol detected in animals with CYP27A1 deficiencies (*Cyp27a1*$^{-/-}$ and *Cyp27a1*$^{-/-}$*Cyp46a1*$^{-/-}$ mice), confirming that these metabolites are indeed the products of CYP46A1 and CYP27A1, respectively [22]. Of importance was that the 24-hydroxycholestanol levels were increased in the cerebellum but not in the whole brain in *Cyp27a1*$^{-/-}$ mice (Fig. 11.5). This was likely a response to the increased cholestanol formation and an indication that in this brain region CYP46A1 could metabolize excess cholestanol. Thus, collectively, the cholestanol metabolite quantifications suggested that CYP46A1 in the cerebellum could metabolize cholestanol and thus should be considered as a potential pharmacologic target for the treatment of CTX.

CYP46A1 as a Pharmacologic Target for CTX

The standard treatment for CTX is replacement therapy with chenodeoxycholic acid either alone or in a combination with one of the statins, drugs that inhibit cholesterol biosynthesis [27]. These pharmacologic interventions usually improve clinical symptoms and lead to CTX stabilization. Yet not all CTX patients respond to the CDCA treatment, and some of them have progressive neurological deterioration [27]. Accordingly, a combination therapeutic strategy should be considered, and one approach could be increasing CYP46A1 activity in the brain as suggested by our in vitro and animal studies [22].

A possibility that CYP46A1 could be a pharmacologic target for treatment of different brain disorders was suggested by a discovery that this enzyme could either be inhibited or allosterically activated by some FDA-approved drugs [28, 29]. The outcomes of the CYP46A1 allosteric activation by low dose anti-HIV drug efavirenz were then evaluated in mouse models of Alzheimer, Niemann-Pick disease type C, and prion diseases as well as depression and glioblastoma and were shown to exert beneficial effects on the disease manifestations [30–35]. A model of how activation of only one enzyme can be beneficial for lessening the symptoms of varied brain disorders was also proposed [36]. Accordingly, a clinical trial was recently carried out to test CYP46A1 activation, safety, and tolerability by low dose efavirenz in geriatric subjects with early Alzheimer disease [37]. Both tested efavirenz doses (50 and 200 mg/day) were found to activate CYP46A1 in the brain and were well tolerated without causing any serious adverse or other events [37]. Another clinical trial is now in progress to evaluate low dose efavirenz (25 mg/day) in adults or more than 14-year old subjects with Niemann-Pick disease type C [38]. This trial will establish efavirenz efficacy, safety, and ability to activate CYP46A1 in a younger population. Collectively, the clinical trial data will help understand whether studies of low dose efavirenz are warranted in CTX patients.

Cholestanol Accumulation in the Retina

CTX leads to ocular abnormalities, affecting the lens (juvenile bilateral cataracts), vitreous (cholesterol-like crystals), and the retina [39–41]. The latter is a multilayered sensory tissue in the back of the eye, which receives photons and transmits visual stimuli to the brain for subsequent processing. The retina is an extension of the brain [42], and it is not surprising that CTX affects the retina as well, leading to premature retinal senescence, drusen, retinal vessel sclerosis, cholesterol-like deposits along the retinal vascular arcades, defects in the retinal pigment epithelium on fluorescein angiography, and optic disc pallor [39–41]. These abnormalities indicate that CYP27A1 plays an important role in the retina, consistent with high retinal CYP27A1 expression and the role as the major retinal cholesterol eliminating enzyme [43, 44]. This is in contrast to the brain, where CYP46A1 is the principal cholesterol hydroxylase, responsible for the majority of the enzymatic cholesterol elimination [19]. Yet, the cholestanol levels have not been reported in human retina; hence, mice were used to fill this gap in our knowledge.

Cholestanol was detected in the retina in all tested mouse genotypes (Fig. 11.6). However, its levels were at least 80-times lower than that of cholesterol. In *Cyp27a1*$^{-/-}$ and *Cyp46a1*$^{-/-}$ mice, the retinal cholestanol content was altered only modestly (up to 1.2-fold), but in *Cyp27a1*$^{-/-}$*Cyp46a1*$^{-/-}$ mice, it was increased up to ten-fold, indicating that both enzymes should be functional to prevent retinal cholestanol accumulation, possibly via the sterol elimination [45]. The cholesterol

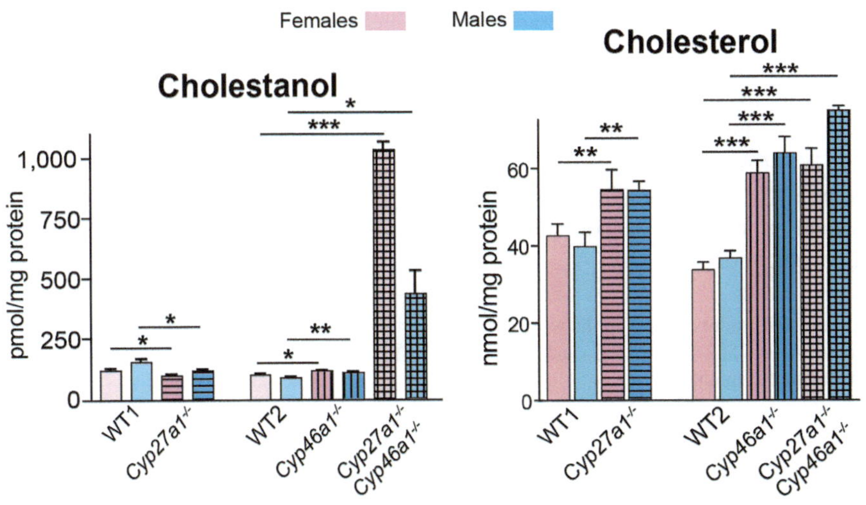

Fig. 11.6 Cholestanol and cholesterol quantifications in mouse retina. The results are mean ± S.D. of the measurements in five mice per genotype and sex. Data were analyzed by two-way ANOVA followed by Bonferroni correction. Asterisks indicate significant changes between mice of the knockout strains and the corresponding wild type (WT) strain. *$P \leq 0.05$; **$P \leq 0.01$; ***$P \leq 0.001$. (Data were taken from Refs. [45, 46])

levels were increased in the *Cyp27a1*$^{-/-}$, *Cyp46a1*$^{-/-}$, and *Cyp27a1*$^{-/-}$ *Cyp46a1*$^{-/-}$ genotypes as well [45] and led in *Cyp27a1*$^{-/-}$ mice to focal cholesterol deposition beneath the retinal pigment epithelium, which underlies the retina [46]. In addition, *Cyp27a1*$^{-/-}$ mice had a pathological neovascularization, which likely arose from both the retina and the choroid and led to the formation of retinal-choroidal anastomoses. Accordingly, the blood vessels became leaky in these areas, and the *Cyp27a1*$^{-/-}$ retina hypoxic [46]. The observed retinal changes were likely reflective of an increase in the retinal cholesterol but not cholestanol levels, although it should be remembered that the manifestations of CYP27A1 deficiency are milder in mice as compared to humans. Although information for the human retina is not available, it was reported that the cholestanol content of a cataractous lens nucleus from a patient with CTX was 4- to 6-fold higher compared to senile cataractous lens nuclei (with a cholestanol-cholesterol ratio of 1.7%, similar to that determined for serum of CTX patient) [40]. Thus, the quantifications on post-mortem human retinal samples are required to ascertain whether there is a cholestanol accumulation in the retina in CTX or the observed abnormalities are due to an increase in the retinal cholesterol levels. Remarkably, retinal-choroidal anastomoses were significantly diminished in a mouse model of Alzheimer disease after low dose efavirenz treatment, thus indicating that the therapeutic effects of low dose efavirenz are not only limited to the brain but also extend to the retina [47].

Conclusions

Studies of *Cyp27a1*$^{-/-}$, *Cyp46a1*$^{-/-}$, and *Cyp27a1*$^{-/-}$ *Cyp46a1*$^{-/-}$ mice suggest that CYP27A1 and CYP46A1 are important enzymes involved in cholestanol elimination from the brain and retina. These studies also indicate that cholestanol metabolism in the brain is region-specific and, in the cerebellum, is preferentially mediated by CYP46A1. A clinical trial of low dose efavirenz in CTX patients might demonstrate if CYP46A1 activation is useful as a potential treatment approach for CTX patients who are non-responsive to the standard CDCA therapy or unable to tolerate the medication.

Acknowledgments Some of the work described in this chapter was supported in part by the NIH grants AG067552, EY018383, and EY011373 (I.A.P.). Irina A. Pikuleva is a Carl F. Asseff Professor of Ophthalmology.

References

1. Oftebro H, Bjorkhem I, Skrede S, Schreiner A, Pederson JI. Cerebrotendinous xanthomatosis: a defect in mitochondrial 26-hydroxylation required for normal biosynthesis of cholic acid. J Clin Invest. 1980;65(6):1418–30.
2. Cali JJ, Hsieh CL, Francke U, Russell DW. Mutations in the bile acid biosynthetic enzyme sterol 27-hydroxylase underlie cerebrotendinous xanthomatosis. J Biol Chem. 1991;266(12):7779–83.

3. Wikvall K. Hydroxylations in biosynthesis of bile acids. Isolation of a cytochrome P-450 from rabbit liver mitochondria catalyzing 26-hydroxylation of C27-steroids. J Biol Chem. 1984;259(6):3800–4.
4. Masumoto O, Ohyama Y, Okuda K. Purification and characterization of vitamin D 25-hydroxylase from rat liver mitochondria. J Biol Chem. 1988;263(28):14256–60.
5. Koyama S, Sekijima Y, Ogura M, Hori M, Matsuki K, Miida T, Harada-Shiba M. Cerebrotendinous xanthomatosis: molecular pathogenesis, clinical spectrum, diagnosis, and disease-modifying treatments. J Atheroscler Thromb. 2021;28(9):905–25.
6. Menkes JH, Schimschock JR, Swanson PD. Cerebrotendinous xanthomatosis. The storage of cholestanol within the nervous system. Arch Neurol. 1968;19(1):47–53.
7. Skrede S, Bjorkhem I, Buchmann MS, Hopen G, Fausa O. A novel pathway for biosynthesis of cholestanol with 7 alpha-hydroxylated C27-steroids as intermediates, and its importance for the accumulation of cholestanol in cerebrotendinous xanthomatosis. J Clin Invest. 1985;75(2):448–55.
8. Skrede S, Bjorkhem I, Buchmann MS, Midtvedt T. Biosynthesis of cholestanol from bile acid intermediates in the rabbit and the rat. J Biol Chem. 1985;260(1):77–81.
9. Bjorkhem I, Skrede S, Buchmann MS, East C, Grundy S. Accumulation of 7 alpha-hydroxy-4-cholesten-3-one and cholesta-4,6-dien-3-one in patients with cerebrotendinous xanthomatosis: effect of treatment with chenodeoxycholic acid. Hepatology. 1987;7(2):266–71.
10. Panzenboeck U, Andersson U, Hansson M, Sattler W, Meaney S, Bjorkhem I. On the mechanism of cerebral accumulation of cholestanol in patients with cerebrotendinous xanthomatosis. J Lipid Res. 2007;48(5):1167–74.
11. Bjorkhem I, Hansson M. Cerebrotendinous xanthomatosis: an inborn error in bile acid synthesis with defined mutations but still a challenge. Biochem Biophys Res Commun. 2010;396(1):46–9.
12. Bjorkhem I. Cerebrotendinous xanthomatosis. Curr Opin Lipidol. 2013;24(4):283–7.
13. Bjorkhem I, Karlmar KE. Biosynthesis of cholestanol: conversion of cholesterol into 4-cholesten-3-one by rat liver microsomes. Biochim Biophys Acta. 1974;337(1):129–31.
14. Buchmann MS, Bjorkhem I, Skrede S. Metabolism of the cholestanol precursor cholesta-4,6-dien-3-one in different tissues. Biochim Biophys Acta. 1987;922(2):111–7.
15. Skrede S, Buchmann MS, Bjorkhem I. Hepatic 7 alpha-dehydroxylation of bile acid intermediates, and its significance for the pathogenesis of cerebrotendinous xanthomatosis. J Lipid Res. 1988;29(2):157–64.
16. Bjorkhem I, Buchmann M, Bystrom S. Mechanism and stereochemistry in the sequential enzymatic saturation of the two double bonds in cholesta-4,6-dien-3-one. J Biol Chem. 1992;267(28):19872–5.
17. Bavner A, Shafaati M, Hansson M, Olin M, Shpitzen S, Meiner V, et al. On the mechanism of accumulation of cholestanol in the brain of mice with a disruption of sterol 27-hydroxylase. J Lipid Res. 2010;51(9):2722–30.
18. Lund EG, Xie C, Kotti T, Turley SD, Dietschy JM, Russell DW. Knockout of the cholesterol 24-hydroxylase gene in mice reveals a brain-specific mechanism of cholesterol turnover. J Biol Chem. 2003;278(25):22980–8.
19. Bjorkhem I, Lutjohann D, Diczfalusy U, Stahle L, Ahlborg G, Wahren J. Cholesterol homeostasis in human brain: turnover of 24S-hydroxycholesterol and evidence for a cerebral origin of most of this oxysterol in the circulation. J Lipid Res. 1998;39(8):1594–600.
20. Dubrac S, Lear SR, Ananthanarayanan M, Balasubramaniyan N, Bollineni J, Shefer S, et al. Role of CYP27A in cholesterol and bile acid metabolism. J Lipid Res. 2005;46(1):76–85.
21. Rosen H, Reshef A, Maeda N, Lippoldt A, Shpizen S, Triger L, et al. Markedly reduced bile acid synthesis but maintained levels of cholesterol and vitamin D metabolites in mice with disrupted sterol 27-hydroxylase gene. J Biol Chem. 1998;273(24):14805–12.
22. Mast N, Anderson KW, Lin JB, Li Y, Turko IV, Tatsuoka C, et al. Cytochrome P450 27A1 deficiency and regional differences in brain sterol metabolism cause preferential cholestanol accumulation in the cerebellum. J Biol Chem. 2017;292(12):4913–24.

23. Mast N, Norcross R, Andersson U, Shou M, Nakayama K, Bjorkhem I, Pikuleva IA. Broad substrate specificity of human cytochrome P450 46A1 which initiates cholesterol degradation in the brain. Biochemistry. 2003;42(48):14284–92.
24. von Bahr S, Movin T, Papadogiannakis N, Pikuleva I, Ronnow P, Diczfalusy U, Bjorkhem I. Mechanism of accumulation of cholesterol and cholestanol in tendons and the role of sterol 27-hydroxylase (CYP27A1). Arterioscler Thromb Vasc Biol. 2002;22(7):1129–35.
25. Mast N, White MA, Björkhem I, Johnson EF, Stout CD, Pikuleva IA. Crystal structures of substrate-bound and substrate-free cytochrome P450 46A1, the principal cholesterol hydroxylase in the brain. Proc Natl Acad Sci USA. 2008;105(28):9546–51.
26. Mast N, Murtazina D, Liu H, Graham SE, Björkhem I, Halpert JR, et al. Distinct binding of cholesterol and 5-cholestane-3 alpha,7 alpha,12 alpha-triol to cytochrome P450 27A1: evidence from modeling and site-directed mutagenesis studies. Biochemistry. 2006;45(14):4396–404.
27. Mignarri A, Magni A, Del Puppo M, Gallus GN, Bjorkhem I, Federico A, Dotti MT. Evaluation of cholesterol metabolism in cerebrotendinous xanthomatosis. J Inherit Metab Dis. 2015;39:75–83.
28. Shafaati M, Mast N, Beck O, Nayef R, Heo GY, Bjorkhem-Bergman L, et al. The antifungal drug voriconazole is an efficient inhibitor of brain cholesterol 24S-hydroxylase in vitro and in vivo. J Lipid Res. 2010;51(2):318–23.
29. Mast N, Li Y, Linger M, Clark M, Wiseman J, Pikuleva IA. Pharmacologic stimulation of cytochrome P450 46A1 and cerebral cholesterol turnover in mice. J Biol Chem. 2014;289(6):3529–38.
30. Mast N, Saadane A, Valencia-Olvera A, Constans J, Maxfield E, Arakawa H, et al. Cholesterol-metabolizing enzyme cytochrome P450 46A1 as a pharmacologic target for Alzheimer's disease. Neuropharmacology. 2017;123:465–76.
31. Patel TK, Patel VB, Rana DG. Possible anti-depressant effect of efavirenz and pro-depressive-like effect of voriconazole in specified doses in various experimental models of depression in mice. Pharmacol Rep. 2017;69(5):1082–7.
32. Petrov AM, Mast N, Li Y, Pikuleva IA. The key genes, phosphoproteins, processes, and pathways affected by efavirenz-activated CYP46A1 in the amyloid-decreasing paradigm of efavirenz treatment. FASEB J. 2019;33(8):8782–98.
33. Mitroi DN, Pereyra-Gomez G, Soto-Huelin B, Senovilla F, Kobayashi T, Esteban JA, Ledesma MD. NPC1 enables cholesterol mobilization during long-term potentiation that can be restored in Niemann-Pick disease type C by CYP46A1 activation. EMBO Rep. 2019:e48143.
34. Han M, Wang S, Yang N, Wang X, Zhao W, Saed HS, et al. Therapeutic implications of altered cholesterol homeostasis mediated by loss of CYP46A1 in human glioblastoma. EMBO Mol Med. 2020;12(1):e10924.
35. Ali T, Hannaoui S, Nemani S, Tahir W, Zemlyankina I, Cherry P, et al. Oral administration of repurposed drug targeting Cyp46A1 increases survival times of prion infected mice. Acta Neuropathol Commun. 2021;9(1):58.
36. Pikuleva IA. Targeting cytochrome P450 46A1 and brain cholesterol 24-hydroxylation to treat neurodegenerative diseases. Explor Neuroprotective Ther. 2021;1(3):159–72.
37. Lerner AJ, Arnold SE, Maxfield E, Koenig A, Toth ME, Fortin B, et al. CYP46A1 activation by low-dose efavirenz enhances brain cholesterol metabolism in subjects with early Alzheimer's disease. Alzheimers Res Ther. 2022;14(1):198.
38. Gascón-Bayarri J, Simon PC, Llop R, Carnaval T, Ledesma MD, Rico I, et al. Efficacy and safety clinical trial with efavirenz in patients diagnosed with adult Niemann-pick type C with cognitive impairment. Medicine (Baltimore). 2022;101(48):e31471.
39. Cruysberg JR, Wevers RA, van Engelen BG, Pinckers A, van Spreeken A, Tolboom JJ. Ocular and systemic manifestations of cerebrotendinous xanthomatosis. Am J Ophthalmol. 1995;120(5):597–604.

40. Morgan SJ, McKenna P, Bosanquet RC. Case of cerebrotendinous xanthomatosis. I: unusual ophthalmic features. Br J Ophthalmol. 1989;73(12):1011–4.
41. Dotti MT, Rufa A, Federico A. Cerebrotendinous xanthomatosis: heterogeneity of clinical phenotype with evidence of previously undescribed ophthalmological findings. J Inherit Metab Dis. 2001;24(7):696–706.
42. London A, Benhar I, Schwartz M. The retina as a window to the brain—from eye research to CNS disorders. Nat Rev Neurol. 2013;9(1):44–53.
43. Liao WL, Heo GY, Dodder NG, Reem RE, Mast N, Huang S, et al. Quantification of cholesterol-metabolizing P450s CYP27A1 and CYP46A1 in neural tissues reveals a lack of enzyme-product correlations in human retina but not human brain. J Proteome Res. 2011;10(1):241–8.
44. Mast N, Reem R, Bederman I, Huang S, DiPatre PL, Björkhem I, Pikuleva IA. Cholestenoic acid is an important elimination product of cholesterol in the retina: comparison of retinal cholesterol metabolism with that in the brain. Invest Ophthalmol Vis Sci. 2011;52(1):594–603.
45. Saadane A, Mast N, Charvet CD, Omarova S, Zheng W, Huang SS, et al. Retinal and nonocular abnormalities in *Cyp27a1*$^{-/-}$*Cyp46a1*$^{-/-}$ mice with dysfunctional metabolism of cholesterol. Am J Pathol. 2014;184(9):2403–19.
46. Omarova S, Charvet CD, Reem RE, Mast N, Zheng W, Huang S, et al. Abnormal vascularization in mouse retina with dysregulated retinal cholesterol homeostasis. J Clin Invest. 2012;122(8):3012–23.
47. El-Darzi N, Mast N, Buchner DA, Saadane A, Dailey B, Trichonas G, Pikuleva IA. Low-dose anti-HIV drug efavirenz mitigates retinal vascular lesions in a mouse model of Alzheimer's disease. Front Pharmacol. 2022;13:902254.

Role of Bile Acid Pathway Intermediates in Pathology of Cerebrotendinous Xanthomatosis (CTX)

12

William J. Griffiths, Eylan Yutuc, Mohsen Ali Asgari, and Yuqin Wang

Introduction

The identification of sterol 27-hydroxylase (cytochrome P450 family 27 subfamily A member 1, CYP27A1, MIM 606530) as the deficient enzyme in the autosomal recessive genetic disorder cerebrotendinous xanthomatosis (CTX) was made thanks to the pioneering work of Ingemar Björkhem and David Russell in the 1980s and 1990s [1–3]. CYP27A1 represents the first enzyme of the acidic pathway of bile acid synthesis introducing a hydroxy group at the terminal carbon of the sterol side-chain with resultant R stereochemistry at C-25 and further converts this primary alcohol to a carboxylic acid (Fig. 12.1) [4]. The enzymatic products 27-hydroxycholesterol (27-HC), systematically but less commonly named (25R)26-hydroxycholesterol [5], and 3β-hydroxycholest-5-en-(25R)26-oic acid (3β-HCA) are then metabolised through multiple steps to primary bile acids, mostly chenodeoxycholic acid (CDCA) [4]. (Note that stereochemistry at C-25 in C_{27} sterols is assumed to be 25R unless stated otherwise). CYP27A1 also appears in the neutral pathway of bile acid biosynthesis converting 7α,12α-dihydroxycholesterol (7α,12α-diHC), 7α,12α-dihydroxycholest-4-en-3-one (7α,12α-diHCO), and their reduced metabolite 5β-cholestan-3α,7α,12α-triol to their respective C_{27} carboxylic acids ready for side-chain shortening to ultimately yield cholic acid (Fig. 12.1). CDCA can also be formed via the neutral pathway crossing over to the acidic pathway and also through reduction of 7α-hydroxycholest-4-en-3-one (7α-HCO) prior to C_{27} carboxylation by CYP27A1 and side-chain shortening. The pathology of CTX is often attributed to a build-up of toxic intermediates up-stream of CYP27A1 in the neutral pathway, and indeed, many of the clinical features of CTX can be resolved by treatment with CDCA if

W. J. Griffiths (✉) · E. Yutuc · M. A. Asgari · Y. Wang
Swansea University Medical School, Swansea, Wales, UK
e-mail: w.j.griffiths@swansea.ac.uk

A. Federico et al. (eds.), *Cerebrotendinous Xanthomatosis*,
https://doi.org/10.1007/978-3-031-92526-9_12

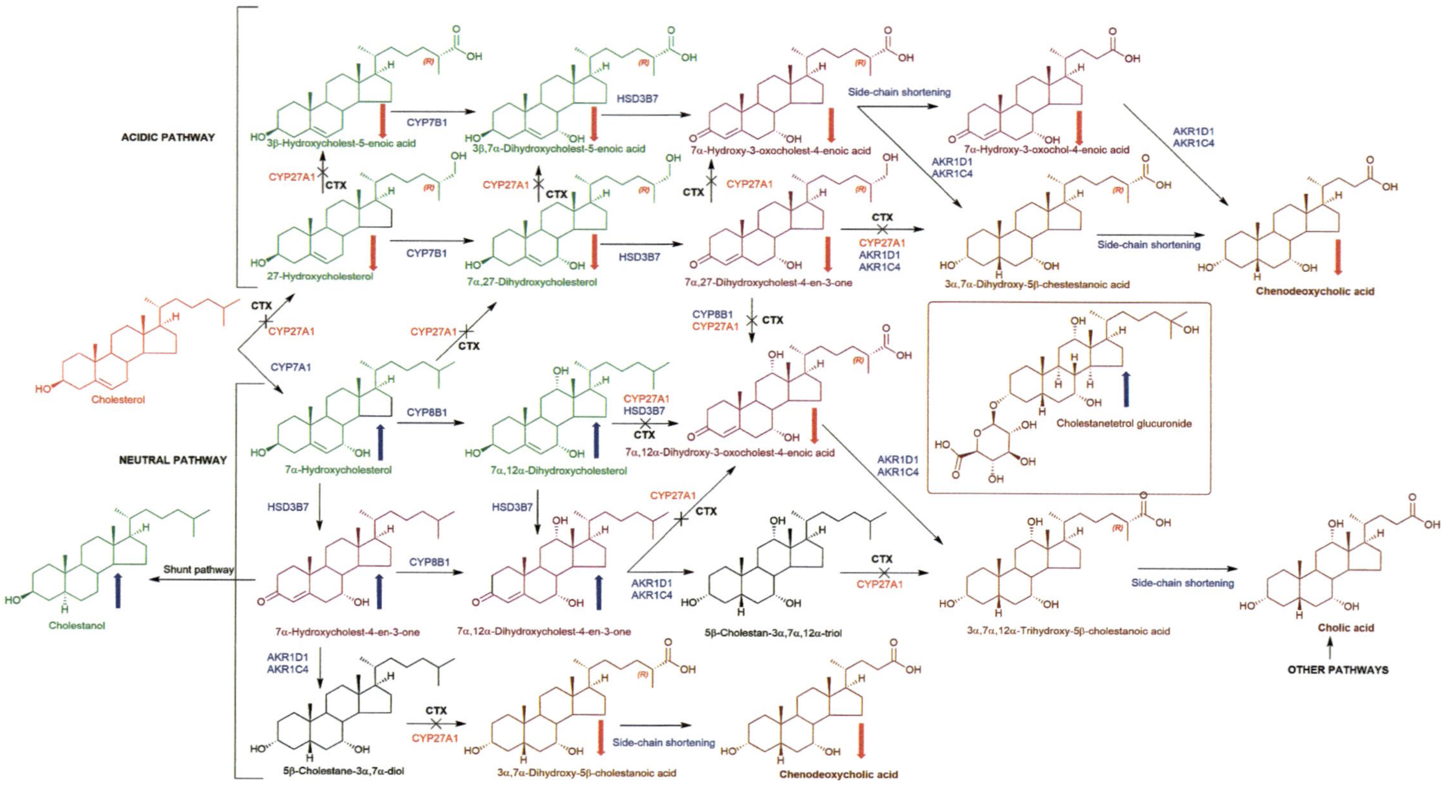

Fig. 12.1 Abbreviated versions of the acidic and neutral pathways of bile acid biosynthesis. Metabolites absent or greatly diminished in plasma from CTX patients are indicated by a downward pointing thick red arrow, those elevated by an upward pointing thick blue arrow. The enzyme CYP27A1 is shown in red, other enzymes in blue. Defective reactions in CTX are shown by a crossed arrow. Cholesterol is drawn in red, its metabolites detected by positive-ion LC-ESI-MS^n following treatment with cholesterol oxidase and deuterium labelled Girard-P derivatisation reagent [$^2H_5$]GP (Fr-1A) are in green, those detected following unlabelled [$^2H_0$]GP derivatisation in the absence of cholesterol oxidase treatment (Fr-1B) are in claret, and those with a 5α-hydroxy plus carboxylic acid group detected by negative-ion LC-ESI-MS^n are shown in brown. A cholestanetetrol GlcA is shown in the inset with the GlcA drawn attached to C-3

instituted early enough [6]. However, CDCA does not appear to be effective in treating some of the neurological aspects of CTX especially if treatment is delayed and alternative strategies to restore the functional enzyme may have merit.

CTX is an autosomal recessive genetic disorder, and in cases where pathogenic variants are present in both alleles of *CYP27A1* resulting in a largely inactive enzyme, diagnosis can be made by gene sequencing or by mass spectrometry (MS). This can be done by gas-chromatography (GC)-MS detecting an elevation in cholestanol (5α-cholestane-3β-ol) in plasma or by detecting an increase in urinary or plasma bile alcohol glucuronides (GlcA), e.g. cholestanetetrol-, cholestanepentol-, cholestanehexol-GlcA, accompanied by a fall in CDCA by direct infusion (DI)-MS or liquid chromatography (LC)-MS [7–10]. A disadvantage of cholestanol as a diagnostic biomarker of CTX is that it can be elevated in other genetic disorders like familial hypercholesterolemia and sitosterolaemia, as well as liver disease [10, 11]. Diagnosis may be more difficult in cases where some enzyme activity is maintained, in which case it may be prudent to monitor additional metabolites such as 27-HC and 3β-HCA which will be almost absent when the enzyme is inactive but present at a reduced concentration where partial activity is maintained, or 7α-HCO and 7αH,12α-diHCO and bile alcohols which are highly elevated when CYP27A1 activity is deficient [12, 13].

Analytical Techniques to Detect CTX Biomarkers

GC-MS is applicable for measurement of cholestanol, 7α-hydroxycholesterol (7α-HC) and 7α-HCO, all of which are elevated in CTX plasma, and Lütjohann et al. have recommended the latter two compounds as optimal markers in plasma for monitoring the response to therapy and their ratio to 27-HC, also measured in the same GC-MS run, as a good CTX diagnostic biomarker [10]. While GC-MS is routinely used in dedicated mass spectrometry laboratories, the additional requirement of derivatisation has, over the decades, led to a shift to more direct analysis methods. Historically elevated levels of bile alcohol glucuronides in urine or plasma/serum have also been used to diagnose CTX, first by fast atom bombardment (FAB)-MS and later by electrospray ionisation (ESI)-MS [7–9]. Here there is no requirement for derivatisation, just a simple sample clean-up, often by solid-phase extraction (SPE). Currently there is a move towards the use of ESI-tandem-MS (MS/MS or MS^2) in the screening for CTX from dried blood spots. Vaz et al. have generated convincing data using ESI-MS/MS to demonstrate the ratio of cholestanetetrol-GlcA to taurochenodeoxycholic acid (TCDCA) as a screening biomarker for CTX, where cholestanetetrol-GlcA is elevated and TCDCA diminished [14]. By also measuring the ratio of taurotrihydroxycholestanoic acid to cholestanetetrol-GlcA, confusion with peroxisomal disorders can be avoided where cholestanetetrol-GlcA and taurotrihydroxycholestanoic acid are both elevated, but taurotrihydroxycholestanoic acid will be greatly diminished in CTX. Hong et al. have added LC separation to the ESI-MS/MS diagnostic method, concluding that both cholestanetetrol-GlcA and the ratio of cholestanetetrol-GlcA to TCDCA are excellent CTX biomarkers suitable for newborn screening [15].

Measuring Multiple Bile Acid Precursors in CTX in a Single Analysis

The deficiency in CYP27A1 shifts cholesterol metabolism from the acidic to the neutral pathway; this is accentuated by a lack in production of CDCA, resulting in reduced negative feedback via the farnesoid X receptor (FXR) on CYP7A1 expression, the first enzyme of the neutral pathway of bile acid biosynthesis (Fig. 12.1), driving enhanced production of 7α-HC [8]. Additionally, the block in the neutral pathway by deficient CYP27A1 results in an elevation in plasma of the early metabolites of the pathway, i.e. 7α-HC, 7α-HCO, 7α,12α-diHC and 7α,12α-diHCO. These four metabolites fall into the family of molecules called oxysterols, i.e. oxidised forms of cholesterol, which also include 27-HC, 7α,27-dihydroxycholesterol (7α,27-diHC), 7α,27-dihydroxycholest-4-en-3-one (7α,27-diHCO) and the cholestenoic acids all of which are diminished in CTX [16–18]. While these molecules can be detected by GC-MS, it requires multiple different derivatisation steps, often with and without additional saponification necessary to hydrolyse sterol esters [19].

To optimise detection of these bile acid precursors, we have developed a simple derivatisation strategy which allows the detection of most of the bile acid precursors in a single LC-ESI-MS^n experiment (Fig. 12.1) [20]. In brief, oxysterols including cholestenoic acids are extracted from plasma into ethanol and after dilution with water passed through a C_{18} SPE column. Cholesterol and other highly lipophilic components are retained by the column leaving an eluent rich in oxysterols including cholestenoic acids. This eluate is divided into two equal fractions, Fr-1A and Fr1-B. Both fractions are dried down then reconstituted in propan-2-ol. To Fr-1A bacterial cholesterol oxidase enzyme in phosphate buffer is added. This converts sterols with a 3β-hydroxy group to equivalents 3-ones via the classical Richmond reaction (Fig. 12.2a) [21, 22]. [$^2H_5$]Girard P ([$^2H_5$]GP) reagent is then added in methanol; this reacts with the 3-oxo group to give a GP-hydrazone. The reaction mixture can be cleaned up on a second reversed-phase SPE column to remove excess derivatisation reagent or injected directly onto a trap column preceding the LC column linked to the MS. The derivatised sterols give greatly improved ESI response and intense fragment ions useful for both quantification and identification (Fig. 12.2) [16, 20, 23]. However, some oxysterols and cholestenoic acids, e.g. 7α-HCO, 7α,12α-diHCO, 7α-hydroxy-3-oxocholest-4-en-(25R/S)26-oic acid (7αH,3O-CA), naturally possess a native 3-oxo group and do not require an oxidation step prior to derivatisation. These can be analysed directly from Fr-1B which is treated as Fr-1A but in the absence of cholesterol oxidase and with the use of [$^2H_0$]GP instead of [$^2H_5$]GP (Fig. 12.2b). The use of different isotopic GP reagents means that after the second SPE step, equal aliquots of Fr-1A and Fr-1B can be combined and analysed in combination by LC-ESI-MS^n providing complementary information on cholesterol metabolites. Sterols derivatised with [$^2H_5$]GP can be differentiated from those derivatised with [$^2H_0$]GP by virtue of their difference in mass (5.0314 Da). This protocol allows the identification of all major cholesterol metabolites in the bile acid biosynthesis pathway with a 3β-hydroxy or 3-oxo group (Fig. 12.1) and, with the inclusion of internal standards, absolute quantification [20].

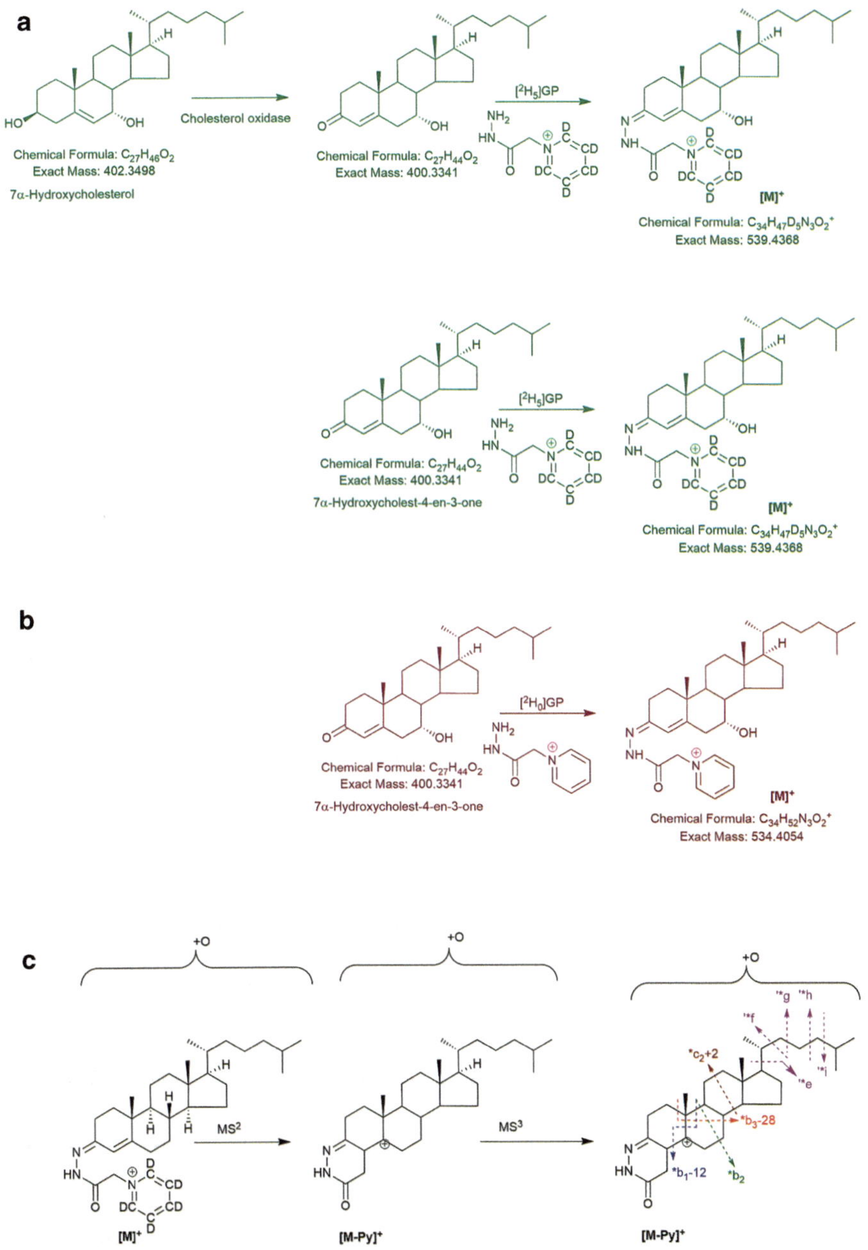

Fig. 12.2 Measuring multiple bile acid precursors via simple derivatisation and LC-ESI-MS^n. (**a**) Cholesterol metabolites with a 3β-hydroxy-5-ene structure are converted by bacterial cholesterol oxidase in the Richmond reaction to the equivalent 3-oxo-4-enes which are then derivatised with [$^2H_5$]GP (i.e. Fr-1A). (**b**) Metabolites with a native 3-oxo group are derivatised directly with [$^2H_0$]GP (i.e. Fr-1B). Fr-1A and Fr-1B are combined and analysed by LC-ESI-MS^n. Note that positive-negative ion switching allows the detection of bile acid precursor with a 3α-hydroxy group which are transparent to this derivatisation, providing they also have a carboxylic acid group. (**c**) Derivatised metabolites fragment by MS^2 to give abundant fragment-ions valuable for multiple-reaction monitoring and by MS^3 to give structural information

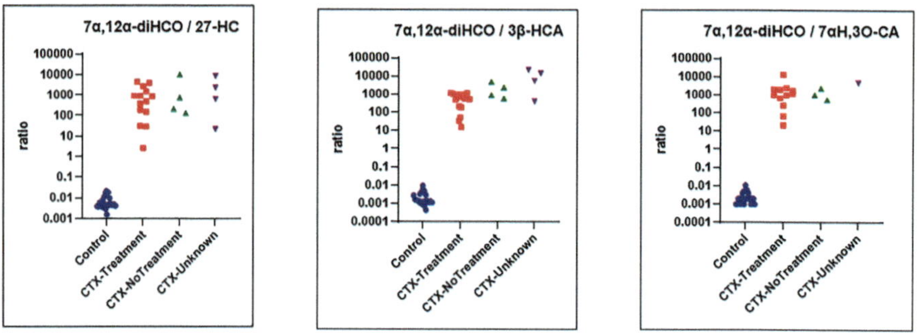

Fig. 12.3 Concentration ratios of bile acid precursors in plasma provide unequivocal diagnosis of CTX. Ratios are shown on a log scale. Data from control samples are shown in blue ($n = 24$), from CTX patients on bile acid therapy are shown in red ($n = 14$), from untreated CTX patients in green ($n = 4$), and from CTX patients where treatment is unknown in purple ($n = 4$). In the case of 7αH,3O-CA measurements were made from 12 CTX patients on bile acid therapy, three patients not on treatment, and one patient where the treatment regime was not known. (Data from Griffiths et al. [16], Theofilopoulos et al. [17], Abdel-Khalik et al. [24] and Hoflinger et al. [18])

From data generated using this methodology, the optimal CTX diagnostic biomarkers in plasma are the concentration ratios of 7α,12α-diHCO to 27-HC, 7α,12α-diHCO to 3β-HCA and 7α,12α-diHCO to 7αH,3O-CA (Fig. 12.3) [16–18, 24]. In each case, there is no overlap in the measured ratios between control and CTX plasma, and for the latter two ratios, the controls differ from CTX by about three orders of magnitude. An advantage of the 7α,12α-diHCO to 7αH,3O-CA ratio is that both metabolites can be analysed in Fr-1B, i.e. Fr-1A does not require preparation or analysis.

As discussed, LC-ESI-MS^n following GP-derivatisation allows the detection of all abundant bile acid precursors with a 3β-hydroxy-5-ene, 3β-hydroxy-5α-hydrogen or 3-oxo structure. This is performed in the positive-ion MS mode. However, primary bile acids and their immediate precursors possess a 3α-hydroxy group and are transparent to cholesterol oxidase treatment and GP-derivatisation. However, these metabolites often possess a carboxylic acid group or are conjugated with GlcA and can be readily analysed in the negative-ion MS mode. So, if we follow the cholesterol oxidase and GP-derivatisation protocol with positive-negative ion switching, bile acid pathway intermediates with a 3β-hydroxy, 3-oxo or 3α-hydroxy group can be detected providing the latter have also a carboxylic group. This covers almost the entire bile acid biosynthesis pathway plus a shunt to the bile alcohol glucuronides and cholestanol (Fig. 12.1). For those cholesterol metabolites with a 3α-hydroxy group, an alternative strategy is treatment with 3α-hydroxysteroid dehydrogenase to introduce a 3-oxo group for subsequent derivatisation with GP-reagent [25].

Unexpected Bile Acid Precursors Present in Plasma and CSF in CTX

CYP27A1 introduces the 27-hydroxy and 27-carboxylate groups onto the side-chain of cholesterol and other sterols, leading to R-stereochemistry at the asymmetric centre at C-25. Other CYP enzymes can also hydroxylate the terminal carbon of sterols including CYP46A1 and CYP3A [26, 27], and we have found that CYP3A4 will 27-hydoxylate 7α-HC to 7α,27-diHC to specifically give S-stereochemistry at C-25, i.e. 7α,27-diHC(25S) [28].

When plasma or CSF is analysed from control individuals, the cholestenoic acid 7αH,3O-CA is observed as both the 25R and 25S isomers, the latter being about 10–20% of the abundance of the former, with the two isomers being interconvertible via their CoA-thioesters by the enzyme alpha-methylacyl-CoA-racemase (AMACR) [4, 20]. Interestingly, in CTX, we also find both isomers at very low levels but of quite similar abundance [18, 20]. This leads to the hypothesis that in CTX elevated, 7α-HC can be hydroxylated by CYP3A4 to 7α,27-diHC(25S) which can then undergo oxidation by 3β-hydroxy-Δ^5-steroid oxidoreductase (HSD3B7) and further oxidation, perhaps by CYP3A4 or another oxygenase, at the terminal carbon to give 7αH,3O-CA(25S). This acid can undergo side-chain shortening and may account for the presence of low levels of CDCA sometimes observed in CTX. Alternatively, 7αH,3O-CA(25S) can isomerise to 7αH,3O-CA(25R) [4].

Bile Acid Precursors in Human Brain and Their Potential Role in Pathophysiology of CTX

In human brain, the major cholesterol metabolite is 24S-hydroxycholesterol (24S-HC), which can be exported from the brain and transported in the circulation to the liver for conversion to bile acids [29]. Unlike cholesterol, oxysterols can cross the blood brain barrier; in this way, 24S-HC is exported from, while 27-HC is imported into the brain. We have analysed brain tissue samples from a single CTX patient [18]. Levels of 24S-HC were similar to controls, but 27-HC was absent in CTX, while 7α-HCO and 7α,12α-diHCO were both elevated in CTX, as was cholestanol [18]. Presumably both 7α-HCO and 7α,12α-diHCO enter the brain from the circulation as the necessary 7α- and 12α-hydroxylases (CYP7A1 and CYP8B1) are not expressed in brain [30]. Interestingly, 7α,12α-diHCO and cholestanol were not found to be toxic to a neuronal-like cell line, suggesting that some of the neurological problems associated with CTX may not be a consequence of toxic metabolites but rather an absence of neuroprotective metabolites [18, 31]. In this regard, 27-HC, although toxic towards neurons at high concentration [32], may also be important to maintain cholesterol homeostasis in brain [18]. 27-HC is one of a number of side-chain oxysterols that binds to the endoplasmic reticulum anchor protein INSIG (insulin induced gene) causing a conformational change and the resultant binding of INSIG to the transport protein SCAP (SREBP cleavage activating protein), with the result that SCAP is unable to transport SREBP-2 (sterol regulatory element-binding protein-2), the master transcription for genes coding the enzymes of the cholesterol biosynthesis pathway and of the LDL-receptor, to the Golgi for processing to its active form [33]. An absence of 27-HC could lead to a failure of this feedback mechanism and enhanced formation of cholesterol in brain and ultimately potentially toxic metabolites. In addition, 27-HC is a ligand to the liver X receptors (LXRs) [34], activation of which leads to transcription of the *ABCA1* and *APOE* genes coding for cholesterol transport and carrier proteins, respectively [35]. Thus, an absence of 27-HC could enhance cholesterol synthesis in brain and also impair cholesterol export from brain cells, resulting in ineffective cholesterol homeostasis.

Besides being the enzyme that generates 27-HC from cholesterol, CYP27A1 is essential for the normal formation of the cholestenoic acids, e.g. 3β,7α-dihydroxycholest-5-en-(25R/S)-oic acid (3β,7α-diHCA) and 7αH,3O-CA. 7αH,3O-CA can be synthesised in brain and exported from brain. Although it is mostly considered as providing a route for removal of 27-HC from brain [36], it also offers a route for the removal of cholesterol, its absence in CTX could also lead to ineffective cholesterol homeostasis. 3β,7α-diHCA is a precursor of 7αH,3O-CA and likewise is synthesised in brain. This acid has been shown to promote neuronal survival in an LXR-dependent fashion [17]. 3β,7α-diHCA is a normal constituent of blood and its supplementation could provide a pharmacological treatment for CTX as it is likely to pass the blood-brain barrier down a concentration gradient.

Considering the important functions of CYP27A1 in brain, an absence of its catalytic products may be more significant to the pathology of CTX, at least regarding the neurological aspects, than a build-up of toxic bile acid intermediates [18]. We speculate that a successful treatment approach may be pharmacological restoration of its enzyme products or replacement of defective CYP27A1. In principle, this can be via enzyme replacement or adeno-associated virus (AAV) vectors expressing *CYP27A1*. An AAV vector carrying *CYP46A1* is currently being used in a first in-human, phase 1/2 trial for the treatment of Huntington's disease. A word of warning regarding AAV-*CYP27A1* treatment and CTX. While the CYP27A1 metabolic product 3β,7α-diHCA is neuroprotective, other CYP27A1-derived metabolites, 27-HC, 3β-HCA and 3β,7β-diHCA, can be neurotoxic [17], so a careful titration of enzyme would be required.

Conclusions

While genome sequencing can identify pathogenic variants in *CYP27A1*, sequencing often identifies variants of uncertain significance. Biochemical analysis can help to determine the resultant biochemical phenotype and can be performed with comparative ease by currently available MS analytical methods to assist in providing a definitive diagnosis. Improved biochemical methods are likely to become ever more important with the uncovering of a broader clinical and biochemical phenotypic spectrum of disease for CTX than was previously recognised. In addition, MS methods provide an optimal approach to determine a deficiency in CYP27A1 activity in the realm of newborn screening, the next great opportunity for progress in improving the lives of CTX patients.

Acknowledgements This work was supported by funding from the UKRI (grant numbers BB/I001735/1, BB/S019588/1, MR/X012387/1 and MR/Y008057/1 to WJG, BB/L001942/1 to YW), and the European Union, through European Structural Funds (ESF), as part of the Welsh Government funded Academic Expertise for Business project (to WJG and YW). For the purpose of open access, the authors have applied a CC BY public copyright license to any Author Accepted Manuscript version arising. Members of the European Network for Oxysterol Research (ENOR, https://www.oxysterols.net/) are thanked for informative discussions.

Declaration of Competing Interests The authors declare the following financial interests/personal relationships, which may be considered as potential competing interests: WJG and YW are listed as inventors on the patent "Kit and method for quantitative detection of steroids" US9851368B2 and the patent application "Compound and method for the treatment and diagnosis of neurodegenerative conditions" US 2021/0139529 A1. WJG, EY and YW are shareholders in CholesteniX Ltd.

References

1. Skrede S, Björkhem I, Kvittingen EA, Buchmann MS, Lie SO, East C, et al. Demonstration of 26-hydroxylation of C27-steroids in human skin fibroblasts, and a deficiency of this activity in cerebrotendinous xanthomatosis. J Clin Invest. 1986;78(3):729–35.
2. Cali JJ, Hsieh CL, Francke U, Russell DW. Mutations in the bile acid biosynthetic enzyme sterol 27-hydroxylase underlie cerebrotendinous xanthomatosis. J Biol Chem. 1991;266(12):7779–83.
3. Bjorkhem I. Cerebrotendinous xanthomatosis. Curr Opin Lipidol. 2013;24(4):283–7.
4. Russell DW. The enzymes, regulation, and genetics of bile acid synthesis. Annu Rev Biochem. 2003;72:137–74.
5. Fakheri RJ, Javitt NB. 27-hydroxycholesterol, does it exist? On the nomenclature and stereochemistry of 26-hydroxylated sterols. Steroids. 2012;77(6):575–7.
6. Berginer VM, Salen G, Shefer S. Long-term treatment of cerebrotendinous xanthomatosis with chenodeoxycholic acid. N Engl J Med. 1984;311(26):1649–52.
7. Egestad B, Pettersson P, Skrede S, Sjövall J. Fast atom bombardment mass spectrometry in the diagnosis of cerebrotendinous xanthomatosis. Scand J Clin Lab Invest. 1985;45(5):443–6.
8. Clayton PT. Disorders of bile acid synthesis. J Inherit Metab Dis. 2011;34(3):593–604.
9. Setchell KD, Heubi JE. Defects in bile acid biosynthesis--diagnosis and treatment. J Pediatr Gastroenterol Nutr. 2006;43(Suppl 1):S17–22.
10. Lütjohann D, Stellaard F, Björkhem I. Levels of 7alpha-hydroxycholesterol and/or 7alpha-hydroxy-4-cholest-3-one are the optimal biochemical markers for the evaluation of treatment of cerebrotendinous xanthomatosis. J Neurol. 2020;267(2):572–3.
11. Koopman BJ, van der Molen JC, Wolthers BG, de Jager AE, Waterreus RJ, Gips CH. Capillary gas chromatographic determination of cholestanol/cholesterol ratio in biological fluids. Its potential usefulness for the follow-up of some liver diseases and its lack of specificity in diagnosing CTX (cerebrotendinous xanthomatosis). Clin Chim Acta. 1984;137(3):305–15.
12. DeBarber AE, Connor WE, Pappu AS, Merkens LS, Steiner RD. ESI-MS/MS quantification of 7α-hydroxy-4-cholesten-3-one facilitates rapid, convenient diagnostic testing for cerebrotendinous xanthomatosis. Clin Chim Acta. 2010;411(1):43–8.

13. DeBarber AE, Luo J, Giugliani R, Souza CF, Chiang JP, Merkens LS, et al. A useful multi-analyte blood test for cerebrotendinous xanthomatosis. Clin Biochem. 2014;47(9):860–3.
14. Vaz FM, Jamal Y, Barto R, Gelb MH, DeBarber AE, Wevers RA, et al. Newborn screening for Cerebrotendinous Xanthomatosis: a retrospective biomarker study using both flow-injection and UPLC-MS/MS analysis in 20,000 newborns. Clin Chim Acta. 2023;539:170–4.
15. Hong X, Daiker J, Sadilek M, DeBarber AE, Chiang J, Duan J, et al. Toward newborn screening of cerebrotendinous xanthomatosis: results of a biomarker research study using 32,000 newborn dried blood spots. Genet Med. 2020;22(10):1606–12.
16. Griffiths WJ, Crick PJ, Wang Y, Ogundare M, Tuschl K, Morris AA, et al. Analytical strategies for characterization of oxysterol lipidomes: liver X receptor ligands in plasma. Free Radic Biol Med. 2013;59:69–84.
17. Theofilopoulos S, Griffiths WJ, Crick PJ, Yang S, Meljon A, Ogundare M, et al. Cholestenoic acids regulate motor neuron survival via liver X receptors. J Clin Invest. 2014;124(11):4829–42.
18. Hoflinger P, Hauser S, Yutuc E, Hengel H, Griffiths L, Radelfahr F, et al. Metabolic profiling in serum, cerebrospinal fluid, and brain of patients with cerebrotendinous xanthomatosis. J Lipid Res. 2021;62:100078.
19. Axelson M, Mork B, Sjovall J. Occurrence of 3 beta-hydroxy-5-cholestenoic acid, 3 beta,7 alpha-dihydroxy-5-cholestenoic acid, and 7 alpha-hydroxy-3-oxo-4-cholestenoic acid as normal constituents in human blood. J Lipid Res. 1988;29(5):629–41.
20. Yutuc E, Dickson AL, Pacciarini M, Griffiths L, Baker PRS, Connell L, et al. Deep mining of oxysterols and cholestenoic acids in human plasma and cerebrospinal fluid: quantification using isotope dilution mass spectrometry. Anal Chim Acta. 2021;1154:338259.
21. Richmond W. Use of cholesterol oxidase for assay of total and free cholesterol in serum by continuous-flow analysis. Clin Chem. 1976;22(10):1579–88.
22. MacLachlan J, Wotherspoon AT, Ansell RO, Brooks CJ. Cholesterol oxidase: sources, physical properties and analytical applications. J Steroid Biochem Mol Biol. 2000;72(5):169–95.
23. Karu K, Hornshaw M, Woffendin G, Bodin K, Hamberg M, Alvelius G, et al. Liquid chromatography-mass spectrometry utilizing multi-stage fragmentation for the identification of oxysterols. J Lipid Res. 2007;48(4):976–87.
24. Abdel-Khalik J, Yutuc E, Crick PJ, Gustafsson JA, Warner M, Roman G, et al. Defective cholesterol metabolism in amyotrophic lateral sclerosis. J Lipid Res. 2017;58(1):267–78.
25. Abdel-Khalik J, Crick PJ, Yutuc E, Wang Y, Griffiths WJ. Developing an enzyme-assisted Derivatization method for analysis of C27 bile alcohols and acids by electrospray ionization-mass spectrometry. Molecules. 2019;24(3):597.
26. Mast N, Norcross R, Andersson U, Shou M, Nakayama K, Bjorkhem I, et al. Broad substrate specificity of human cytochrome P450 46A1 which initiates cholesterol degradation in the brain. Biochemistry. 2003;42(48):14284–92.
27. Honda A, Salen G, Matsuzaki Y, Batta AK, Xu G, Leitersdorf E, et al. Side chain hydroxylations in bile acid biosynthesis catalyzed by CYP3A are markedly up-regulated in Cyp27−/− mice but not in cerebrotendinous xanthomatosis. J Biol Chem. 2001;276(37):34579–85.
28. Griffiths WJ, Crick PJ, Meljon A, Theofilopoulos S, Abdel-Khalik J, Yutuc E, et al. Additional pathways of sterol metabolism: evidence from analysis of Cyp27a1−/− mouse brain and plasma. Biochim Biophys Acta Mol Cell Biol Lipids. 2019;1864(2):191–211.
29. Bjorkhem I. Rediscovery of cerebrosterol. Lipids. 2007;42(1):5–14.
30. Baloni P, Funk CC, Yan J, Yurkovich JT, Kueider-Paisley A, Nho K, et al. Metabolic network analysis reveals altered bile acid synthesis and metabolism in Alzheimer's disease. Cell Rep Med. 2020;1(8):100138.
31. Theofilopoulos S, Wang Y, Kitambi SS, Sacchetti P, Sousa KM, Bodin K, et al. Brain endogenous liver X receptor ligands selectively promote midbrain neurogenesis. Nat Chem Biol. 2013;9(2):126–33.
32. Schols L, Rattay TW, Martus P, Meisner C, Baets J, Fischer I, et al. Hereditary spastic paraplegia type 5: natural history, biomarkers and a randomized controlled trial. Brain. 2017;140(12):3112–27.

33. Radhakrishnan A, Ikeda Y, Kwon HJ, Brown MS, Goldstein JL. Sterol-regulated transport of SREBPs from endoplasmic reticulum to Golgi: oxysterols block transport by binding to Insig. Proc Natl Acad Sci USA. 2007;104(16):6511–8.
34. Fu X, Menke JG, Chen Y, Zhou G, MacNaul KL, Wright SD, et al. 27-hydroxycholesterol is an endogenous ligand for liver X receptor in cholesterol-loaded cells. J Biol Chem. 2001;276(42):38378–87.
35. Tontonoz P. Transcriptional and posttranscriptional control of cholesterol homeostasis by liver X receptors. Cold Spring Harb Symp Quant Biol. 2011;76:129–37.
36. Meaney S, Heverin M, Panzenboeck U, Ekstrom L, Axelsson M, Andersson U, et al. Novel route for elimination of brain oxysterols across the blood-brain barrier: conversion into 7alpha-hydroxy-3-oxo-4-cholestenoic acid. J Lipid Res. 2007;48(4):944–51.

Part IV

Neuroimaging in Cerebrotendinous Xanthomatosis (CTX)

Overview of Neuroimaging in Cerebrotendinous Xanthomatosis (CTX)

13

Rosa Cortese, Carlo Manco, and Nicola De Stefano

Introduction

Cerebrotendinous xanthomatosis (CTX) is a rare autosomal recessive disorder caused by a deficiency in the enzyme sterol 27-hydroxylase, leading to the accumulation of cholestanol and cholesterol in various tissues, including the brain [1, 2]. This accumulation may give neurological involvement and result in a wide range of neurological signs and symptoms, including intellectual disability, ataxia, spasticity, seizures, psychiatric disturbances, and progressive cognitive decline [2, 3]. Notably, approximately 84% of cases are concomitant with abnormalities in neuroimaging investigations [3–5]. Given the diverse clinical presentation, timely and accurate diagnosis of CTX is essential for effective management and treatment. Among the diagnostic tools available, brain magnetic resonance imaging (MRI) plays a pivotal role in identifying characteristic abnormalities associated with CTX [3]. In this overview, we will explore how brain MRI contributes to the diagnosis and monitoring of cerebrotendinous xanthomatosis, including the key findings and their clinical significance.

The Role of Conventional MRI in CTX

Brain MRI is a valuable diagnostic tool in the evaluation of cerebrotendinous xanthomatosis. It allows clinicians to visualize and assess structural abnormalities, which are characteristic of this disorder. The key findings in brain MRI of CTX patients include the following (Figs. 13.1 and 13.2).

R. Cortese (✉) · C. Manco · N. De Stefano
Department of Medicine, Surgery and Neuroscience University of Siena, Siena, Italy
e-mail: rosa.cortese@unisi.it; destefano@unisi.it

A. Federico et al. (eds.), *Cerebrotendinous Xanthomatosis*,
https://doi.org/10.1007/978-3-031-92526-9_13

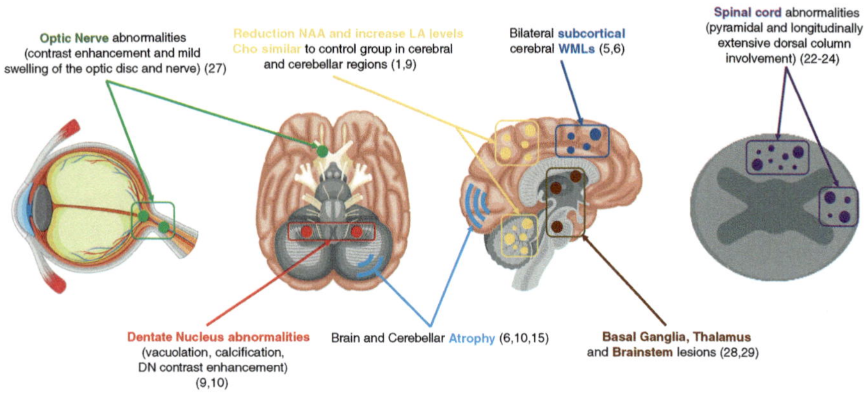

Fig. 13.1 Anatomical structures involved in cerebrotendinous xanthomatosis (CTX) disease and their main abnormalities, as detected using conventional and non-conventional magnetic resonance imaging techniques. (The figure was created using Powerpoint, open access images retrieved from the site https://it.freepik.com/ were used). Abbreviations: NAA, N-Acetilaspartate. Cho, cholin. La, lactate. WMLs, white Matter lesions. DN, dentate nucleus

Bilateral Cerebral White Matter Lesions

One of the most prominent features seen on brain MRI in CTX is the presence of bilateral cerebral white matter lesions [6]. These lesions typically involve the subcortical white matter regions, especially in the frontal and parietal lobes [7, 8]. These abnormalities may appear hyperintense on T2-weighted images and hypointense on T1-weighted images [9–11]. The severity and extent of white matter involvement can vary among individuals [12]. Similar to other CTX-related abnormalities, cerebral white matter lesions tend to be progressive, worsening over time if not effectively managed through treatment [12]. The extent of white matter involvement can vary among CTX patients. Some individuals may exhibit minimal lesions, while others may have more extensive and debilitating changes in cerebral white matter (Table 13.1).

Dentate Nucleus Abnormalities

One of the distinctive neuroimaging features of CTX is the presence of dentate nucleus abnormalities [4, 12]. The dentate nucleus is a structure located within the cerebellum, specifically within the white matter core of the cerebellar hemisphere. In CTX, this region is particularly vulnerable to pathological changes. Dentate nucleus abnormalities in CTX are often characterized by hyperintensity on T2-weighted MRI images [11, 12]. This hyperintensity reflects altered tissue properties, likely due to the accumulation of cholestanol and cholesterol. In some cases, contrast-enhanced MRI may reveal enhancement of the dentate nucleus [12]. This enhancement can be attributed to inflammatory or vascular changes associated with

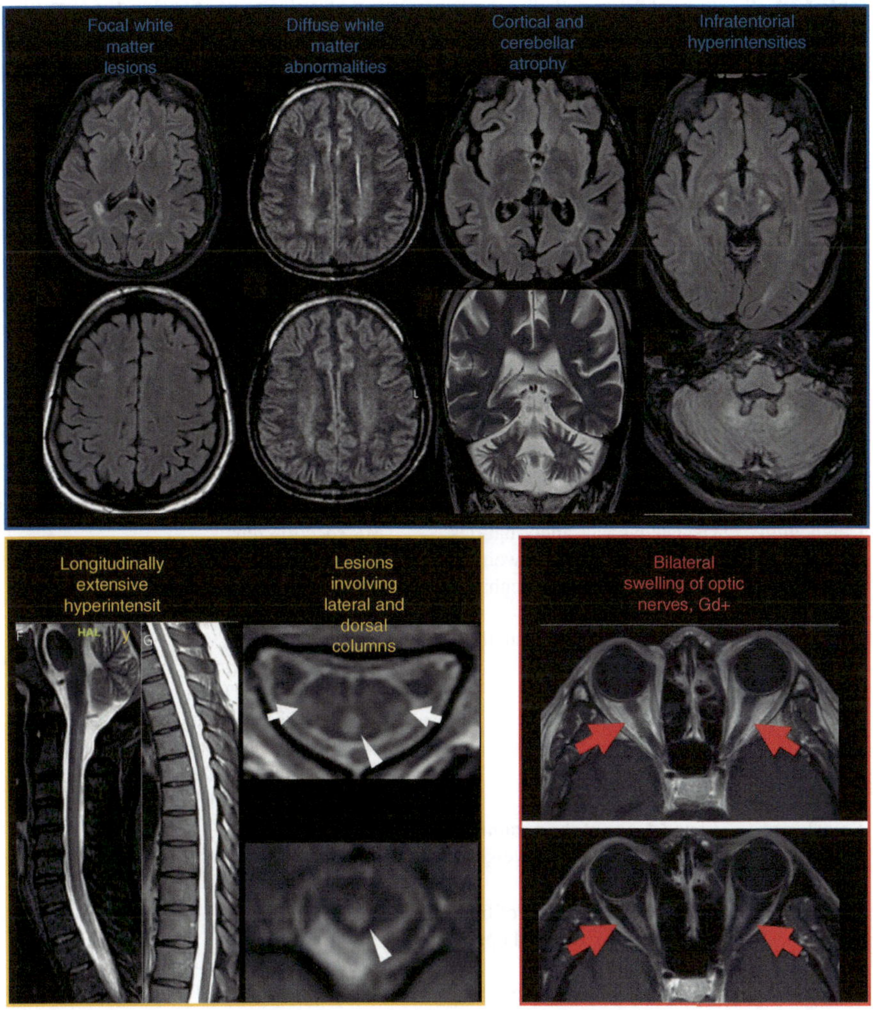

Fig. 13.2 Main characteristics identified on magnetic resonance imaging (MRI) associated with cerebrotendinous xanthomatosis (CTX), particularly focusing on the brain (blue box), spinal cord (yellow box), and optic nerve (red box). The images are sourced from the references [1, 12, 25, 28]. Abbreviations: Gd, gadolinium

the disease process [13]. A large CTX population has been analysed in Siena (Italy) to redefine the spectrum of brain lesions, with particular attention to those involving the cerebellum. In 37 CTX patients, four different MRI patterns involving the dentate nuclei were observed: (i) T2W and FLAIR hyperintensities suggesting cholestanol accumulation, (ii) T1W and FLAIR hypointensities consistent with vacuolation due to neuroaxonal loss, (iii) T1W, FLAIR and SWI hypointensities consistent with calcifications as confirmed by computerized tomography (CT), (iv) or alternatively absence of signal alterations [12]. Dentate nucleus abnormalities on MRI can aid in

Table 13.1 Summary of the main findings from previous study using conventional and non-conventional magnetic resonance imaging techniques in different central nervous system compartments

CNS compartments	Conventional MRI	Advanced MRI
Brain	Subcortical white matter lesions, especially in the frontal and parietal lobe [5, 6] Basal ganglia, thalamus, and brainstem lesions [28, 29] Brain atrophy (visually detected) [10, 15]	*Atrophy using SIENAX*: Detection of brain atrophy [15] *MR spectroscopy*: Reduction of NAA levels (related to clinical disability), almost stable Cho resonance intensities and increase in La [1, 9] *Magnetization transfer imaging*: Differences in MT ratio and peak heights in the whole brain between CTX patients and HC related to EDSS scores and composite scores [41] *Diffusion tensor imaging*: Widespread reductions of FA compared to HC [44]
Cerebellum	Dentate nucleus abnormalities (hyperintensity on T2-weighted MRI images, contrast-enhanced MR) [9, 10] Cerebellar atrophy (visually detected) [6, 15]	*MR spectroscopy*: Reduction of NAA levels (related to clinical disability), almost stable Cho resonance intensities and increase in La [1, 9] *Magnetization transfer imaging*: Differences in MT ratio and peak heights between CTX patients and HC related to EDSS scores and composite scores [41] *Diffusion tensor imaging*: Reduction of FA [44]
Spinal cord	Long lesions of the pyramidal and dorsal column on T2-weighted image [22–24]	
Optic nerve	Contrast enhancement of both peripapillary retina and optic nerve [27] Swelling of bilateral optic disc and nerve on T1-weighted images [27]	

Abbreviations: *CTX* cerebrotendinous xanthomatosis, *NAA* N-Acetilaspartate, *Cho* Cholin, *La* lactate, *HC* healthy control, *FA* fractional anisotropy, *MT* magnetization transfer

the differential diagnosis of CTX [14]. They are a distinctive feature that, when observed in conjunction with other clinical and imaging findings, can help differentiate CTX from other neurological disorders.

A long-term follow-up of a subset of these patients found worsened condition in vacuolated baseline patients; non-vacuolated subjects remained stable clinically and neuroradiologically [12]. These findings suggested that the replacement of FLAIR hyperintensities with FLAIR hypointense areas consistent with vacuolation or calcification (or presence of vacuolation/calcification at onset) is a marker of disease progression and poor response to therapy [12]. Therefore, cerebellar lesions on FLAIR images followed over time might represent "two sides of the same coin": while hyperintensities are probably the initial result of abnormal lipid storage, hypointense areas may be due to cerebellar degeneration caused by cholestanol-induced apoptosis [15] or by other yet undefined mechanisms leading to neuroaxonal loss [13]. Finally, monitoring dentate nucleus abnormalities through neuroimaging can assist in evaluating the response to treatment, particularly chenodeoxycholic acid (CDCA) therapy [12]. Improvements in dentate nucleus abnormalities may correlate with better clinical outcomes [12].

The most notable clinical consequence of dentate nucleus abnormalities in CTX is ataxia [12], a neurological symptom characterized by impaired coordination and balance. Ataxia can significantly impact an individual's mobility and ability to perform daily tasks.

In addition to ataxia, motor dysfunction can manifest as muscle weakness, tremors, and incoordination.

Brain Cortical and Cerebellar Atrophy

Among the hallmark features of CTX observed through neuroimaging, brain cortical and cerebellar atrophy are significant findings that hold clinical importance, especially in those with long-standing or untreated disease. Brain atrophy in CTX is typically progressive [16]. Over time, affected individuals often experience a gradual loss of brain tissue, particularly in specific regions like the frontal and parietal lobes [16]. The presence and extent of brain and cerebellar atrophy in CTX have clinical significance, as they are associated with specific neurological manifestations. This includes progressive cognitive decline, ataxia, spasticity, and other motor and cognitive deficits [16]. The severity of atrophy can vary among individuals with CTX. Some may exhibit minimal atrophy, while others may experience more pronounced and debilitating changes in brain and cerebellar structure. The mechanisms driving brain and cerebellar atrophy in CTX are not fully understood, but they are likely related to the accumulation of cholestanol and cholesterol in neural tissues [15]. Some proposed mechanisms include: (a) inflammatory processes, as the accumulation of cholestanol and cholesterol in neural tissues may trigger inflammatory responses, leading to tissue damage and atrophy [17]; (b) oxidative stress, as the excess sterols may induce oxidative stress, which can damage neurons and their supporting structures, contributing to atrophy [18]; (c) demyelination, as cholesterol accumulation can disrupt myelin, the protective covering of nerve fibres [19, 20], which can lead to impaired neural communication and contribute to brain atrophy [8]; (d) the prolonged presence of cholesterol deposits may result in neurodegeneration, causing the gradual loss of neural cells and overall brain and cerebellar volume.

Spinal Cord Abnormalities

In CTX, the spinal cord can also be affected, either independently or concurrently with brain-related complications [21, 22]. It is noteworthy that certain patients may exhibit a gradual development of myelopathy (the so-called "spinal xanthomatosis"), a condition characterized by spinal cord abnormalities, accompanied by distinctive pyramidal and dorsal column signs [23–25]. Interestingly, these manifestations often present in a milder form compared to the classic CTX neurological profile [25]. When subjected to magnetic resonance imaging (MRI), these individuals' scans frequently unveil the presence of longitudinally extensive lesions localized within the dorsal columns of the spinal cord [21].

Optic Nerve Abnormalities

Regarding ophthalmological signs and symptoms, aside from cataract, optic nerve abnormalities in CTX are a significant aspect of the disease that can have a profound impact on an individual's visual function [20, 26, 27]. Lesions typically affect both eyes and may be associated with contrast enhancement and mild swelling of the optic disc at funduscopic examination [28]. Similar to other neurological manifestations in CTX, optic nerve abnormalities tend to be progressive. Over time, there can be a gradual worsening of visual function if left untreated.

The severity and presentation of optic nerve abnormalities can vary among individuals with CTX. Some may experience milder visual disturbances, while others may suffer more profound vision loss [28].

Lesions in Other Brain Regions

In addition to the characteristic findings mentioned above, CTX can manifest with lesions in various brain regions, including the basal ganglia, thalamus, and brainstem [29, 30]. The location and extent of these lesions may correlate with specific clinical symptoms [31].

Summary

Conventional brain MRI is a crucial tool in the diagnosis and management of cerebrotendinous xanthomatosis. The characteristic findings of bilateral cerebral white matter lesions, dentate nucleus abnormalities, and cortical atrophy not only help lead to the diagnosis but also help guide treatment decisions and provide valuable prognostic information. Given the rarity of CTX and its diverse clinical presentation, the use of brain MRI is instrumental in achieving timely and accurate diagnoses, ultimately improving the outcomes and quality of life for affected individuals. As our understanding of this rare disorder continues to evolve, advances in neuroimaging techniques and their application in CTX diagnosis will further enhance our ability to diagnose and manage this condition effectively.

The Role of Non-conventional Advanced MRI in CTX

While conventional MRI plays a crucial role in diagnosing and monitoring CTX, non-conventional MRI techniques have emerged as valuable tools for gaining deeper insights into the disease's pathophysiology and progression. By employing these advanced MRI modalities, we can readily assess crucial factors such as myelin integrity, axonal health, and cerebral oxidative metabolism directly within living organisms. This innovative approach holds the potential to usher in a more comprehensive comprehension of the intricate dynamics underlying pathological changes in rare metabolic disorders like CTX, thus paving the way for enhanced diagnostic precision and therapeutic strategies. In this part of the chapter, we will explore some of the non-conventional advanced MRI techniques employed in CTX research and their potential clinical applications.

Brain Atrophy

In CTX, brain atrophy is a prevailing characteristic of the disease, often becoming particularly conspicuous in patients with advanced stages of the condition [30]. While the visible signs of atrophy can be observed through conventional MRI, advanced software-based techniques offer a more objective means of quantification. The significance of these atrophy measures becomes apparent when we delve into their implications for both diagnosis and understanding disease progression [16].

A previous study showed a striking disparity when comparing brain volumes, including whole brain, cortical, and cerebellar volumes, between a group of 24 CTX patients and a cohort of 22 healthy controls (HC) using SIENAX software [16]. It is noteworthy that all measurements in the CTX group consistently exhibited significantly lower values compared to those in the HC group. This stark contrast underscores the profound impact of CTX on brain structure and highlights the potential utility of these quantitative measures in diagnostic settings. Furthermore, the reduction in grey matter volumes was found to be closely associated with the clinical status of CTX patients [16]. In other words, the more significant the atrophy, the more pronounced the neurological deficits experienced by patients. This correlation underscores the clinical relevance of these measurements and their potential role as biomarkers for disease progression and treatment response [12, 16]. Conversely, in this study, no differences in white matter volumes between groups were found.

However, it is essential to recognize that brain atrophy may represent the end result of earlier pathological processes that inflict damage to the brain. These preliminary mechanisms, which culminate in atrophy, may not always be apparent through conventional neuroimaging scans. Hence, the importance of other advanced imaging techniques becomes even more evident, as they allow for the detection of subtle changes in brain structure that may precede the visible signs of atrophy.

In essence, the ability to objectively quantify brain atrophy in CTX not only aids in the diagnosis and monitoring of the disease but also provides valuable insights into the underlying neurodegenerative processes. It is a powerful tool that enhances our understanding of CTX, paving the way for more effective clinical management and potential interventions aimed at mitigating the neurological impact of this rare metabolic disorder.

Magnetic Resonance Spectroscopy (MRS)

MRS is a non-invasive technique that provides information about biochemical assay of living proton MR spectra acquired from two different volumes tissues, relative to a selective volume of interest [32]. In CTX, MRS can help quantify the levels of cholestanol and cholesterol in the brain, providing insights into the metabolic alterations associated with the disease [33, 34]. This technique can aid in treatment monitoring and assessing the effectiveness of therapies aimed at reducing sterol accumulation [1].

In previous studies, proton MRS demonstrated a notable reduction in N-acetylaspartate (NAA) levels across the brains of CTX patients, while brain Choline (Cho) resonance intensities closely resembled those of the control group. Alterations in Cho resonance intensities are typically associated with shifts in phosphocholine and glycerol phosphocholine levels, often reflecting changes in cell membrane integrity [1]. These shifts are commonly observed during the initial stages of myelin breakdown, signifying active demyelination [35]. In contrast, chronic and gradual demyelinating processes generally do not exhibit Cho resonance intensity changes. Consequently, although the presence of chronic demyelination in the brains of CTX patients could not be excluded, the widespread NAA reduction observed in the study strongly supports the hypothesis that the underlying enzymatic deficiency in this disorder leads to the accumulation of neurotoxic brain metabolites, potentially initiating primary neuroaxonal pathology [36].

In addition, an increase in Lactate (La) was observed within the cerebral and cerebellar regions of CTX patients [11]. The detection of La resonance intensity via in vivo MRS encompasses both intracellular and extracellular sources [35, 37]. Therefore, it may serve as indicator of either primary or secondary disturbances in mitochondrial metabolism or the infiltration of macrophages and inflammatory cells [37]. In instances involving the latter scenario, the intensities of resonance increase temporarily within regions of pathological activity in the brain, usually confined to the lesion site and its immediate vicinity [38, 39]. By contrast, a widespread and diffuse pathological increase in brain La likely signifies underlying cerebral mitochondrial dysfunction [40, 41]. These findings contribute to the existing body of data, further supporting the notion of a widespread disruption in mitochondrial oxidative metabolism among individuals with CTX [1]. Remarkably, a noteworthy correlation emerged, indicating a strong link between declining NAA levels and increasing clinical disability [1]. This observation underscores the potential utility of measuring axonal loss through MRS as a dependable surrogate marker for predicting disease outcomes.

Magnetization Transfer Imaging

Proton MR spectroscopy provides valuable insights, but it has limitations such as incomplete brain coverage and the potential for errors in serial studies required for treatment monitoring [42]. Magnetization transfer (MT) imaging addresses these issues effectively.

MT imaging involves selectively saturating protons bound to macromolecules, including myelin, thereby reducing their longitudinal magnetization. This process allows for the creation of MT saturation images (MTsat) and magnetization transfer ratio (MTR) images, which offer information about this specific group of molecules [43]. By doing so, MT imaging overcomes the limitations of proton MR spectroscopy, providing a more comprehensive and accurate assessment of brain tissue changes, particularly important for monitoring treatment efficacy over time.

Inglese et al. [42] employed MT imaging to quantify brain and cerebellar damage in nine CTX patients and ten healthy volunteers. They found significant differences in MT ratio and peak heights between CTX patients and healthy controls in various brain regions, including the whole brain, brain normal-appearing white matter (NAWM), brain normal-appearing gray matter (NAGM), cerebellar NAWM, and cerebellar NAGM. Moreover, the study revealed strong correlations between EDSS scores and composite scores derived from MT ratio histograms of the whole brain and brain white matter. Additionally, a strong correlation was found between the cerebellar functional system score and a composite score derived from cerebellar NAWM. The study suggests that quantitative assessment of brain damage using MT MRI in CTX patients can serve as a powerful measure of disease outcome. This implies that MT MRI may provide valuable insights into the progression and severity of CTX-related brain damage, facilitating better disease management and treatment [42].

Diffusion Tensor Imaging

Diffusion refers to the random movement of molecules in fluid systems, including biological tissue. It is described by tracking a molecule's likelihood to travel a certain distance in a given time. Key diffusion indices are fractional anisotropy (FA) and mean diffusivity (MD). Typically, water molecules in axons and extracellular spaces move parallel to fibres due to cellular and structural barriers, known as anisotropic diffusion. Measuring anisotropic diffusion reveals vital information about tissue microstructure. Reduced anisotropy signifies damage to white matter tracts, enabling freer water molecule diffusion away from the tract's primary orientation [44].

In one CTX family, two siblings with cerebrotendinous xanthomatosis (CTX) were studied using diffusion tensor imaging (DTI) before and after chenodeoxycholic acid (CDCA) therapy (45). They presented with spastic paraparesis, epilepsy, learning difficulties, diarrhoea, and cataracts. CDCA treatment improved diarrhoea, normalized cholestanol levels, EEG and led to better gait, cognition, and seizure control. Before treatment, conventional brain MRI showed no CTX-related abnormalities, but DTI revealed reduced FA in the cerebellum and widespread cerebral FA reductions compared to healthy controls. After CDCA therapy, DTI demonstrated increasing cerebellar tract density and cerebral FA. The study suggests that DTI may detect changes when conventional MRI is uninformative (45), serving as potential neuroimaging biomarkers for monitoring CTX treatment response.

In a study of 14 CTX patients treated with CDCA for around 5 years, plasma cholestanol levels normalized quickly. Significant clinical improvement was observed in patients up to 25 years old, treated within 15 years of symptom onset. Conversely, those treated after 25 years of onset continued deteriorating. Patients with peripheral neuropathy exhibited electrophysiological improvement with CDCA. Despite brain volume remaining stable, a subgroup analysis revealed improved FA in the ponto-cerebellar tract and radial diffusivity in the internal capsule with CDCA (46). This study underscores that diffusion metrics may offer greater sensitivity to change compared to volumetry, as seen in other neurometabolic diseases.

Conclusions

Non-conventional advanced MRI techniques have expanded our understanding of CTX by offering insights into the disease's underlying mechanisms and progression. These advanced imaging modalities enable researchers and clinicians to investigate microstructural, metabolic, and functional alterations associated with CTX, providing valuable information for diagnosis, treatment monitoring, and research studies. Such techniques may provide valuable biomarkers for use in clinical trials, though additional validation with clinical status would be needed. As our knowledge of CTX continues to evolve, non-conventional advanced MRI techniques will likely play an increasingly vital role in improving patient care and advancing our understanding of this rare but treatable metabolic disorder.

References

1. De Stefano N, Dotti MT, Mortilla M, Federico A. Magnetic resonance imaging and spectroscopic changes in brains of patients with cerebrotendinous xanthomatosis. Brain. 2001;124(Pt1):121–31. https://doi.org/10.1093/brain/124.1.121.
2. Nie S, Chen G, Cao X, Zhang Y. Cerebrotendinous xanthomatosis: a comprehensive review of pathogenesis, clinical manifestations, diagnosis, and management. Orphanet J Rare Dis. 2014;9:179. https://doi.org/10.1186/s13023-014-0179-4.
3. Barkhof F, Verrips A, Wesseling P, Van der Knaap MS, Van Engelen BGM, Gabreels FJM, et al. Cerebrotendinous xanthomatosis: the spectrum of imaging findings and the correlation with neuropathologic findings. Radiology. 2000;217(3):869–76. https://pubs.rsna.org/doi/10.1148/radiology.217.3.r00dc03869
4. Ma C, De RY, Wang JC, Wang CJ, Zhao JP, Zhou T, et al. The clinical and imaging features of cerebrotendinous xanthomatosis: a case report and review of the literature. Medicine (Baltimore). 2021;100(9):e24687. https://doi.org/10.1097/MD.0000000000024687.
5. Stelten BML, Raal FJ, Marais AD, Riksen NP, Roeters van Lennep JE, Duell PB, et al. Cerebrotendinous xanthomatosis without neurological involvement. J Intern Med [Internet]. 2021;290(5):1039–47. https://doi.org/10.1111/joim.13277.
6. Dotti MT, Federico A, Signorini E, Caputo N, Venturi C, Filosomi G, et al. Cerebrotendinous Xanthomatosis (van Bogaert-Scherer-Epstein disease): CT and MR findings. AJNR Am J Neuroradiol. 1994;15(9):1721–6.
7. Hokezu Y, Kuriyama M, Kubota R, Nakagawa M, Fujiyama J, Osame M. Cerebrotendinous xanthomatosis: cranial CT and MRI studies in eight patients. Neuroradiology. 1992;34(4):308–12. https://doi.org/10.1007/BF00588188.
8. Chang CC, Lui CC, Wang JJ, Huang SH, Lu CH, Chen C, et al. Multi-parametric neuroimaging evaluation of cerebrotendinous xanthomatosis and its correlation with neuropsychological presentations. BMC Neurol. 2010;10:59. https://doi.org/10.1186/1471-2377-10-59.
9. Swanson PD, Cromwell LD. Magnetic resonance imaging in cerebrotendinous xanthomatosis. Neurology. 1986;36(1):124–6. https://doi.org/10.1212/wnl.36.1.124.
10. Pedley TA, Emerson RG, Warner CL, Rowland LP, Salen G. Treatment of cerebrotendinous xanthomatosis with chenodeoxycholic acid. Ann Neurol. 1985;18(4):517–8. https://doi.org/10.1212/wnl.36.1.124.
11. Zhang Y, Sun YM, Li H. Teaching NeuroImage: symmetric deep cerebellar white matter T2 and susceptibility-weighted imaging Hypointense lesions in a case of Cerebrotendinous Xanthomatosis. Neurology. 2021;97(9):e968–9. https://doi.org/10.1212/WNL.0000000000012154.
12. Mignarri A, Dotti MT, Federico A, De Stefano N, Battaglini M, Grazzini I, et al. The spectrum of magnetic resonance findings in cerebrotendinous xanthomatosis: redefinition and evidence of new markers of disease progression. J Neurol. 2017;264(5):862–74. https://doi.org/10.1007/s00415-017-8440-0.
13. Mignarri A, Dotti MT, Del Puppo M, Gallus GN, Giorgio A, Cerase A, et al. Cerebrotendinous xanthomatosis with progressive cerebellar vacuolation. Neuroradiology. 2012;54(6):649–51. https://doi.org/10.1007/s00234-012-1026-8.
14. Khadilkar S, Jaggi S, Patel B, Yadav R, Hanagandi P, Faria Do Amaral LL. A practical approach to diseases affecting dentate nuclei. Clin Radiol. 2016;71(1):107–19. https://doi.org/10.1016/j.crad.2015.09.010.
15. Inoue K, Kubota S, Seyama Y. Cholestanol induces apoptosis of cerebellar neuronal cells. Biochem Biophys Res Commun. 1999;256(1):198–203. https://doi.org/10.1006/bbrc.1998.9497.
16. Guerrera S, Stromillo ML, Mignarri A, Battaglini M, Marino S, Di Perri C, et al. Clinical relevance of brain volume changes in patients with cerebrotendinous xanthomatosis. J Neurol Neurosurg Psychiatry. 2010;81(11):1189–93. https://doi.org/10.1136/jnnp.2009.203364.

17. Zak A, Zeman M, Slaby A, Vecka M. Xanthomas: clinical and pathophysiological relations. Biomed Papers. 2014;158(2):181–8. https://doi.org/10.5507/bp.2014.016.
18. Gonzalez-Cuyar LF, Hunter B, Harris PLR, Perry G, Smith MA, Castellani RJ. Cerebrotendinous xanthomatosis: case report with evidence of oxidative stress. Redox Rep. 2007;12(3):119–24. https://doi.org/10.1179/135100007X200173.
19. Pilo B, De Blas G, Sobrido MJ, Navarro C, Grandas F, Barrero FJ, et al. Neurophysiological study in cerebrotendinous xanthomatosis. Muscle Nerve. 2011;43(4):531–6. https://doi.org/10.1002/mus.21905.
20. Federico A, Dotti MT. Cerebrotendinous xanthomatosis: clinical manifestations, diagnostic criteria, pathogenesis, and therapy. J Child Neurol. 2003;18(9):13–22. https://doi.org/10.1177/08830738030180091001.
21. Valencia-Sanchez C, Wingerchuk DM, Dhamija R. Teaching NeuroImages: spinal xanthomatosis: a misdiagnosed, treatable cause of progressive myelopathy. Neurology. 2020;95(11):E1615–6. https://doi.org/10.1212/WNL.0000000000010194.
22. Yanagihashi M, Kano O, Terashima T, Kawase Y, Hanashiro S, Sawada M, et al. Late-onset spinal form xanthomatosis without brain lesion: a case report. BMC Neurol. 2016;16(1) https://doi.org/10.1186/s12883-016-0542-2.
23. Verrips A, Lycklama À, Nijeholt GJ, Barkhof F, Van Engelen BGM, Wesseling P, Luyten JAFM, et al. Spinal xanthomatosis: a variant of cerebrotendinous xanthomatosis. Brain. 1999;122(Pt 8):1589–95. https://doi.org/10.1093/brain/122.8.1589.
24. Atallah I, Millán DS, Benoît W, Campos-Xavier B, Superti-Furga A, Tran C. Spinal cerebrotendinous xanthomatosis: a case report and literature review. Mol Genet Metab Rep. 2021;26:100719. https://doi.org/10.1016/j.ymgmr.2021.100719.
25. Abe R, Sekijima Y, Kinoshita T, Yoshinaga T, Koyama S, Kato T, et al. Spinal form cerebrotendinous xanthomatosis patient with long spinal cord lesion. J Spinal Cord Med. 2016;39(6):726–9. https://doi.org/10.1179/1079026815Z.000000000409.
26. Cruysberg JRM, Wevers RA, Van Engelen BGM, Pinckers A, Van Spreeken A, Tolboom JJM. Ocular and systemic manifestations of cerebrotendinous xanthomatosis. Am J Ophthalmol. 1995;120(5):597–604. https://doi.org/10.1016/s0002-9394(14)72206-8.
27. Cruysberg JRM, Wevers RA, Tolboom JJM. Juvenile cataract associated with chronic diarrhea in pediatric cerebrotendinous xanthomatosis. Am J Ophthalmol. 1991;112(5):606–7. https://doi.org/10.1016/s0002-9394(14)76874-6.
28. Miyamoto M, Ishii N, Mochizuki H, Shiomi K, Kaida T, Chuman H, et al. Optic neuropathy with features suggestive of optic neuritis in Cerebrotendinous Xanthomatosis. Case Rep Neurol Med. 2019;2576826 https://doi.org/10.1155/2019/2576826.
29. Agrawal NK, Garg S. Cerebrotendinous xanthomatosis: a rare disorder with a rare presentation. BMJ Case Rep. 2012;2012:bcr2012006202. https://doi.org/10.1136/bcr-2012-006202.
30. Vanrietvelde F, Lemmerling M, Mespreuve M, Crevits L, De Reuck J, Kunnen M. MRI of the brain in cerebrotendinous xanthomatosis (van Bogaert-Scherer-Epstein disease). Eur Radiol. 2000;10(4):576–8. https://doi.org/10.1007/s003300050964.
31. Rubio-Agusti I, Kojovic M, Edwards MJ, Murphy E, Chandrashekar HS, Lachmann RH, et al. Atypical parkinsonism and cerebrotendinous xanthomatosis: report of a family with corticobasal syndrome and a literature review. Mov Disord. 2012;27(14):1769–74. https://doi.org/10.1002/mds.25229.
32. Rhodes CJ. Magnetic resonance spectroscopy. Sci Prog. 2017;100(3):241–92. https://doi.org/10.3184/003685017X14993478654307.
33. Embiruçu EK, Otaduy MCG, Taneja AK, Leite CC, Kok F, Lucato LT. MR spectroscopy detects lipid peaks in cerebrotendinous xanthomatosis. AJNR Am J Neuroradiol. 2010;31(7):1347–9. https://doi.org/10.3174/ajnr.A1885.
34. Makary MS, Kisanuki YY, Amin NN, Slone HW. Teaching NeuroImages: Cerebrotendinous xanthomatosis. Neurology. 2018;90(7):e637–8. https://doi.org/10.1212/WNL.0000000000004967.

35. Matthews PM, Pioro E, Narayanan S, De Stefano N, Fu L, Francis G, et al. Assessment of lesion pathology in multiple sclerosis using quantitative MRI morphometry and magnetic resonance spectroscopy. Brain. 1996;119(Pt 3):715–22. https://doi.org/10.1093/brain/119.3.715.
36. Soffer D, Benharroch D, Berginer V. The neuropathology of cerebrotendinous xanthomatosis revisited: a case report and review of the literature. Acta Neuropathol. 1995;90(2):213–20. https://doi.org/10.1007/BF00294324.
37. Prichard JW. What the clinician can learn from MRS lactate measurements. NMR Biomed. 1991;4(2):99–102. https://doi.org/10.1002/nbm.1940040212.
38. Arnold DL, Matthews PM, Francis GS, O'Connor J, Antel JP. Proton magnetic resonance spectroscopic imaging for metabolic characterization of demyelinating plaques. Ann Neurol. 1992;31(3):235–41. https://doi.org/10.1002/ana.410310302.
39. De Stefano N, Matthews PM, Antel JP, Preul M, Francis G, Arnold DL. Chemical pathology of acute demyelinating lesions and its correlation with disability. Ann Neurol. 1995;38(6):901–9. https://doi.org/10.1002/ana.410380610.
40. Matthews PM, Andermann F, Silver K, Karpati G, Arnold DL. Proton MR spectroscopic characterization of differences in regional brain metabolic abnormalities in mitochondrial encephalomyopathies. Neurology. 1993;43(12):2484–90. https://doi.org/10.1212/wnl.43.12.2484.
41. De Stefano N, Matthews PM, Ford B, Genge A, Karpati G, Arnold DL. Short-term dichloroacetate treatment improves indices of cerebral metabolism in patients with mitochondrial disorders. Neurology. 1995;45(6):1193–8. https://doi.org/10.1212/wnl.45.6.1193.
42. Inglese M, De Stefano N, Pagani E, Dotti MT, Comi G, Federico A, et al. Quantification of brain damage in Cerebrotendinous Xanthomatosis with magnetization transfer MR imaging. AJNR Am J Neuroradiol. 2003;24(3):495–500.
43. Van Waesberghe JHTM, Kamphorst W, De Groot JA, Van Walderveen MAA, Castelijns JA, Ravid R, et al. Axonal loss in multiple sclerosis lesions: magnetic resonance imaging insights into substrates of disability. Ann Neurol. 1999;46(5):747–54. https://doi.org/10.1002/1531-8249(199911)46:5<747::aid-ana10>3.3.co;2-w.
44. Woo ST, Byung JH, Sung BP, Shin HK, Byung JK. Current clinical applications of diffusion-tensor imaging in neurological disorders. J Clin Neurol. 2018;14(2):129–40. https://doi.org/10.3988/jcn.2018.14.2.129.

Novel Neuroimaging Tools to Monitor Cerebrotendinous Xanthomatosis (CTX)

14

Fanny Mochel

Introduction

As discussed in previous chapters, metabolic intervention like chenodeoxycholic acid (CDCA) can halt, and even reverse, neurological dysfunctions in cerebrotendinous xanthomatosis (CTX) if treatment is initiated early enough, i.e., before the occurrence of irreversible damage of the central and peripheral nervous system. However, patient's response to treatment is variable, and there are few existing biomarkers to monitor therapeutic outcomes. Normalization of plasma metabolites like cholestanol reflects the overall metabolic control under treatment like CDCA, but they do not allow to study the therapeutic effect on the brain. Furthermore, given the existence of attenuated forms of CTX in adult patients with no over neuropsychiatric symptoms [1], it is unclear whether all children diagnosed with CTX should be treated. This is especially relevant with the inclusion of CTX in newborn screening in the near future. Therefore, there is a clear unmet medical need for biomarkers that can reflect neurological disease onset and progression.

In a retrospective French cohort study, we showed that diffusion tensor imaging (DTI) techniques may be able to detect white matter alterations and brain response to treatment in patients with CTX [2]. Unlike standard MRI that does not quantify myelin content or axonal injury, quantitative imaging like brain DTI can provide sensitive outcome measures to follow disease progression and therapeutic interventions in patients with leukodystrophies [3–5]. These results are in line with extensive literature showing the relevance of DTI-derived markers to quantify in vivo myelin in humans [6]. However, while the potential interest of MRI diffusion

F. Mochel (✉)
Reference Center for Adult Neurometabolic Diseases and Leukodystrophies,
Department of Medical Genetics of APHP, Sorbonne University, Paris Brain Institute (ICM),
La Pitié-Salpêtrière University Hospital, Paris, France
e-mail: fanny.mochel@icm-institute.org

A. Federico et al. (eds.), *Cerebrotendinous Xanthomatosis*,
https://doi.org/10.1007/978-3-031-92526-9_14

markers has been extensively reported in several clinical applications, such as multiple sclerosis [7], Parkinson disease [8], Alzheimer disease [9], traumatic brain injury [10], or stroke [11], the translation into clinics of these meaningful biomarkers remains a major challenge. The implementation of DTI in clinical practice has thus far been limited by large inter-center measurements variability [12] and bias due to data quality issues, including motion-related artifacts that may lead to wrong DTI metrics [13]. BrainTale-care, a recently CE-marked platform, overcomes these issues by providing standardized DTI parameters and designing fit-for-purpose digital biomarkers. In intensive care unit, these standardized diffusion MRI biomarkers can reliably predict the outcome of comatose patients [14, 15]. Therefore, they may offer the opportunity to efficiently follow drug efficacy in patients with CTX.

We have obtained preliminary data on the relevance of the DTI brainQuant pipeline in two leukodystrophies: a rapidly progressive inflammatory leukodystrophy called cerebral adrenoleukodystrophy (ALD) and metachromatic leukodystrophy (MLD). In cerebral ALD and MLD, active neuroinflammation leads to rapid white matter degeneration and death within years of symptom onset. If performed at the earliest stages of neuroinflammation, hematopoietic stem cell transplantation (HSCT) can be a life-saving treatment through the replacement of the immune component of the brain. Furthermore, Leriglitazone, a PPARγ agonist that has obtained the orphan drug designation from EMA and FDA for the treatment of ALD [16], was tested in the ADVANCE randomized and placebo-controlled trial on 116 male patients with ALD. It confirmed its safety and showed an effect on myelopathy through a reduction of body sway amplitudes, a stabilization of walking aids, and a slower decline of ambulation scores in early-stage patients [17]. Further analyses showed that cerebral lesion progression occurred significantly more often in the placebo group, suggesting a preventive effect on the occurrence of cerebral ALD [17]. Consequently, we tested leriglitazone in adult patients with cerebral ALD, either not eligible to HSCT or awaiting HSCT, who benefitted from a compassionate use of the drug in France. We found that leriglitazone halts neuroinflammation and demyelination in most patients with complete clinical and radiological stabilization over 2 years of treatment [18].

Methods

We tested the DTI brainQuant pipeline in patients with three metabolic leukodystrophies on treatment:

- Cerebral ALD: Three patients who underwent HSCT and 11 patients treated with leriglitazone [18].
- MLD: Two siblings addressed for HSCT but only one was deemed eligible.
- CTX: Four patients on CDCA.

All diffusion MRI exams were processed according to the brainQuant pipeline [19]. Briefly, it includes eddy-current, motion correction, and tensor model fitting to derive maps of tensor parameters: Fractional Anisotropy (FA), Mean Diffusivity

(MD), Axial Diffusivity (AD), and Radial Diffusivity (RD). These maps were then co-registered onto the standard Montreal Neurological Institute (MNI) space to extract averaged diffusion parameters within 19 regions of the deep white matter atlas (Fig. 14.1). For each scanner and magnetic resonance protocol, final

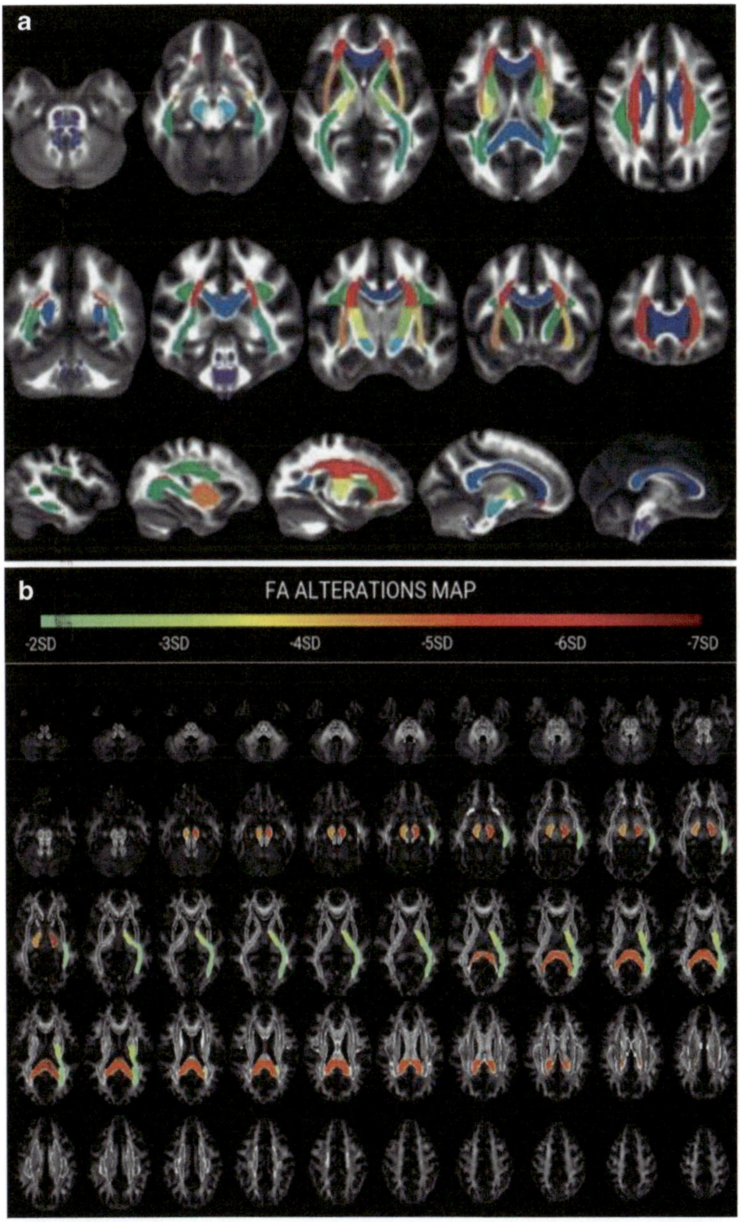

Fig. 14.1 BrainQuant DTI methods. (**a**) Diffusion parameters within 19 regions of the deep white matter atlas indicated by different colors. (**b**) Example of FA alterations map. Colors indicate brain regions with white matter alterations

calibration was achieved by dividing the resulting parameters by mean values obtained from a group of healthy controls acquired in the exact same conditions (same scanner, same acquisition protocol) than those that were used for patients. Each MRI exam and its processing were controlled for quality according to the brainQuant quality control process. This included checks for motion, signal dropout, number of global signal dropouts, vibration artifact, and FA map co-registration in MNI space visual inspection.

Results

In adult patients with cerebral ALD, we compared conventional MRI to DTI brainQuant to monitor white matter alterations in patients undergoing HSCT ($n = 3$). While conventional MRI may lack sensitivity to detect white matter changes, DTI maps showed transient demyelination 3 months after HSCT followed by improvement at 6 months and return to baseline of the DTI maps at 1 year post-transplant (Fig. 14.2). Moreover, in patients with cerebral ALD not eligible to HSCT and treated with leriglitazone, we gathered DTI brainQuant data in 11 patients. brainQuant DTI showed progression of neuroinflammation and demyelination up to 3–6 months of treatments, as indicated by FA, MD, AD, and RD whole brain maps, but then the disease stabilized with maps comparable to baseline (Fig. 14.3). In both therapeutic strategies (HSCT and leriglitazone), patients were clinically remarkably stable ([18] and unpublished data for HSCT).

In adult patients with MLD, we used brainQuant DTI to support decision to perform HSCT. Likewise, we monitored a presymptomatic individual, whose sibling was diagnosed with frontotemporal dementia, with minimal white matter abnormalities in frontal regions. Instead, all DTI maps (FA, MD, AD, and RD) showed diffuse abnormalities (Fig. 14.4a). By the time the patient underwent HSCT (i.e., 3 months to identify a donor and run the pre-transplant assessment), DTI maps revealed a clear aggravation of all parameters (Fig. 14.4b) confirming the timely decision to perform transplant. One year after HSCT, the patient has remained asymptomatic, and his DTI maps (FA, MD, AD, and RD) have returned to initial values.

In adult patients with CTX, we have generated preliminary data showing that brainQuant DTI correlate with clinical evolution. Indeed, in patients with favorable clinical outcome, DTI maps (FA, MD, AD, and RD) improved after 1 year of treatment with CDCA (Fig. 14.5). Instead, in patients with poorer prognosis—especially patients with parkinsonism [20] and extensive alterations on DTI maps— clinical deterioration was associated with further aggravation of DTI maps (Fig. 14.6).

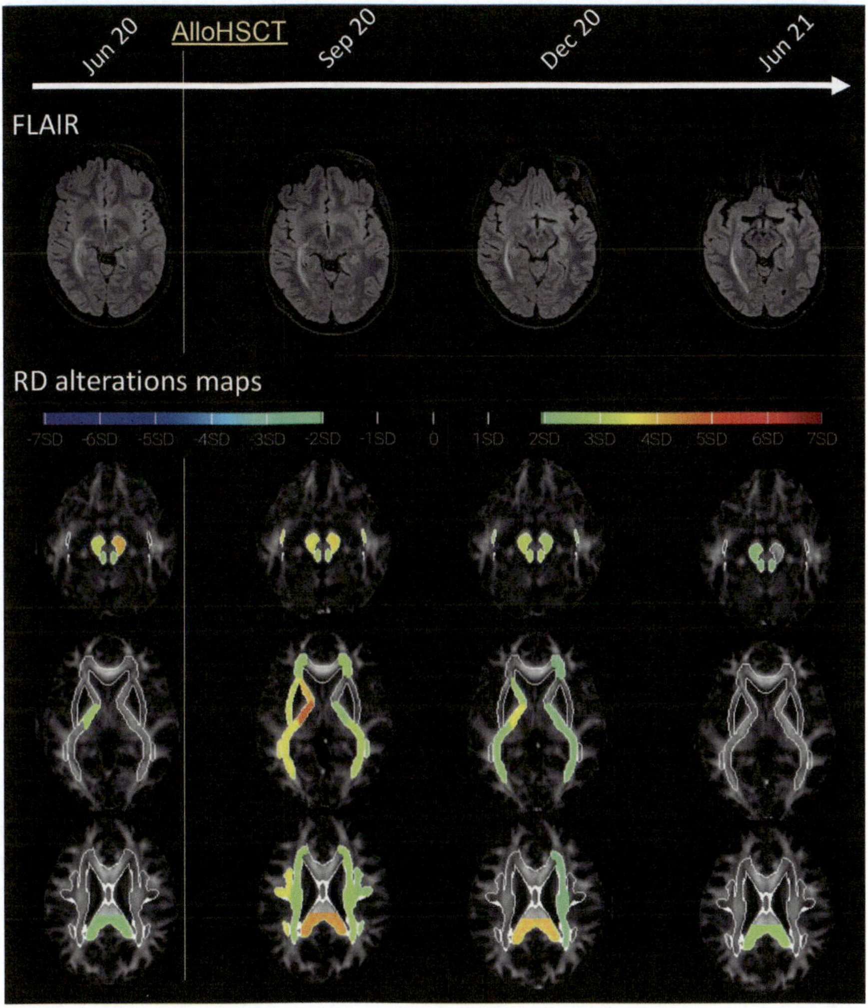

Fig. 14.2 BrainQuant DTI in cerebral adrenoleukodystrophy (ALD). We performed brain DTI analyses in a 22-year-old man with cerebral ALD who underwent hematopoietic stem cell transplant (HSCT). While conventional MRI showed stable hypersignal of the right occipital horn on FLAIR images, RD metrics detected very dynamic changes at 3 months post-transplant that regressed at 6 months and returned to baseline values 1 year after transplant. Colors indicate brain regions with white matter alterations

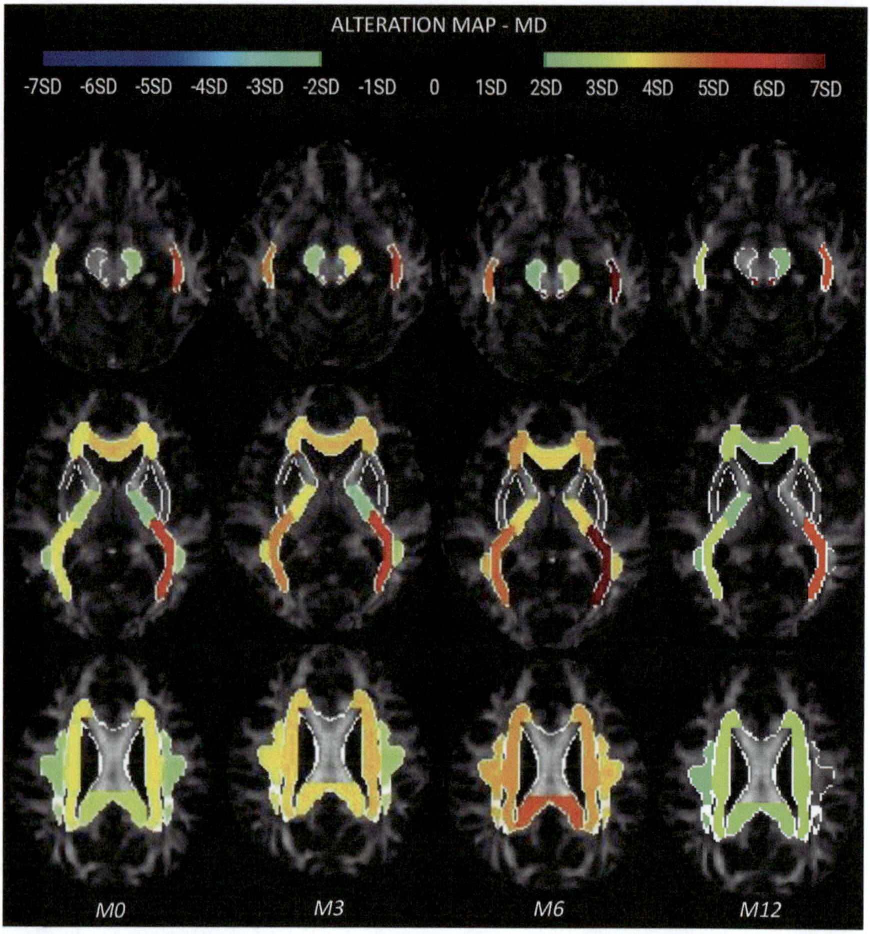

Fig. 14.3 BrainQuant DTI in cerebral adrenoleukodystrophy (ALD). We treated with leriglitazone a 44-year-old man with cerebral ALD not eligible to HSCT. While neuroinflammation and demyelination kept progressing up until 6 months of treatment, leriglitazone led to disease stabilization and MD metric at 1 year returned to baseline levels. Colors indicate brain regions with white matter alterations

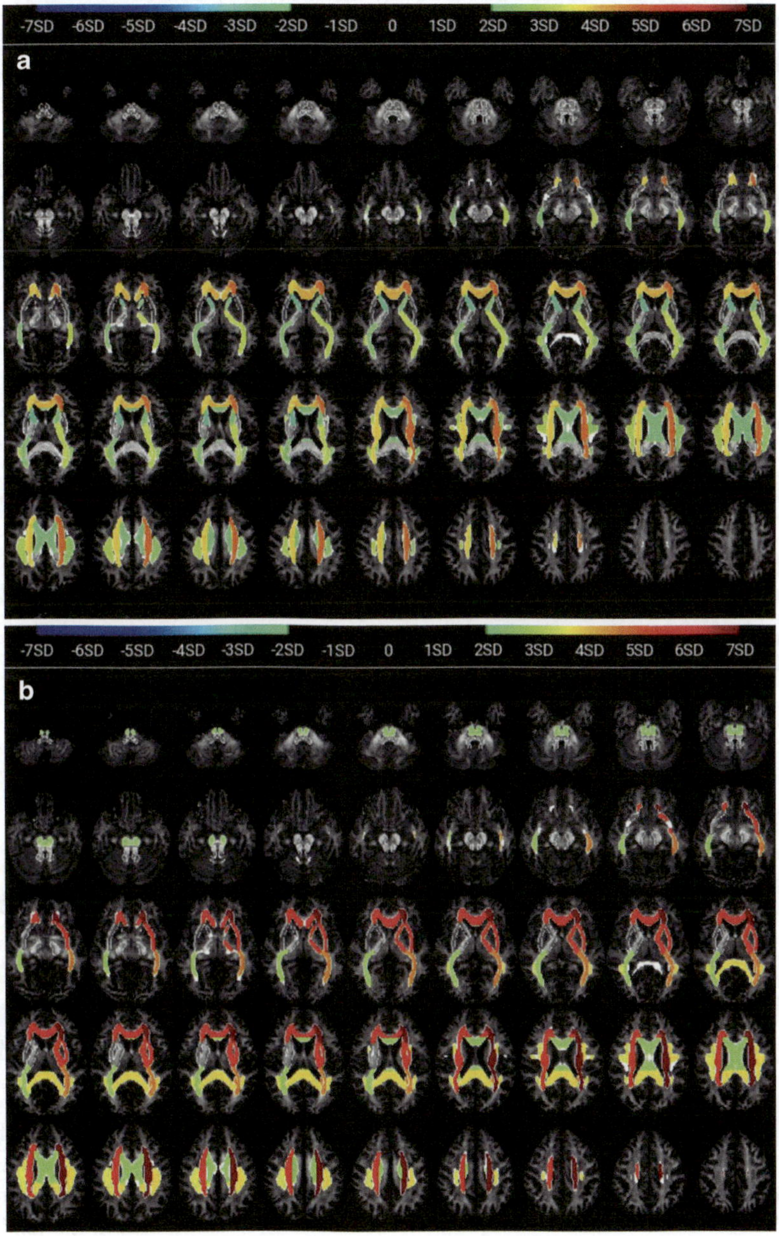

Fig. 14.4 BrainQuant DTI in metachromatic leukodystrophy (MLD). We diagnosed an asymptomatic 28-year-old man with MLD after the diagnosis was made in his sibling who presented with a rapidly progressive frontotemporal dementia. Clinical examination and cognitive testing were strictly normal, and conventional MRI showed very mild FLAIR hypersignal in the periventricular frontal regions. Instead, MD maps showed diffuse alterations reflecting a likely active disease (**a**). Three months later, at the time of HSCT, MD maps revealed a clear progression of neuroinflammation and demyelination (**b**). Colors indicate brain regions with white matter alterations

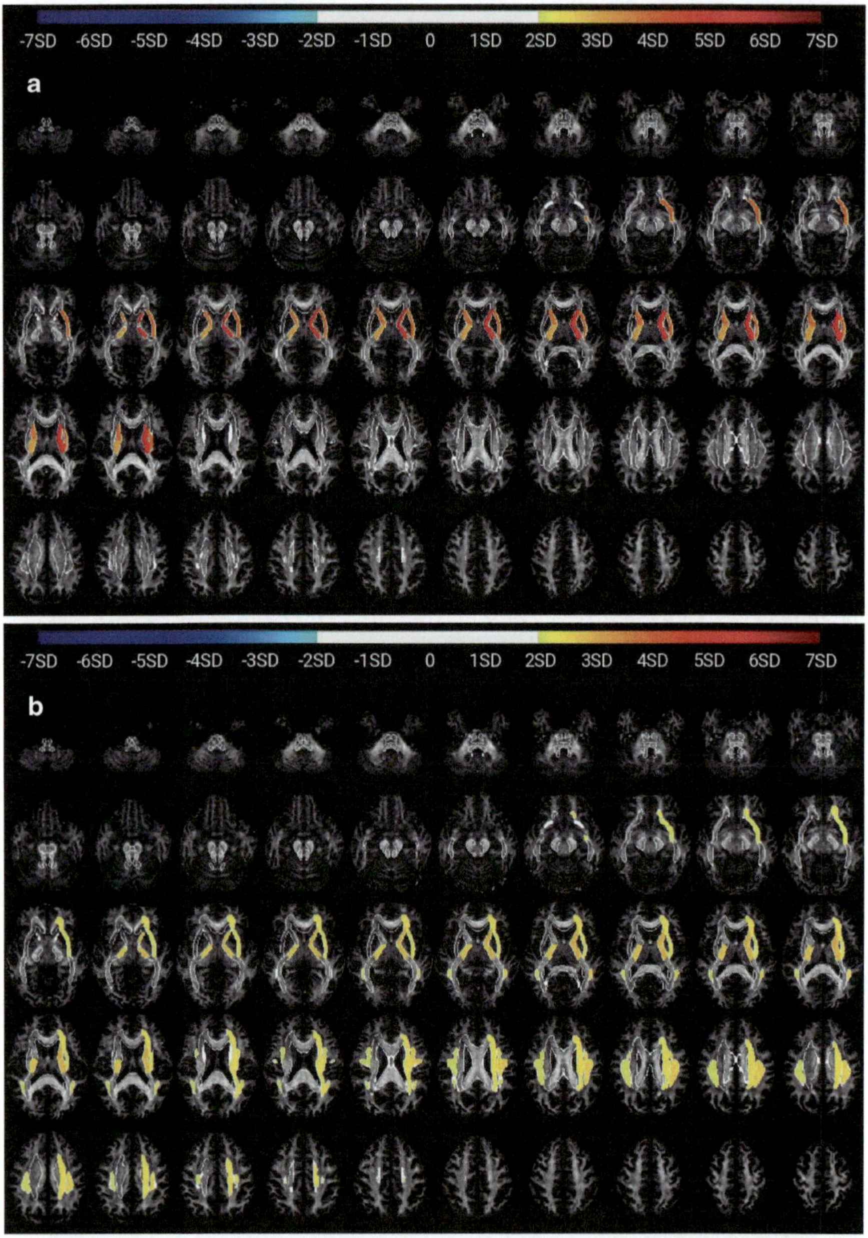

Fig. 14.5 BrainQuant DTI in cerebrotendinous xanthomatosis (CTX). We diagnosed with CTX a 30-year-old woman with mild intellectual disability, moderate cerebellar ataxia, and pyramidal signs. Compared to baseline (**a**), her MD maps improved after 1 year of treatment with chenodeoxycholic acid (**b**), consistent with improvement of her cerebellar syndrome. Colors indicate brain regions with white matter alterations

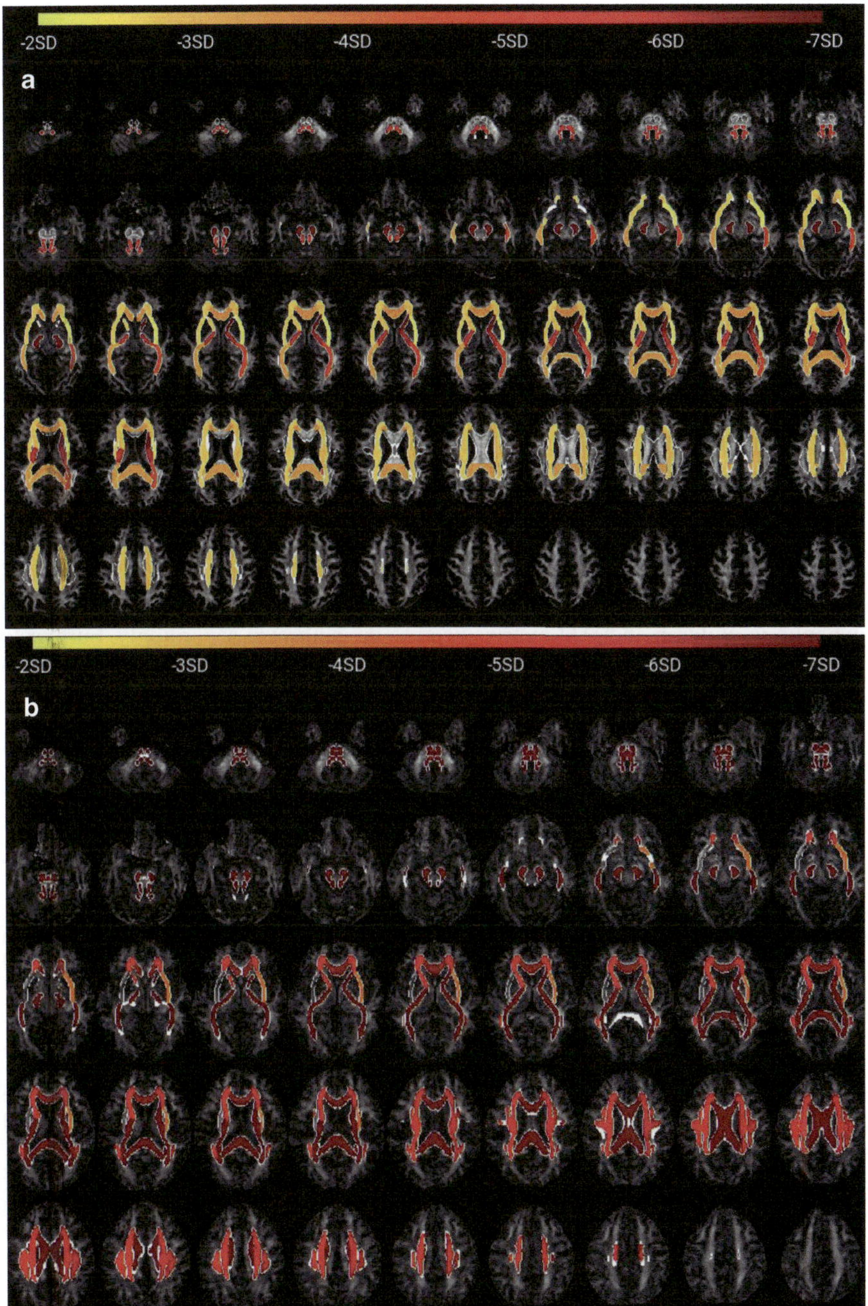

Fig. 14.6 BrainQuant DTI in cerebrotendinous xanthomatosis (CTX). We diagnosed with CTX a 30 year-old man with cognitive decline, parkinsonism, dystonia, and spastic paraparesis. Compared to baseline (**a**), his MD maps aggravated despite 1 year of treatment with chenodeoxycholic acid (**b**), consistent with his continued neurological deterioration. Colors indicate brain regions with white matter alterations

Discussion

This proof-of-concept study showed that standardized DTI markers using the brainQuant pipeline are sensitive to monitor disease progression and treatment response in adult patients with metabolic leukodystrophies. In adults with cerebral ALD, DTI maps correlate closely with clinical outcomes to treatments [18], and they are more sensitive to detect white matter changes than conventional MRI. Furthermore, there are ongoing studies designed to evaluate how brainQuant DTI may help detecting cerebral ALD before conventional MRI (NCT05911919). Indeed, data from the ADVANCE study suggest that RD metrics can detect the onset of cerebral ALD 1 year before the identification of typical demyelinating lesions (data not shown).

In CTX, our preliminary results indicate that brainQuant DTI may allow a better evaluation of the therapeutic benefit on the nervous system of existing treatments like CDCA. This is especially important to assess upcoming add-on or alternative therapies to CDCA. Furthermore, the detection of brain disease onset in CTX using standardized DTI markers will be critical to determine when to start treatment in asymptomatic individuals with CTX as illustrated in the presymptomatic MLD case. Nevertheless, the brainQuant pipeline has yet to be calibrated for children, and according to different age groups. Unlike adults, myelination changes are very dynamic in children and DTI metrics need to be calibrated accordingly. Further to these preliminary data, it will be very important to determine the sensitivity to change of brainQuant DTI in CTX patients with and without treatment.

References

1. Stelten BML, Raal FJ, Marais AD, Riksen NP, Roeters van Lennep JE, Duell PB, et al. Cerebrotendinous xanthomatosis without neurological involvement. J Intern Med. 2021;290(5):1039–47.
2. Amador MDM, Masingue M, Debs R, Lamari F, Perlbarg V, Roze E, et al. Treatment with chenodeoxycholic acid in cerebrotendinous xanthomatosis: clinical, neurophysiological, and quantitative brain structural outcomes. J Inherit Metab Dis. 2018;41(5):799–807.
3. Adanyeguh IM, Branzoli F, Delorme C, Méneret A, Monin ML, Luton MP, et al. Multiparametric characterization of white matter alterations in early stage Huntington disease. Sci Rep. 2021;11(1):13101.
4. Castellano A, Papinutto N, Cadioli M, Brugnara G, Iadanza A, Scigliuolo G, et al. Quantitative MRI of the spinal cord and brain in adrenomyeloneuropathy: in vivo assessment of structural changes. Brain. 2016;139(Pt 6):1735–46.
5. Huffnagel IC, van Ballegoij WJC, Vos JMBW, Kemp S, Caan MWA, Engelen M. Longitudinal diffusion MRI as surrogate outcome measure for myelopathy in adrenoleukodystrophy. Neurology. 2019;93(23):e2133–43.
6. Lazari A, Lipp I. Can MRI measure myelin? Systematic review, qualitative assessment, and meta-analysis of studies validating microstructural imaging with myelin histology. Neuroimage. 2021;230:117744.
7. Roosendaal SD, Geurts JJG, Vrenken H, Hulst HE, Cover KS, Castelijns JA, et al. Regional DTI differences in multiple sclerosis patients. Neuroimage. 2009;44(4):1397–403.
8. Atkinson-Clement C, Pinto S, Eusebio A, Coulon O. Diffusion tensor imaging in Parkinson's disease: review and meta-analysis. Neuroimage Clin. 2017;16:98–110.

9. Mayo CD, Mazerolle EL, Ritchie L, Fisk JD, Gawryluk JR. Alzheimer's Disease Neuroimaging Initiative. Longitudinal changes in microstructural white matter metrics in Alzheimer's disease. Neuroimage Clin. 2017;13:330–8.
10. Bourke NJ, Yanez Lopez M, Jenkins PO, De Simoni S, Cole JH, Lally P, et al. Traumatic brain injury: a comparison of diffusion and volumetric magnetic resonance imaging measures. Brain Commun. 2021;3(2):fcab006.
11. Moura LM, Luccas R, de Paiva JPQ, Amaro E, Leemans A, Leite CDC, et al. Diffusion tensor imaging biomarkers to predict motor outcomes in stroke: a narrative review. Front Neurol. 2019;10:445.
12. Vollmar C, O'Muircheartaigh J, Barker GJ, Symms MR, Thompson P, Kumari V, et al. Identical, but not the same: intra-site and inter-site reproducibility of fractional anisotropy measures on two 3.0T scanners. Neuroimage. 2010;51(4):1384–94.
13. Roalf DR, Quarmley M, Elliott MA, Satterthwaite TD, Vandekar SN, Ruparel K, et al. The impact of quality assurance assessment on diffusion tensor imaging outcomes in a large-scale population-based cohort. Neuroimage. 2016;125:903–19.
14. Velly L, Perlbarg V, Boulier T, Adam N, Delphine S, Luyt CE, et al. Use of brain diffusion tensor imaging for the prediction of long-term neurological outcomes in patients after cardiac arrest: a multicentre, international, prospective, observational, cohort study. Lancet Neurol. 2018;17(4):317–26.
15. Puybasset L, Perlbarg V, Unrug J, Cassereau D, Galanaud D, Torkomian G, et al. Prognostic value of global deep white matter DTI metrics for 1-year outcome prediction in ICU traumatic brain injury patients: an MRI-COMA and CENTER-TBI combined study. Intensive Care Med. 2022;48(2):201–12.
16. Rodríguez-Pascau L, Vilalta A, Cerrada M, Traver E, Forss-Petter S, Weinhofer I, et al. The brain penetrant PPARγ agonist leriglitazone restores multiple altered pathways in models of X-linked adrenoleukodystrophy. Sci Transl Med. 2021;13(596):eabc0555.
17. Köhler W, Engelen M, Eichler F, Lachmann R, Fatemi A, Sampson J, et al. Safety and efficacy of leriglitazone for preventing disease progression in men with adrenomyeloneuropathy (ADVANCE): a randomised, double-blind, multi-centre, placebo-controlled phase 2-3 trial. Lancet Neurol. 2023;22(2):127–36.
18. Golse M, Weinhofer I, Blanco B, Barbier M, Yazbeck E, Huiban C, et al. Leriglitazone halts disease progression in adult patients with early cerebral adrenoleukodystrophy. Brain. 2024:awae169.
19. van der Eerden AW, Khalilzadeh O, Perlbarg V, Dinkel J, Sanchez P, Vos PE, et al. White matter changes in comatose survivors of anoxic ischemic encephalopathy and traumatic brain injury: comparative diffusion-tensor imaging study. Radiology. 2014;270(2):506–16.
20. Stelten BML, van de Warrenburg BPC, Wevers RA, Verrips A. Movement disorders in cerebrotendinous xanthomatosis. Parkinsonism Relat Disord. 2019;58:12–6.

Part V

Epidemiology

Epidemiology of Cerebrotendinous Xanthomatosis (CTX)

15

Tiziano Pramparo and Celia Jenkinson

Abbreviations

23S-Pentol	5β-cholestane-3α,7α,12α,23,25-pentol
7α12αC4	7α,12α-hydroxy-4-cholsten-3-one
7αC4	7α-hydroxy-4-cholesten-3-one
AFR	African/African American
AMR	Latino/Admixed American
CDCA	Chenodeoxycholic acid
CTX	Cerebrotendinous xanthomatosis
DBS	Dried blood spots
EAS	East Asian
EUR	Non-Finnish European
ExAC	Exome Aggregation Consortium
FIN	Finnish
gnomAD	Genome Aggregation Database
HCP	Healthcare provider
HGMD	Human Gene Mutation Database
HWE	Hardy-Weinberg Equilibrium

T. Pramparo (✉)
Travere Therapeutics, Inc., San Diego, CA, USA

Mirum Pharmaceuticals, Foster City, CA, USA
e-mail: Tiziano.Pramparo@mirumpharma.com

C. Jenkinson
Travere Therapeutics, Inc., San Diego, CA, USA
e-mail: celia.jenkinson@travere.com

A. Federico et al. (eds.), *Cerebrotendinous Xanthomatosis*,
https://doi.org/10.1007/978-3-031-92526-9_15

SAS	South Asian
Tetrol	5β-Cholestane-3a,7a,12a,25-tetrol
VOUS	Variants of uncertain significance
VSI	VarSome Insights

In this chapter, we provide a broad understanding of the epidemiology of cerebrotendinous xanthomatosis (CTX) with emphasis on disease frequency and geographic distribution, as reviewed from published studies and unpublished work. We will preface this chapter by discussing inherent challenges that make CTX a difficult disease to recognize and diagnose, in order for the reader to have a contextual understanding of the limitations of accurately estimating its frequency in the general population.

Challenges in CTX Recognition

There are various challenges that limit the understanding and recognition of CTX, even beyond it being an ultra-rare disease. Here, we highlight key obstacles including clinical presentation heterogeneity especially in the first 2–3 decades of life, atypical CTX presentation in a small subset of cases without significant cholestanol elevation, and suboptimal physician education and awareness. We also address genetic testing, newborn screening, and the absence of an international CTX registry or patient database.

The clinical presentation of CTX is highly heterogeneous. Affected individuals may exhibit a wide range of signs, symptoms, and manifestations that can differ in severity, frequency, and age of onset. This may be partially due to the slow and progressive nature of the disease and by the different combinations of neurologic and non-neurologic manifestations that may affect patients at any age. Some individuals may develop neurological symptoms, pyramidal and cerebellar in nature, such as cognitive impairment, psychiatric disturbances, and movement disorders, while others may primarily exhibit non-neurological features like diarrhea and juvenile-onset bilateral cataracts. Still others may experience both significant neurologic and non-neurologic manifestations. Neurological symptoms typically become more prominent with age, and a range of neurological issues can emerge. Non-neurological symptoms, that is, chronic diarrhea or bilateral cataracts often present at an early age, whereas tendon xanthomas usually develop from adolescence onward. This concept is well described by Salen and Steiner (2017) and illustrated in Fig. 2 of the same paper [1] summarizing the variable nature of symptoms and their frequencies spanning across about five decades. Although genotype-phenotype relationships have not been well established, heterogeneity in clinical manifestations may be attributed to specific pathogenic variants in the *CYP27A1* gene, the extent of enzyme deficiency, and/or individual variations in the metabolism of sterols. The heterogeneity of CTX symptoms leads to patients seeking care from various therapeutic specialists, for example, gastroenterologists, ophthalmologists, and neurologists. Thus, in many cases, these challenges lead to an underdiagnosis or misdiagnosis and delayed diagnosis of CTX patients as compared to other neurological or metabolic disorders that are more common. To provide an example, tendon xanthomas, considered one of the four clinically recognizable hallmarks of CTX and sufficient to prompt measurement of serum cholestanol, are found in about 70% of patients [1]. This evidence suggests that approximately the remaining 30% of CTX patients may be mis-diagnosed as having another more common disease and/or remain undiagnosed. In fact, even when present, xanthomas may be associated with other conditions similar to CTX, such as familial hypercholesterolemia and sitosterolemia [2]. Improving awareness of CTX and a better understanding of its clinical heterogeneity is therefore crucial for timely recognition and accurate diagnosis by healthcare professionals.

Complicating the heterogeneous clinical picture even more, variability may be found also at the biochemical level. Historically CTX is biochemically diagnosed by elevations in plasma cholestanol levels [3, 4]; however, there is a growing body of case studies in which genetically confirmed CTX patients have normal or only slightly elevated plasma cholestanol levels [5–8]. These atypical CTX patients may be likely missed, if a holistic evaluation of the clinical course is not performed. Adoption of determination of additional biomarkers in the dysregulated bile acid metabolism pathway would help in the diagnosis of these patients. For example, a biochemical panel that includes metabolites that have been shown be elevated in CTX may help lead to a diagnosis in patients without an increase in cholestanol. Such a panel could include 7αC4, 7α12αC4, and urinary bile alcohols including 23S-Pentol [8–12]. It is also plausible to hypothesize that these atypical cases as well as those cases with a milder CTX phenotype are likely to be overlooked by less informed or experienced physicians.

In Europe, CDCA has been approved for the treatment of CTX since 2017. In the United States, CDCA treatment was until 2025 available only by medical necessity, limiting physician awareness and education, but was approved by the FDA (February 2025) for the treatment of CTX in adults. Also, cholic acid in some instances, particularly in very young patients, due to the lower risk of hepatoxicity, has been successfully used for decades [4, 13, 14]. While a test has been developed for newborn screening using dried blood spots both in the United States and in Europe, the test has not yet been approved for inclusion on the newborn screening panel in either region [7, 9, 15, 16].

New tools are indeed being developed that can help close the gaps between progress in the scientific or clinical understanding of disease and the actual implementation of this knowledge in disease recognition. One example is the democratization of scientific information to help share the knowledge related to diseases. In the last few years, free access databases or tools (some of which are fee-based) such as ClinVar, LOVD, VarSome, Mastermind, and many others have become available to assist clinicians in overcoming the challenges of diagnoses and treatment decisions. In recent work, we have leveraged such resources to provide a more accurate prevalence estimate of CTX and a first geographical map of the disease using retrospective user queries for the *CYP27A1* gene. Altogether, these tools may translate into opportunities to improve the poor recognition of disease and delay in diagnosis [17–19].

Additional challenges may be related to the mutational landscape, genetic testing, and biallelic confirmation of disease. Heterogeneity in pathogenic variants leading to a deficiency in the enzyme sterol 27-hydroxylase is well described. We queried the HGMD database to get an account of the current molecular landscape based on a literature review for CTX and found 121 disease-causing variants (labeled as "DM") and 21 likely disease-causing variants (labeled as "DM?", as of 11/2023, professional version 2023.2). This genetic variability has not been associated with any specific clinical feature or profile; thus, there is a lack of genotype-phenotype relationship which further complicates the identification of potential patients for genetic testing. To help the evaluation of patients, Mignarri et al. (2014), suggested that clinicians may follow a suspicion index [20] and consider genetic testing even in cases with less typical clinical presentations. Second, access and costs to genetic diagnostic testing may be a challenge especially in regions with limited resources and where specialty clinics and diagnostic labs may not be readily available. Third, once genetic testing is performed, there are scenarios where biallelic confirmation is not achieved due to either technical limitations that reduce our sensitivity to detect variants or due to the presence of variants of uncertain significance (VUS) for which there is a lack of scientific or clinical evidence to determine whether a variant is causing disease. A better understanding of patient's disease progression could be derived from a publicly available international patient database which currently does not exist. Among the goals of the US-based patient advocacy organization CTX Alliance https://ctxalliance.org/ are to connect patients and their families and to help support the effort to gain approval to have CTX added to the Recommended Universal Newborn Screen Panel (RUSP) in the United States.

CTX Prevalence Estimates

There is strong scientific consensus that CTX remains severely underdiagnosed. This is clearly seen by the discrepancy between the number of reported cases worldwide and estimates based on carrier allele frequency calculations in populations of healthy individuals or individuals without Mendelian conditions. For instance, according to a systematic review of the literature, only 568 CTX cases have been reported worldwide between 2000 and 2021 [19]. The estimated number of cases however is greatly surpassed even when applying a conservative disease frequency in the US population alone. This phenomenon has also been described outside the United States, as the number of Japanese CTX patients predicted from ExAC allele frequencies were found to be 50 times higher than those seen in a nationwide survey of CTX in Japan [21].

Prevalence estimates vary considerably depending on the population genetic background or ancestry, size, geographic location, and on the assessment methodology. If a population-based approach is used, estimates will also depend on the number of disease-causing variants included in the calculation and the size of the database or reference population used to derive the pooled carrier allele frequencies (see additional limitations below).

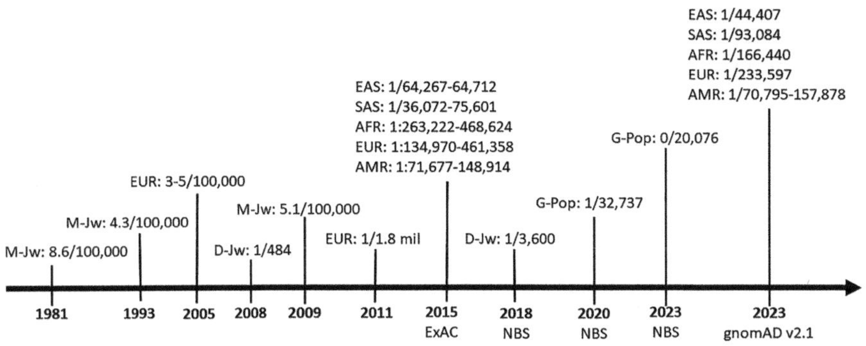

Fig. 15.1 CTX prevalence estimates. Chronological timeline of studies providing insights into CTX prevalence based on case reports or allele frequencies of variants in the *CYP27A1* gene. M-Jw, Moroccan Jews; D-Jw, Druze; G-Pop, general population; AFR, African/African American; AMR, Latino-Admixed American; EAS, East Asian; EUR, European non-Finnish; FIN, European Finnish; SAS, South Asian; NBS, Newborn Screening; ExAC, Exome Aggregation Consortium; gnomAD, Genome Aggregation Database

It is unsurprising that much higher estimates have been described in areas where consanguinity and cultural resistance to pregnancy termination are more common. Examples of this phenomenon can be seen in the Moroccan Jewish [22–24] and Druze [25] populations. In addition, higher prevalence has been reported in subpopulations preselected for a particular symptom, such as individuals with juvenile bilateral cataract as discussed in detail in the next chapter section. In Fig. 15.1, we summarize the chronological order of the main estimates of CTX prevalence from global studies utilizing both case reports and calculations using allele frequencies.

In 1981, Berginer and Abeliovich reported 6 Sephardic Jews patients from 3 families yielding an estimated gene frequency of 1 in 108 or a prevalence of 6 in 70,000 (or 8.6 in 100,000), which represented the size of the Jewish population of Moroccan origin in the Beer-Sheba region [22]. In 1993, Leitersdorf reported slightly lower estimates with 5 patients from four unrelated Moroccan Jewish families estimating a gene frequency to be 1 in 152 or a prevalence of 3 in 70,000 (or 4.3 in 100,000) based on the assessment of a frameshift and a splice-junction variant in the sterol 27-hydroxylase gene [23]. Lorincz et al. (2005) reported a prevalence estimate of 3–5 in 100,000 based on carrier allele frequency of the most common European variant (p.Arg395Cys) from a small group of healthy white individuals and first described CTX as an underdiagnosed disease [26]. With a population screening, Falik-Zaccai et al. in 2008 identified CTX carriers in the Druze population with a carrier frequency at the highest rate currently known of 1 in 11, which corresponds to a prevalence of 1 in 484 [25]. In 2009, Rosner et al., provided supporting information on the Moroccan Jews carrier frequency of 1 in 70 which translates to a prevalence of 3.6 in 70,000 (or 5.1 in 100,000) [24]. In 2011, Pilo-de-la-Fuente et al. reported 25 CTX patients with a high frequency of the same European variant (p.Arg395Cys) used by Lorincz et al. (2005); however, the observed prevalence was significantly smaller with 1 in 1.8 million, as the entire

Spanish population of 45 million individuals was considered [27]. In 2015, Appadurai et al., for the first time, provided disease incidence across multiple populations of different genetic backgrounds by analyzing the ExAC genomic database. Estimates ranged from 1 in 64,000 in the Asian populations to 1 in 468,000 in the African/African American, Latino-admixed American, and European non-Finnish populations [28]. In addition to demonstrate the large variability of such estimates across ancestries, this study strengthened the notion that CTX was underdiagnosed. In a newborn screening of dried bloodspots (DBS), DeBarber et al. (2018) identified heterozygosity in 1 in 30 which estimated a prevalence of 1 in 3600 CTX patients in the Druze population [10]. In 2020, Hong et al. reported the findings of a newborn screening study conducted in the United States in which 1 genetically confirmed CTX case was identified from a cohort of 32,000 samples [29]. More recently, a similar newborn screening of 20,000 DBS in the Dutch population reported no cases with genetically confirmed CTX [16]. A follow-up analysis of prevalence calculation, using carrier allele frequencies of the larger gnomAD v2.1 genomic database, provided an opportunity to update the estimates of the ExAC study [28] across multiple ancestries. Results largely supported and refined previous genetic estimates showing that prevalence ranges from 1 in 44,000 in the Asian populations to 1 in 233,000 in the African/African American, Latino-admixed American, and European populations [30].

At the time of writing this chapter, a new version of gnomAD has been released (version 4). While it is outside the scope of this chapter to describe the analysis of this new dataset, it is reasonable to expect that CTX prevalence estimates will change and be refined due to the much larger number of individuals and more diversified populations included in this gnomAD v4 release. An additional resource currently in development that can help with calculating prevalence estimates across main and subcontinental populations, as well as carrier frequencies, is GeniE (https://genie.broadinstitute.org/). This tool provides a simplified framework to include (likely) pathogenic variants and easily modify the selection of additional variants to calculate estimates in real time.

While the use of carrier allele frequencies from large genomic databases is a powerful approach to calculating prevalence estimates for monogenic recessive conditions that are likely underestimated based on clinical reports, there are important limitations that need to be taken into consideration when referring to such estimates [30]. Several assumptions are being made in order to apply the Hardy-Weinberg Equilibrium (HWE) principle which allows us to sum and square the disease-associated alleles. Among other assumptions are the mutual independence and full penetrance of the rare variants. Since this method is based on an additive model, the number and types of variants included in the calculation will have an impact on the final prevalence numbers. Similarly, of careful consideration is the size of a population used to calculate the carrier allele frequencies. For instance, we have highlighted that the allele frequency of the most common European variant (p.Arg395Cys) has been greatly over-estimated in a small cohort of healthy individuals [26], at a time when large genomic databases were not available, thus leading to an over-estimation of the number of CTX patients. Lastly, we need to be aware that there is a potential bias in estimates from those populations for which clinical variation has been most intensively studied.

CTX Prevalence in Patients with Bilateral Cataracts

Much greater CTX prevalence has been reported in subpopulations of individuals with early-onset, apparently idiopathic, bilateral cataracts [31]. In fact, the consequences of accumulation of cholestanol in the eye provide an excellent opportunity to diagnose this disease early [32, 33]. The PREVALENCE observational study (clinicaltrials.gov identifier NCT02638220) was designed to identify patients with early-onset bilateral cataracts that also had elevated plasma cholestanol and urinary bile alcohol. The diagnosis of CTX in patients that met the pre-set criteria for elevated cholestanol and urinary bile alcohols was followed by eligibility to receive genetic confirmation of CTX. Following the final analysis, a prevalence of CTX of 0.9% in a cohort 426 patients aged 2–21 years with early-onset bilateral cataract was found; notably 15.4% of the patients met the criteria for genetic testing [34, 35]. In a similar study in the Turkish population, 7 cases from a total of 452 patients were genetically confirmed to have CTX providing an estimate of 1.55% [36]. An even higher estimate of CTX in patients with juvenile-onset unexplained bilateral cataracts of 3.3% was found by Fernandez-Eulate et al., although this was from a single patient identified from a small cohort of 30 patients [37]. These findings highlight and stress the critical role of ophthalmologists to be aware and informed about CTX as a possible underlying condition.

CTX Geographic Distribution

Defining the global geographic distribution of diseases is critical to our understanding of genetic diversity at the population level, disease susceptibility, and evolutionary patterns. In the context of disease prevalence, it helps to identify regions or countries where genetic risk and liabilities are most pronounced, which may guide intervention strategies and potentially address health disparities tailored to specific populations. Moreover, a growing number of tools are becoming available to share and democratize critical information to disease recognition and diagnosis. Such tools can also be leveraged to raise awareness among different communities, in particular scientists and medical professionals. We have recently described the use of one of these tools, VarSome Insights (VSI), to generate an estimated CTX disease map based on the raw number of unique queries from professionals designated as healthcare providers (HCPs) [30]. We performed this analysis under the assumption that HCPs queries were potentially linked to clinical activity ultimately leading to the diagnosis or care of prospective CTX patients. From the analysis of about 1200 queries collected in 2021, we identified Spain, Iran, Italy, the United States, and Turkey as top countries for clinical activity related to CTX disease. Here we

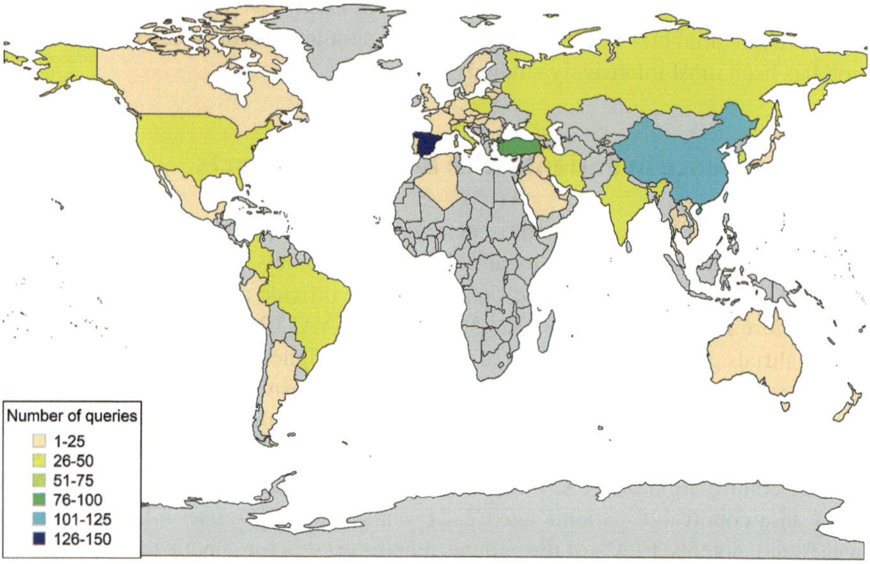

Fig. 15.2 *CYP27A1* pathogenic variants world map. Geographic distribution of *CYP27A1* gene variants queries performed by HCPs of selected clinical/medical professions using the VarSome search engine. The map represents a proxy for clinical activity by country potentially linked to the diagnosis and care of prospective CTX patients. Gray color indicates no queries reported

propose an updated map using an expanded dataset of global raw queries collected in VSI from Jan 2021 to May 2023. This new analysis included 4300 total queries, of which 67% were from designated HCPs. Following the same methods of our previous study [30], we qualified 2500 queries of which 42% were from clinical geneticists and genetic counselors. We next mapped all the VarSome pathogenic HCPs queries (N = 880) to obtain a global geographic distribution of CTX. Also in this expanded analysis, we identified Spain as the top country with the highest number of *CYP27A1* variant queries, followed by China and Turkey (Fig. 15.2). Additional countries with a sizable number of queries were Poland, Korea, Iran, Columbia, Italy, and the United States (Fig. 15.2). For limitations of this approach, please refer to the original publication [30].

Conclusions, Future Perspectives

CTX is a treatable disease. Administration of bile acid replacement in the form of CDCA [4, 13, 14] both in Europe and the United States (approved in adults by the FDA in February 2025) along with the knowledge that earlier treatment is associated with better prognosis [38, 39] provides an urgent drive to identify patients as early as possible. With the increase in genetic testing and expansion of genetic databases, our understanding of the prevalence of CTX has underscored the degree of underdiagnosis, misdiagnosis, and delayed diagnosis based on the variability, onset, and severity of the disease. The hope for the future as we envisage inclusion of CTX in newborn screening panels in the United States and Europe is the ability to diagnose patients much earlier and with increased physician awareness to have the chance to provide treatment and a much better chance of an improved quality of life with absent or minimal symptoms for this currently life-changing disease.

Acknowledgments We would like to thank Steve Rodems, Sika Dunyoh, Rana Dutta, Jolan Terner-Rosenthal, Pam Vig, and Andrea Goldstein for critical reading of the manuscript and providing feedback. We thank the VarSome team, C. Kopanos et al. [40], for sharing the raw queries data for the CTX geographic distribution analysis and mapping.

Competing Interests TP was an employee of and shareholder in Travere Therapeutics, Inc. TP is currently an employee of and shareholder in Mirum Pharmaceuticals, Inc. CJ is a full-time employee of Travere Therapeutics, Inc., and may have an equity or other financial interest in Travere Therapeutics.

References

1. Salen G, Steiner RD. Epidemiology, diagnosis, and treatment of cerebrotendinous xanthomatosis (CTX). J Inherit Metab Dis. 2017;40(6):771–81.
2. Moghadasian MH. Cerebrotendinous xanthomatosis: clinical course, genotypes and metabolic backgrounds. Clin Invest Med. 2004;27(1):42–50.
3. Bjorkhem I, Hansson M. Cerebrotendinous xanthomatosis: an inborn error in bile acid synthesis with defined mutations but still a challenge. Biochem Biophys Res Commun. 2010;396(1):46–9.
4. Berginer VM, Salen G, Shefer S. Long-term treatment of cerebrotendinous xanthomatosis with chenodeoxycholic acid. N Engl J Med. 1984;311(26):1649–52.
5. Bonnet JB, Couvert P, Di-Filippo M, Boissiere F, Cristol JP, Sutra T, et al. Tuberous xanthomatosis is not necessarily associated with increased plasma concentrations of cholestanol in cerebrotendinous xanthomatosis. J Intern Med. 2023;293(1):121–3.
6. Alexandria Van Grouw SG, Jeffries KM, Duell PB, DeBarber AE. Presented at SMD 2023. Quantification of urinary 5β-Cholestane-3α,7α,12α,23S,25-Pentol as a diagnostic test for Cerebrotendinous Xanthomatosis (CTX) poster presentation at SIMD. Salt Lake City; 2023.
7. John A, Bernat GR, Redder S, Fowler M, Orvidas M, Duell PB, DeBarber AE. Quantification of bile acid pathway intermediate/bile alcohol biomarkers as a biochemical diagnostic test for Cerebrotendinous Xanthomatosisand to monitor therapeutic efficacy: comparison to cholestanol. Poster presentation at SSIEM. Jerusalem; 2023.
8. DeBarber AE, Schaefer EJ, Do J, Ray JW, Larson A, Redder S, Fowler M, Duell PB. Genetically and clinically confirmed atypical cerebrotendinous xanthomatosis with normal cholestanol and marked elevations of bile acid precursors and bile alcohols. J Clin Lipidol. 2024;18(3):e465–e476. https://doi.org/10.1016/j.jacl.2024.03.004. Epub 2024 Mar 15. PMID: 38637260.
9. DeBarber AE, Luo J, Star-Weinstock M, Purkayastha S, Geraghty MT, Chiang JP, et al. A blood test for cerebrotendinous xanthomatosis with potential for disease detection in newborns. J Lipid Res. 2014;55(1):146–54.
10. DeBarber AE, Kalfon L, Fedida A, Fleisher Sheffer V, Ben Haroush S, Chasnyk N, et al. Newborn screening for cerebrotendinous xanthomatosis is the solution for early identification and treatment. J Lipid Res. 2018;59(11):2214–22.
11. Panzenboeck U, Andersson U, Hansson M, Sattler W, Meaney S, Bjorkhem I. On the mechanism of cerebral accumulation of cholestanol in patients with cerebrotendinous xanthomatosis. J Lipid Res. 2007;48(5):1167–74.

12. Bove KE, Heubi JE, Balistreri WF, Setchell KD. Bile acid synthetic defects and liver disease: a comprehensive review. Pediatr Dev Pathol. 2004;7(4):315–34.
13. Salen G, Berginer V, Shore V, Horak I, Horak E, Tint GS, et al. Increased concentrations of cholestanol and apolipoprotein B in the cerebrospinal fluid of patients with cerebrotendinous xanthomatosis. Effect of chenodeoxycholic acid. N Engl J Med. 1987;316(20):1233–8.
14. Mandia D, Chaussenot A, Besson G, Lamari F, Castelnovo G, Curot J, et al. Cholic acid as a treatment for cerebrotendinous xanthomatosis in adults. J Neurol. 2019;266(8):2043–50.
15. Bleyle L, Huidekoper HH, Vaz FM, Singh R, Steiner RD, DeBarber AE. Update on newborn dried bloodspot testing for cerebrotendinous xanthomatosis: an available high-throughput liquid-chromatography tandem mass spectrometry method. Mol Genet Metab Rep. 2016;7:11–5.
16. Vaz FM, Jamal Y, Barto R, Gelb MH, DeBarber AE, Wevers RA, et al. Newborn screening for Cerebrotendinous Xanthomatosis: a retrospective biomarker study using both flow-injection and UPLC-MS/MS analysis in 20,000 newborns. Clin Chim Acta. 2023;539:170–4.
17. DeBarber AE, Duell PB. Update on cerebrotendinous xanthomatosis. Curr Opin Lipidol. 2021;32(2):123–31.
18. Fraidakis MJ. Psychiatric manifestations in cerebrotendinous xanthomatosis. Transl Psychiatry. 2013;3:e302.
19. Badura-Stronka M, Hirschfeld AS, Winczewska-Wiktor A, Budzynska E, Jakubiuk-Tomaszuk A, Piontek A, et al. First case series of polish patients with cerebrotendinous xanthomatosis and systematic review of cases from the 21st century. Clin Genet. 2022;101(2):190–207.
20. Mignarri A, Gallus GN, Dotti MT, Federico A. A suspicion index for early diagnosis and treatment of cerebrotendinous xanthomatosis. J Inherit Metab Dis. 2014;37(3):421–9.
21. Sekijima Y, Koyama S, Yoshinaga T, Koinuma M, Inaba Y. Nationwide survey on cerebrotendinous xanthomatosis in Japan. J Hum Genet. 2018;63(3):271–80.
22. Berginer VM, Abeliovich D. Genetics of cerebrotendinous xanthomatosis (CTX): an autosomal recessive trait with high gene frequency in Sephardim of Moroccan origin. Am J Med Genet. 1981;10(2):151–7.
23. Leitersdorf E, Reshef A, Meiner V, Levitzki R, Schwartz SP, Dann EJ, et al. Frameshift and splice-junction mutations in the sterol 27-hydroxylase gene cause cerebrotendinous xanthomatosis in Jews or Moroccan origin. J Clin Invest. 1993;91(6):2488–96.
24. Rosner G, Rosner S, Orr-Urtreger A. Genetic testing in Israel: an overview. Annu Rev Genomics Hum Genet. 2009;10:175–92.
25. Falik-Zaccai TC, Kfir N, Frenkel P, Cohen C, Tanus M, Mandel H, et al. Population screening in a Druze community: the challenge and the reward. Genet Med. 2008;10(12):903–9.
26. Lorincz MT, Rainier S, Thomas D, Fink JK. Cerebrotendinous xanthomatosis: possible higher prevalence than previously recognized. Arch Neurol. 2005;62(9):1459–63.
27. Pilo-de-la-Fuente B, Jimenez-Escrig A, Lorenzo JR, Pardo J, Arias M, Ares-Luque A, et al. Cerebrotendinous xanthomatosis in Spain: clinical, prognostic, and genetic survey. Eur J Neurol. 2011;18(10):1203–11.
28. Appadurai V, DeBarber A, Chiang PW, Patel SB, Steiner RD, Tyler C, et al. Apparent underdiagnosis of Cerebrotendinous Xanthomatosis revealed by analysis of ~60,000 human exomes. Mol Genet Metab. 2015;116(4):298–304.
29. Hong X, Daiker J, Sadilek M, DeBarber AE, Chiang J, Duan J, et al. Toward newborn screening of cerebrotendinous xanthomatosis: results of a biomarker research study using 32,000 newborn dried blood spots. Genet Med. 2020;22(10):1606–12.
30. Pramparo T, Steiner RD, Rodems S, Jenkinson C. Allelic prevalence and geographic distribution of cerebrotendinous xanthomatosis. Orphanet J Rare Dis. 2023;18(1):13.
31. Verrips A, van Engelen BG, Wevers RA, van Geel BM, Cruysberg JR, van den Heuvel LP, et al. Presence of diarrhea and absence of tendon xanthomas in patients with cerebrotendinous xanthomatosis. Arch Neurol. 2000;57(4):520–4.
32. Monson DM, DeBarber AE, Bock CJ, Anadiotis G, Merkens LS, Steiner RD, et al. Cerebrotendinous xanthomatosis: a treatable disease with juvenile cataracts as a presenting sign. Arch Ophthalmol. 2011;129(8):1087–8.

33. Tibrewal S, Duell PB, DeBarber AE, Loh AR. Cerebrotendinous xanthomatosis: early diagnosis on the basis of juvenile cataracts. J AAPOS. 2017;21(6):505–7.
34. Freedman SF, Del Monte MA, Diva U, Donahue SP, Drack AV, Dutta R, et al. Prevalence of cerebrotendinous xanthomatosis among patients diagnosed with early-onset idiopathic bilateral cataracts: final analysis. J AAPOS. 2023;27(4):208–11.
35. Freedman SF, Brennand C, Chiang J, DeBarber A, Del Monte MA, Duell PB, et al. Prevalence of Cerebrotendinous Xanthomatosis among patients diagnosed with acquired juvenile-onset idiopathic bilateral cataracts. JAMA Ophthalmol. 2019;137(11):1312–6.
36. Atilla H, Coskun T, Elibol B, Kadayifcilar S, Altinel S, Group G-E-IW. Prevalence of cerebrotendinous xanthomatosis in cases with idiopathic bilateral juvenile cataract in ophthalmology clinics in Turkey. J AAPOS. 2021;25:269.e1.
37. Fernandez-Eulate G, Martin GC, Dureau P, Speeg-Spatz C, Brassier A, Gillard P, et al. Prospective cholestanol screening of cerebrotendinous xanthomatosis among patients with juvenile-onset unexplained bilateral cataracts. Orphanet J Rare Dis. 2022;17(1):434.
38. Yahalom G, Tsabari R, Molshatzki N, Ephraty L, Cohen H, Hassin-Baer S. Neurological outcome in cerebrotendinous xanthomatosis treated with chenodeoxycholic acid: early versus late diagnosis. Clin Neuropharmacol. 2013;36(3):78–83.
39. Stelten BML, Huidekoper HH, van de Warrenburg BPC, Brilstra EH, Hollak CEM, Haak HR, et al. Long-term treatment effect in cerebrotendinous xanthomatosis depends on age at treatment start. Neurology. 2019;92(2):e83–95.
40. Kopanos C, Tsiolkas V, Kouris A, Chapple CE, Albarca Aguilera M, Meyer R, et al. VarSome: the human genomic variant search engine. Bioinformatics. 2019;35(11):1978–80.

Part VI

Treatments for Cerebrotendinous Xanthomatosis (CTX); Present and Future

Chenodeoxycholic Acid Treatment in the Italian Cohort of Cerebrotendinous Xanthomatosis (CTX) Patients

16

Antonio Federico

Introduction

Cerebrotendinous xanthomatosis (CTX) is an autosomal recessive lipid storage disease caused by pathogenic variants in the *CYP27A1* gene.

The biochemical defect is due to the deficiency of sterol-27-hydroxylase, a mitochondrial enzyme involved in the first step of degradation of the sterol side chain of bile acid biosynthesis.

CTX is biochemically characterized by high plasma and tissue concentration of cholestanol and other bile acid precursors, decreased levels of chenodeoxycholic acid (CDCA) and 27-hydroxycholesterol (27-OHC), and markedly increased excretion of 25-hydroxylated bile alcohols in urine, bile, and feces [1].

The Background for CDCA Therapy

The research group of Salen and colleagues from 1971 to 1975 provided the basic background to consider cholestanol accumulation and abnormalities in bile acids as one of the pathogenetic factors in CTX and started to consider chenodeoxycholic acid treatment as a possible therapy for this disorder.

Table 16.1 reports the basic articles by this group on cholestanol and bile acid metabolism in CTX, indicating the possible pathogenetic role of these substances in the CTX pathogenesis.

A. Federico (✉)
Department of Medicine, Surgery and Neurosciences, Medical School, University of Siena, Siena, Italy
e-mail: federico@unisi.it

A. Federico et al. (eds.), *Cerebrotendinous Xanthomatosis*,
https://doi.org/10.1007/978-3-031-92526-9_16

Table 16.1 Published literature from the Salen research group articles which opened up the possibility to use chenodeoxycholic acid for CTX therapy

Cholestanol deposition in cerebrotendinous xanthomatosis. A possible mechanism. Salen G. Ann Intern Med. 1971;75(6):843–51.
Biosynthesis of 5 -cholestan-3 -ol in cerebrotendinous xanthomatosis. Salen G, Polito A. J Clin Invest. 1972;51(1):134–40.
The metabolism of cholestanol, cholesterol, and bile acids in cerebrotendinous xanthomatosis. Salen G, Grundy SM. J Clin Invest. 1973;52(11):2822–35.
Transformation of 5 alpha-cholest-7-en-3 beta-ol to cholesterol and cholestanol in cerebrotendinous xanthomatosis. Tint GS, Salen G. J Lipid Res. 1974;15(3):256–62.
A biochemical abnormality in cerebrotendinous xanthomatosis. Impairment of bile acid biosynthesis associated with incomplete degradation of the cholesterol side chain. Setoguchi T, Salen G, Tint GS, Mosbach EH. J Clin Invest. 1974;53(5):1393–401.
Increased formation of ursodeoxycholic acid in patients treated with chenodeoxycholic acid. Salen G, Tint GS, Eliav B, Deering N, Mosbach EH. J Clin Invest. 1974;53(2):612–21.
Chenodeoxycholic acid inhibits increased cholesterol and cholestanol synthesis in patients with cerebrotendinous xanthomatosis. Salen G, Meriwether TW, Nicolau G. Biochem Med. 1975;14(1):57–74.
Identification of pentahydroxy bile alcohols in cerebrotendinous xanthomatosis: characterization of 5beta-cholestane-3alpha, 7alpha, 12alpha, 24xi, 25-pentol and 5beta-cholestane-3alpha, 7alpha, 12alpha, 23xi, 25-pentol. Shefer S, Dayal B, Tint GS, Salen G, Mosbach EH. J Lipid Res. 1975; 16(4):280–6.
Bile alcohol metabolism in man. Conversion of 5beta-cholestane-3alpha, 7alpha,12alpha, 25-tetrol to cholic acid. Salen G, Shefer S, Setoguchi T, Mosbach EH. J Clin Invest. 1975; 56(1):226–31.

All these data prompted Berginer et al. [2] to use CDCA therapy in 17 CTX patients, with a 1-year follow-up, reporting marked clinical improvements in neuropsychologic abnormalities, in cerebellar, pyramidal, and peripheral nerve symptoms, in EEG and head CT scans, associated with decreased cholestanol levels, indicating that this therapy is able to correct the biochemical defect and improve the different clinical signs.

Evidence that cholestanol may be neurotoxic is supported by the finding of cholestanol deposition and apoptosis in neuronal cells, most notably in Purkinje cells, in the cerebellum of rats fed a 1% cholestanol diet [3]. CDCA also blocks and antagonizes GABA and NMDA receptors [4].

Given the reduced synthesis of CDCA and high level of cholestanol in blood and tissues in CTX, as well as the recent evidence that cholestanol may be neurotoxic, CDCA treatment became and remains the standard of care for CTX patients.

The same group of Salen-Berginer investigated the CDCA effect on sterol and protein composition in six CTX patients, showing that this therapy is able to normalize the selective permeability of the blood-brain barrier and the concentrations of sterol and apolipoproteins in the cerebrospinal fluid [5].

Our Experience with CDCA Therapy

We used the classical recommended dosing for CDCA ranging from 5 to 15 mg/kg per day in children (usually the dose remains 5 mg/day) and 750 mg per day, in three divided doses, in adults. In adults, we utilized a slowly progressive dosing introduction with 500 mg per day for 2 weeks, followed by a weekly increase of 250 mg per day until the recommended dose is reached. In patients in which serum cholestanol or urine bile alcohols remain elevated after 3 months, CDCA may be increased to 1000 mg per day.

In infants and young children, it is recommended to start with 5 mg/kg/day, in three divided doses. If needed, the dose can be increased, controlling liver function. Older children and adolescents may need dosages up to 10 to 15 mg/kg/day divided in three dosages to obtain adequate metabolic control.

Our first reported experience was a significant improvement in nerve conduction velocities, N13 to N20 interpeak latencies, and visual evoked potential latencies with no changes in brainstem auditory evoked potentials in ten CTX patients treated by CDCA [6].

In a larger number of patients (35), peripheral neuropathy was detected in 74.2% of cases, consisting of sensory-motor axonal neuropathy in 10 patients (38.4%), motor axonal neuropathy in 10 (38.4%), motor demyelinating neuropathy in 4 (15.3%), and sensory-motor demyelinating neuropathy in 2 (7.7%). CDCA treatment improved nerve conduction velocities, whereas most nerve amplitudes remained unchanged [7].

Mignarri et al. [8] reported that transcranial magnetic stimulation (TMS) was capable of detecting corticospinal tract damage, monitoring the effects of CDCA replacement therapy in nine patients who started CDCA therapy at baseline and neurophysiological follow-up. All patients showed signs of pyramidal damage with spastic paraparesis. TMS revealed corticospinal alterations even in subjects with mild clinical signs of corticospinal tract involvement. After CDCA treatment, serum cholestanol decreased to normal concentrations in all patients. Clinical findings were unchanged in seven out of nine cases; in two others, pyramidal signs disappeared. A reduction in abnormal neurophysiological parameters was also found [8].

Further evidence that CDCA therapy may change brain metabolism and structure detected by PET imaging have been reported by Caroppo et al. [9] in 2013 and by diffusion tensor imaging and tractography, with normalization of findings correlated with improvement of clinical symptoms [10].

In 1993, we reported a pathophysiologic study on bone metabolism in CTX patients [11]; in the same year, Berginer et al. (1993) also reported osteoporosis and increased bone fractures in their patients [12].

In 2013, we investigated 11 CTX patients aged 13–43 years with dual-energy X-ray absorptiometry and assessed serum cholestanol and 25-hydroxyvitamin D (25-OHD) concentrations both at the time of diagnosis and after long-term treatment with CDCA. We showed at baseline low BMD in nine patients, cholestanol elevation in all subjects, and 25-OHD decreases in nine patients. After a 30-month follow-up, no clinical changes including bone fractures occurred; both planar and volumetric bone mineral density improved with normalization of plasma cholestanol levels and increase of serum 25-OHD. Our study confirmed the presence of low bone mass in CTX showing that long-term CDCA treatment increases bone mineral content [13].

In 2016, we studied the biochemical effect of CDCA therapy in a cohort of 19 CTX patients which at baseline showed an increase of cholestanol, 7α-hydroxy-4-cholesten-3-one (7αC4), lathosterol, and plant sterols, whereas 27-hydroxycholesterol (27-OHC) was extremely low or absent. CDCA treatment at a daily dose of 750 mg normalized all biochemical parameters except for 7αC4 which persisted slightly higher than normal in most patients. 27-OHC was not modified by therapy. Biochemical evaluation did not reveal significant differences between stable and worsening patients [14].

We collaborated with 28 patients diagnosed at 35.0 (±11.4 SD) years on average (median duration of CDCA treatment: 5.75 [range: 0.0–25.0] years) in a long-duration study on safety and effectiveness of CDCA therapy in CTX showing that signs and symptoms of disease resolved, improved, or remained stable in many patients, with concomitant improvements in biochemical marker levels (serum cholestanol, $p < 0.001$; 7α-hydroxy-4-cholesten-3-one, $p < 0.001$ [IT study]) [15].

The outcomes of these retrospective cohort studies indicate that CDCA is effective in the long-term treatment of CTX, with an acceptable safety profile.

CDCA has been used for more than 40 years as an off-label drug for CTX; in 2014, this substance received by EMA a designation of "orphan drug" and in 2017 a patent in Europe for CTX therapy [16].

CDCA Side Effects

Hepatotoxicity is the major side effect with CDCA therapy, in most cases only with minor serum transaminases increase. This is particularly important in young children in which it is important to start at 5 mg/kg/day in three daily divided dosages followed eventually by a further increase of dose [17]. It is useful in such cases to monitor these parameters and if transaminases persist to be elevated, it is necessary to decrease the dose of the drug, or discontinue it. In the majority of cases, the increase of serum transaminase completely normalizes after 6 months of drug discontinuation. Patients with higher levels of serum transaminases (three times the upper normal limit) or with recurrence of the transaminase abnormality after reintroduction of CDCA either discontinue therapy or utilize a lower dose which is usually well tolerated. If therapy is discontinued, the disease will likely progress; in such cases, therapy with cholic acid can be considered.

In patients presenting with persistent diarrhea or severe gastrointestinal complaints, transient reduction of the recommended dosing is employed until improvement of symptoms, when effective dosage is restarted.

CDCA therapy is contraindicated in patients with moderate to severe hepatic dysfunction, intrahepatic cholestasis, primary biliary cirrhosis, sclerosing cholangitis, biliary pancreatitis, biliary gastrointestinal fistula, acute cholecystitis or cholangitis, or biliary tract obstruction.

In one patient poorly responding to CDCA, we evaluated a combined treatment with simvastatin and plasmapheresis with poor efficacy in controlling the clinical signs, besides the normalization of cholestanol [18].

Finally, in one case with neonatal diagnosis, early therapy was able to improve neonatal cholestasis and prevent all subsequent symptoms which at the age of 15 years old are absolutely absent [19].

Conclusions

Based on our experience of CDCA therapy in CTX, we can underline the following points:

- In a follow-up of 25–30 years, we have seen 1/3 of patients showing clinical progression despite CDCA treatment. Motor and cognitive/psychiatric disturbances are the major causes of disability.
- *In relationship to cholesterol metabolism*, we have seen that CDCA restores serum levels of cholestanol (normalization) and 7αC4 (from 200-fold increased to tenfold increased) by inhibiting CYP7A1 (classic pathway); serum levels of 27-OHC (very low or absent) are not influenced by CDCA therapy.
- We did not find statistically relevant biochemical differences between stable and worsening patients.
- *Electrophysiological parameters* of nerve conduction velocities and evoked potentials analyses showed that CDCA improves the conduction of the myelinated fibers of both central nervous system (corticospinal tract) and peripheral nervous system.
- CDCA increases bone mineral density and serum vitamin D levels, decreasing the risk of bone fractures. *In brain MRI studies*, presence/development of vacuolation or calcification of cerebellar dentate nuclei seems to be a negative prognostic factor [20]. In patients in whom treatment was not possible to be continued for side effects or unavailability of drug, we register a more rapid motor and mental deterioration. In some patients, as previously reported [18] we tried sinvastatin associated with plasmapheresis or sinvastatin alone. Cholic acid may also be considered in such cases.
- The possible causes of disease progression despite CDCA treatment may be summarized in Table 16.2.

Table 16.2 Possible causes of disease progression despite CDCA therapy

Delay of diagnosis and treatment (longer exposure to toxic metabolites)
Presence of neurological impairment at diagnosis (encouraging collection and dissemination of follow up data of patients treated since childhood/adolescence)
Dentate nuclei degeneration (vacuolation/calcification) at diagnosis
Persistent high levels of 7αC4 over time (about tenfold increase)
Altered homeostasis of brain oxysterols due to reduced 27-OHC

An early diagnosis and early therapy seems to prevent the severe neurologic and psychiatric symptoms, but more prolonged follow-up of treated children will confirm these observations, reported at present time in few articles [19, 21–23]

Acknowledgments I thank all people who enthusiastically collaborated with me in the different projects on CTX during more than 30 years and all patients and families.

References

1. Gallus GN, Federico A. Cerebrotendinous Xanthomatosis. In: GeneReviews, (2003 Jul 16 [Updated 2022 Mar 17), Adam MP, Feldman J, Mirzaa GM, Pagon RA, Wallace SE, Bean LJH, Gripp KW, Amemiya A, editors. Seattle: University of Washington; 1993–2023.
2. Berginer VM, Salen G, Shefer SN. Long-term treatment of cerebrotendinous xanthomatosis with chenodeoxycholic acid. New Engl J Med. 1984;311(26):1649–52.
3. Inoue K, Kubota S, Seyama Y. Cholestanol induces apoptosis of cerebellar neuronal cells. Biochem Biophys Res Commun. 1999;256:198–203.
4. Schubring SR, Fleischer W, Lin JS, Haas HL, Sergeeva OA. The bile steroid chenodeoxycholate is a potent antagonist at NMDA and GABA(A) receptors. Neurosci Lett. 2012;506:322–6.
5. Salen G, Berginer V, Shore V, Horak I, Horak E, Tint GS, Shefer S. Increased concentrations of cholestanol and apolipoprotein B in the cerebrospinal fluid of patients with cerebrotendinous xanthomatosis. Effect of chenodeoxycholic acid. N Engl J Med. 1987;316(20):1233–8.
6. Mondelli M, Rossi A, Scarpini C, Dotti MT, Federico A. Evoked potentials in cerebrotendinous xanthomatosis and effect induced by chenodeoxycholic acid. Arch Neurol. 1992;49(5):469–75.
7. Ginanneschi F, Mignarri A, Mondelli M, Gallus GN, Del Puppo M, Giorgi S, Federico A, Rossi A, Dotti MT. Polyneuropathy in cerebrotendinous xanthomatosis and response to treatment with chenodeoxycholic acid. J Neurol. 2013;260(1):268–74.
8. Mignarri A, Rossi S, Ballerini M, Gallus GN, Del Puppo M, Galluzzi P, Federico A, Dotti MT. Clinical relevance and neurophysiological correlates of spasticity in cerebrotendinous xanthomatosis. J Neurol. 2011;258(5):783–90.
9. Caroppo P, D'Agata F, Mignarri A, Stromillo ML, Dotti MT, Mongini T. Brain metabolism changes after therapy with chenodeoxycholic acid in a case of cerebrotendinous xanthomatosis. Neurol Sci. 2013;34(9):1693–6.
10. Catarino CB, Vollmar C, Küpper C, Seelos K, Gallenmüller C, Bartkiewicz J, Biskup S, Hörtnagel K, Klopstock T. Brain diffusion tensor imaging changes in cerebrotendinous xanthomatosis reversed with treatment. J Neurol. 2018;265(2):388–93.
11. Federico A, Dotti MT, Lore F, Nuti R. Cerebrotendinous xanthomatosis: pathophysiological study on bone metabolism. J Neurol Sci. 1993;115:67–70.
12. Berginer VM, Shany S, Alkalay D, Berginer J, Dekel S, Salen G, Tint GS, Gazit D. Osteoporosis and increased bone fractures in cerebrotendinous xanthomatosis. Metabolism. 1993;42(1):69–74.
13. Martini G, Mignarri A, Ruvio M, Valenti R, Franci B, Del Puppo M, Federico A, Nuti R, Dotti MT. Long-term bone density evaluation in cerebrotendinous xanthomatosis: evidence of improvement after chenodeoxycholic acid treatment. Calcif Tissue Int. 2013;92(3):282–6.
14. Mignarri A, Magni A, Del Puppo M, Gallus GN, Björkhem I, Federico A, Dotti MT. Evaluation of cholesterol metabolism in cerebrotendinous xanthomatosis. J Inherit Metab Dis. 2016;39(1):75–83.
15. Verrips A, Dotti MT, Mignarri A, Stelten BML, Verma S, Federico A. The safety and effectiveness of chenodeoxycholic acid treatment in patients with cerebrotendinous xanthomatosis: two retrospective cohort studies. Neurol Sci. 2020;41(4):943–9.
16. https://www.ema.europa.eu/en/medicines/human/EPAR/chenodeoxycholic-acid-leadiant#authorisation-details-section

17. Huidekoper HH, Vaz FM, Verrips A, Bosch AM. Hepatotoxicity due to chenodeoxycholic acid supplementation in an infant with cerebrotendinous xanthomatosis: implications for treatment. Eur J Pediatr. 2016;175(1):143–6.
18. Dotti MT, Lütjohann D, von Bergmann K, Federico A. Normalisation of serum cholestanol concentration in a patient with cerebrotendinous xanthomatosis by combined treatment with chenodeoxycholic acid, simvastatin and LDL apheresis. Neurol Sci. 2004;25(4):185–91.
19. Degassi I, Amoruso C, Giordano G, Del Puppo M, Mignarri A, Dotti MT, Naturale N, Nebbia G. Case report: early treatment with Chenodeoxycholic acid in Cerebrotendinous Xanthomatosis presenting as neonatal cholestasis. Front Pediatr. 2020;8:382.
20. Rosini F, Pretegiani E, Mignarri A, Optican LM, Serchi V, De Stefano N, Battaglini M, Monti L, Dotti MT, Federico A, Rufa A. The role of dentate nuclei in human oculomotor control: insights from cerebrotendinous xanthomatosis. J Physiol. 2017;595(11):3607–20.
21. Zhang P, Zhao J, Peng XM, Qian YY, Zhao XM, Zhou WH, Wang JS, Wu BB, Wang HJ. Cholestasis as a dominating symptom of patients with CYP27A1 mutations: an analysis of 17 Chinese infants. J Clin Lipidol. 2021;15(1):116–23.
22. Van Heijst AFJ, Verrips A, Wevers RA, Cruysberg JRM, Renier WO, Tolboom JJM. Treatment and follow up of children with cerebrotendinous xanthomatosis. Eur J Pediatr. 1998;157:313–6.
23. Zubarioglu T, Kıykım E, Aktuglu-Zeybek C. Cerebrotendinous Xanthomatosis (CTX) pediatric presentation (Chap. 23). In: Federico A, DeBarber AE, Falik-Zaccai TC, Huidekoper HH, Steiner RD, editors. Cerebrotendinous Xanthomatosis. Cham: Springer; this volume.

17 Long-Term Treatment Effect in Cerebrotendinous Xanthomatosis (CTX) Depends on Age at Treatment Start

Bianca M. L. Stelten and Aad Verrips

Cerebrotendinous xanthomatosis is an autosomal recessive inborn error of metabolism associated with the deficiency of the enzyme sterol 27-hydroxylase, encoded by the CYP27A1 gene [1]. The deficiency of the enzyme sterol 27-hydroxylase results in the deficiency of the primary bile acids chenodeoxycholic acid (CDCA) and cholic acid (CA), and accumulation of bile acid precursors, like 7α-hydroxy-4-cholesten-3-one, upstream of the metabolic block. The production of cholestanol from the bile acid precursor 7α-hydroxy-4-cholesten-3-one is thought to be of major importance for the accumulation of cholestanol in patients with CTX [2, 3]. Accumulation of cholestanol in the central and peripheral nervous system is postulated to be responsible for the neurological symptoms and disability seen in CTX [4]. Clinical manifestations of CTX range from being nearly asymptomatic in early childhood, to neonatal cholestasis, diarrhea, or cataract as most prominent symptoms, up to severe disability due to psychiatric and neurological symptoms at adult age. Neurological dysfunction is the most disabling feature in CTX. Recognition of CTX may be difficult because of its clinical heterogeneity and the absence of consistent genotype-phenotype correlations, even within families [5]. Although the first signs and symptoms of CTX already appear in infancy or childhood, the actual diagnosis is often delayed by 17 to 25 years [6–8].

Early diagnosis of CTX is crucial because CTX is a treatable disease, and early and long-term treatment with CDCA improves clinical outcomes substantially. The standard of care treatment is oral CDCA, which has been used as a therapy for CTX since 1975 [9]. CDCA treatment has shown to normalize or almost normalize the

B. M. L. Stelten (✉)
Catharina Hospital, Department of Neurology, Eindhoven, The Netherlands
e-mail: bianca.stelten@catharinaziekenhuis.nl

A. Verrips
Canisius-Wilhelmina Hospital, Department of Neurology, Nijmegen, The Netherlands
e-mail: a.verrips@cwz.nl

A. Federico et al. (eds.), *Cerebrotendinous Xanthomatosis*, https://doi.org/10.1007/978-3-031-92526-9_17

biochemical abnormalities in CTX [10]. CDCA therapy is generally given as 250 mg orally 3 times daily in adults and 15 mg/kg/day in children, also in divided doses [11]. Studies on the optimal treatment dose in CTX are lacking. CA is suggested as an alternative treatment for CTX in patients that have side effects related to CDCA [12]. Elevated liver enzymes and hepatotoxicity have been rarely described in CDCA treatment [13–15]. Although CA may be a suitable alternative treatment for CTX, only a few studies have investigated the effect of CA in CTX, with conflicting results [16, 17]. Unfortunately, long-term data are not available.

Many studies have already reported positive effects of CDCA treatment on the disease course of CTX, changing the natural history in a positive way, with stabilization and/or improvement of clinical symptoms. In an important study, 17 patients with already serious neurologic impairments before start of treatment were treated for 1 to 11 years. No signs of neurologic deterioration were observed during follow-up [10]. Several other studies reported stabilization or improvement of neurologic symptoms during follow-up in patients on CDCA therapy [6, 11, 18–27].

Three smaller studies suggested that age at diagnosis and start of CDCA treatment is correlated with prognosis [6, 19, 26]. In the first study, describing a group of 25 patients with a relatively late mean age at diagnosis of 38 years and all with neurologic symptoms at diagnosis, only 28% stabilized, while the majority continued to deteriorate despite treatment [6]. In a second study, describing 6 patients diagnosed before the age of 18, improvement or at least stabilization of neurologic symptoms was seen in all patients [26]. The third study showed that in a cohort of 18 patients, patients diagnosed and treated before the age of 25 had a significantly better outcome, compared with those who started treatment after that age [19]. The effect of CDCA treatment on neurologic symptoms is greater when treatment is started earlier in the disease course [19]. That early start of CDCA treatment not only arrests deterioration but may also result in prevention of the neurologic phenotype was first suggested in a case report describing two pre-symptomatic patients, in whom CDCA treatment was started at the age of 2 and 7 who did not develop any neurologic or other symptoms of CTX during a follow-up period of 14 years [21].

In this chapter, the largest retrospective study reporting clinical long-term follow-up and MRI characteristics of Dutch patients with CTX is discussed [28, 29].

Long-Term Treatment Effect in Cerebrotendinous Xanthomatosis, the Dutch Cohort Study [28]

This retrospective cohort study describes the clinical characteristics of a large Dutch CTX cohort ($n = 56$) during long-term follow-up (maximum follow-up of 31.5 years), evaluating the role and timing of CDCA treatment in relation to improvement, stabilization, or deterioration of clinical characteristics, especially with respect to neurologic symptoms and degree of disability. Diagnosis of CTX was confirmed in all patients by the demonstration of elevated blood (serum) levels of cholestanol and/or elevated urine bile alcohol excretion and finally by genetic analysis of the *CYP27A1* gene (except in 2 siblings). No correlations were found between genotype and clinical characteristics. The clinical condition was assessed with the modified Rankin Scale (mRS) and Expanded Disability Status Scale (EDSS).

Age at diagnosis was correlated with clinical characteristics and the course (improvement, stabilization, or deterioration) of mRS and EDSS scores at follow-up. Treatment adherence was based on history taking and biochemical evaluations. Patients who did not interrupt CDCA treatment for >6 weeks during the follow-up period and always had normal urinary bile acid excretion and plasma cholestanol levels lower than 2 times the upper reference range limit were considered compliant. Patients with plasma cholestanol levels more than twice the upper reference range limit on >1 occasion after 1 year of therapy were considered non-compliant. Mean age at time of diagnosis was 25.6 ± 14.6 years. If the suspicion index of Mignarri [8] was applied, there still is a substantial mean diagnostic delay of 8 years. After diagnosis, all patients were treated with CDCA. The initial therapy dose ranged from 5 to 15 mg/kg/d in children (<16 years of age) and up to 750 mg/d in adult patients. Dose adjustments were based on body weight, serum cholestanol levels, and increased urine bile alcohol excretion. The biochemical evaluation was the reason for dose adjustment to 1000 mg/d in 9 patients. The median follow-up time was 8 years (range 6 months-31.5 years).

Figure 17.1 shows a box-and-whisker plot representing age at diagnosis and the course of mRS and EDSS scores at follow-up (concerning all patients with good treatment adherence). This plot shows that patients diagnosed and treated before the age of 24 years had significantly better outcome with respect to mRS and EDSS scores. Deterioration was only seen in patients diagnosed and treated after the age

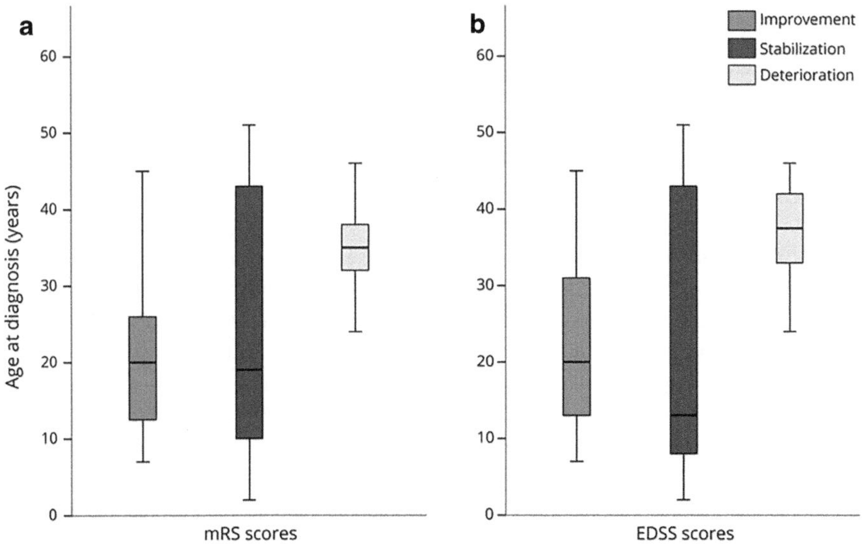

Fig. 17.1 Age at diagnosis and the course of (**a**) mRS and (**b**) EDSS scores during follow-up ($n = 42$). Bottom and top of the box are the first and third quartiles; band inside the box is the median. Ends of the whiskers represent the minimum and maximum of all the data

of 24. This age was therefore used as a cutoff to compare patients diagnosed and treated before and after this age. Twenty-four patients (43%) were diagnosed before the age of 24, and 32 patients (57%) after the age of 24.

Diarrhea during infancy and childhood, present in 39 patients (70%) at the time of diagnosis, disappeared completely shortly after the start of CDCA therapy in the majority of these patients (85%). Nine patients (16%) reported neonatal cholestatic jaundice. At the time of diagnosis, 33 patients (59%) had already had a lens extraction because of cataract and an additional 16 patients (29%) were diagnosed with cataract. Ten patients needed lens extraction during follow-up, in 3 patients cataract resolved during CDCA treatment. Tendon xanthomas were present in 19 patients (34%), at follow-up in 21 patients (38%). Neurologic symptoms were less common in patients diagnosed and treated before the age of 24 years, 25% vs. 88% in those treated after the age of 24, with pyramidal and cerebellar symptoms as the most common neurologic features. Intellectual disability was seen in 50% of patients diagnosed and treated before the age of 24 and in 78% of patients diagnosed and treated after the age of 24. Psychiatric manifestations consisted of mysophobia, hypochondria, mania, depression, functional disorder, frontal disturbances, attention-deficit/hyperactivity disorder, autism spectrum disorder, and obsessive-compulsive disorder.

Neurologic manifestations (epilepsy, pyramidal signs, and cerebellar signs) completely disappeared in all patients ($n = 5$) diagnosed and treated before the age of 24 when considering only patients with good treatment adherence ($n = 43$). Moreover, none of these patients developed new neurologic symptoms during follow-up. Intellectual disability stabilized or improved in 100% of patients in this group, and psychiatric manifestations stabilized or improved in 89% of patients. In patients diagnosed and treated after the age of 24, neurologic symptoms deteriorated in 61% of patients, with parkinsonism as a treatment-resistant feature. In the patients with mRS and EDSS scores at baseline and last clinical visit, and good treatment adherence, there was an improvement or stabilization in favor of patients diagnosed and treated before the age of 24: 100% in patients <24 years vs. 58% in patients ≥24 years for mRS scores and 100% vs. 50%, respectively, for EDSS scores (Fig. 17.2).

In conclusion, treatment start at an early age can reverse or even prevent development of neurologic symptoms in CTX, emphasizing the importance of early diagnosis in CTX. Early treatment start changes the disease course in a positive way, alleviating both the systemic and neurological symptoms of CTX.

In 1994, the first study was published describing MRI findings in CTX patients prior to and upon treatment with CDCA [25]. They found no significant changes on repeated brain MRI after 2–3 years of treatment with CDCA in 11 patients despite neurological and biochemical improvement. Another study described repeat MRI after 4 years with no change in a patient who had shown some neurological deterioration, despite treatment [30]. In another study [31], brain MRI was repeated after 2–5 years CDCA therapy in 7 out of 24 patients, with stable findings on imaging. A study describing MRI findings in 16 CTX patients with a follow-up time of 24–48 months showed that cerebellar white matter alterations correlated with

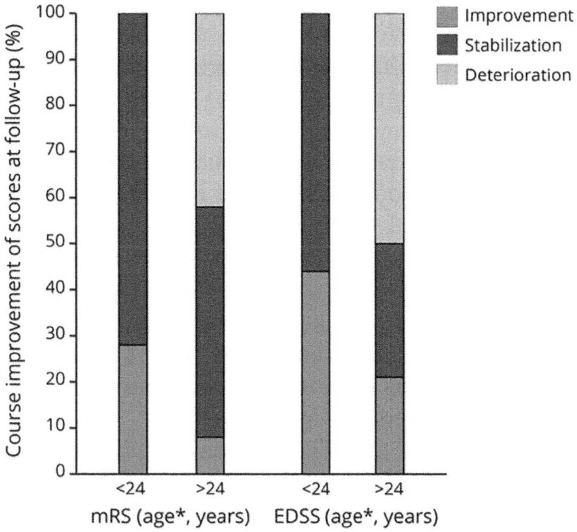

Fig. 17.2 Course (improvement, stabilization, or deterioration) of mRS and EDSS scores at follow-up (%). EDSS = Expanded Disability Status Scale. mRS = modified Rankin Scale. * Age at diagnosis and treatment start

neurological progression. The presence of cerebellar vacuolation was thereby suggested as marker for disease progression and lack of therapy response [32]. In patients who suffer from neurological symptomatology and abnormalities on brain MRI at diagnosis, the effect of therapy on clinical and radiological progression is minimal [33]. The six patients described by Mignarri et al. [32] with cerebellar vacuolation at baseline were patients aged 32, 33, 40, 45, 46, and 54 years, at time of diagnosis. Possibly, the relatively late age of diagnosis and, consequently, late start of treatment may have played a role in the therapy resistance of these patients. Mignarri et al. [32] also suggested that the absence of signal abnormalities of the dentate nuclei at baseline should be considered as an indicator of better prognosis.

Long-Term MRI Findings in Cerebrotendinous Xanthomatosis, the Dutch Cohort Study [29]

Early treatment start changes the disease course in a positive way, as seen in different studies. There are several case reports/series published on brain MRI findings in CTX, but with only a limited follow-up time of maximally 6 years. In 12 patients, brain MRI findings of patients were reviewed before start of treatment and after a follow-up time ranging from 7 to 27 years on CDCA therapy. In all patients, the diagnosis of CTX was biochemically and genetically confirmed, and CDCA treatment was started directly after the diagnosis. The presence of cortical and cerebellar atrophy, abnormalities in the periventricular white matter, basal ganglia, brainstem, cerebellar white matter, and dentate nuclei (hyperintensity, calcification, and vacuolation) were scored, with a maximum total score of 9 (1 point each).

As described earlier, patients diagnosed and treated before the age of 24 have a significantly better clinical outcome after follow-up than patients diagnosed at a later age. Therefore, this age was used as a cutoff to compare patients regarding MRI findings at long-term follow-up [27]. MRI abnormalities showed progression in all 7 patients diagnosed at 24 years or older, and only in 1 out of 5 patients diagnosed before the age of 24 years (Fig. 17.3). In this last patient, MRI at baseline already showed minor cerebellar atrophy and cerebral/periventricular hyperintensities. MRI in the other 4 patients diagnosed before the age of 24 years were normal at baseline, and remained normal even after follow-up of more than 25 years. At baseline, the total MRI score was 2 in the group of patients diagnosed before the age of 24 years, and 19 in the group of patients diagnosed at 24 years or older. At follow-up, these scores were 4 and 37, respectively. At diagnosis, 5 out of 7 patients diagnosed at 24 years or older had dentate nuclei hyperintensity on brain MRI, but at follow-up, this hyperintensity was observed in all 7 patients. Patients with cerebellar vacuolation on MR imaging at baseline showed evident progression of mRS and EDSS scores at follow-up.

In conclusion, early start of adequate treatment prevents brain MRI abnormalities in adult life in CTX. In addition to the age at which treatment is started, the absence or extent of dentate nuclei signal abnormalities at diagnosis seems to be an additional prognostic marker in CTX.

Data reported from two retrospective cohort studies conducted in the Netherlands and Italy show that CDCA is effective at reducing cholestanol levels and stabilizing or improving the progression of disability in the long-term treatment of CTX, with an acceptable safety profile [34]. In CTX patients, CDCA treatment does not always result in reversing (most of) the neurological deficits. Nonstructural "issues" like epilepsy or metabolic encephalopathy can reverse relative quickly, but structural lesions, may be beyond "the point of no return." In adult CTX patients, cholestanol and cholesterol containing crystal clefts within the brain can be found, with neuronal loss and demyelination [5]. It is not expected that these structural lesions will resolve after CDCA treatment start. When there is severe tissue damage and

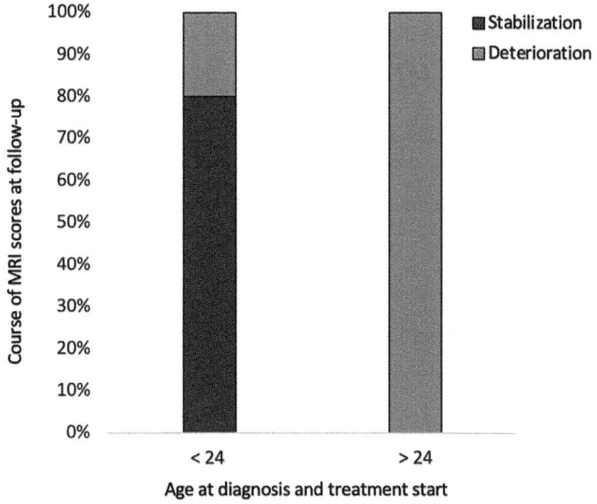

Fig. 17.3 Course of MRI scores (stabilization or deterioration) at follow-up correlated with age at diagnosis and treatment start (<24 years $n = 5$, ≥24 years $n = 7$)

significant cerebral atrophy, reversibility upon treatment is less likely. Some patients experience progression of neurological deficits, despite normalization of serum cholestanol levels, during follow-up, suggestive of ongoing neurodegeneration. In CTX, there might be a "point of no return" regarding the onset of neurological deterioration, emphasizing the importance of early diagnosis in CTX and treatment start.

References

1. Cali JJ, Hsieh CL, Francke U, Russell DW. Mutations in the bile acid biosynthetic enzyme sterol 27-hydroxylase underlie cerebrotendinous xanthomatosis. J Biol Chem. 1991;266(12):7779–83.
2. Björkhem I, Hansson M. Cerebrotendinous xanthomatosis: an inborn error in bile acid synthesis with defined mutations but still a challenge. Biochem Biophys Res Commun. 2010;396(1):46–9.
3. Panzenboeck U, Andersson U, Hansson M, Sattler W, Meaney S, Björkhem I. On the mechanism of cerebral accumulation of cholestanol in patients with cerebrotendinous xanthomatosis. J Lipid Res. 2007;48(5):1167–74.
4. Bhattacharyya AK, Lin DS, Conner WE. Cholestanol metabolism in patients with cerebrotendinous xanthomatosis: absorption, turnover, and tissue deposition. J Lipid Res. 2007;48(1):185–92.
5. Verrips A, Hoefsloot LH, Steenbergen GC, et al. Clinical and molecular genetic characteristics of patients with cerebrotendinous xanthomatosis. Brain. 2000;123(Pt 5):908–19.
6. Pilo-de-la-Fuente B, Jimenez-Escrig A, Lorenzo JR, et al. Cerebrotendinous xanthomatosis in Spain: clinical, prognostic, and genetic survey. Eur J Neurol. 2011;18(10):1203–11.
7. Verrips A, van Engelen BG, Wevers RA, et al. Presence of diarrhea and absence of tendon xanthomas in patients with cerebrotendinous xanthomatosis. Arch Neurol. 2000;57(4):520–4.
8. Mignarri A, Gallus GN, Dotti MT, Federico A. A suspicion index for early diagnosis and treatment of cerebrotendinous xanthomatosis. J Inherit Metab Dis. 2014;37(3):421–9.
9. Salen G, Meriwether TW, Nicolau G. Chenodeoxycholic acid inhibits increased cholesterol and cholestanol synthesis in patients with cerebrotendinous xanthomatosis. Biochem Med. 1975;14(1):57–74.
10. Berginer VM, Salen G, Shefer S. Long-term treatment of cerebrotendinous xanthomatosis with chenodeoxycholic acid. N Engl J Med. 1984;311(26):1649–52.
11. Van Heijst AF, Verrips A, Wevers RA, Cruysberg JR, Renier WO, Tolboom JJ. Treatment and follow-up of children with cerebrotendinous xanthomatosis. Eur J Pediatr. 1998;157(4):313–6.
12. Mandia D, Chaussenot A, Besson G, et al. Cholic acid as a treatment for cerebrotendinous xanthomatosis in adults. J Neurol. 2019;266(8):2043–50.
13. Duell PB, Salen G, Eichler FS, et al. Diagnosis, treatment, and clinical outcomes in 43 cases with cerebrotendinous xanthomatosis. J Clin Lipidol. 2018;12(5):1169–78.
14. Waterreus RJ, Koopman BJ, Wolthers BG, Oosterhuis HJ. Cerebrotendinous xanthomatosis (CTX): a clinical survey of the patient population in The Netherlands. Clin Neurol Neurosurg. 1987;89(3):169–75.
15. Huidekoper HH, Vaz FM, Verrips A, Bosch AM. Hepatotoxicity due to chenodeoxycholic acid supplementation in an infant with cerebrotendinous xanthomatosis: implications for treatment. Eur J Pediatr. 2016;175(1):143–6.
16. Pierre G, Setchell K, Blyth J, Preece MA, Chakrapani A, McKiernan P. Prospective treatment of cerebrotendinous xanthomatosis with cholic therapy. J Inherit Metab Dis. 2008;31(Suppl 2):S241–5.
17. Koopman BJ, Wolthers BG, van der Molen JC, Waterreus RJ. Bile acid therapies applied to patients suffering from cerebrotendinous xanthomatosis. Clin Chim Acta. 1985;152(1–2):115–22.

18. Mignarri A, Rossi S, Ballerini M, et al. Clinical relevance and neurophysiological correlates of spasticity in cerebrotendinous xanthomatosis. J Neurol. 2011;258(5):783–90.
19. Yahalom G, Tsabari R, Molshatzki N, Ephraty L, Cohen H, Hassin-Baer S. Neurological outcome in cerebrotendinous xanthomatosis treated with chenodeoxycholic acid: early versus late diagnosis. Clin Neuropharmacol. 2013;36(3):78–83.
20. Ginanneschi F, Mignarri A, Mondelli M, et al. Polyneuropathy in cerebrotendinous xanthomatosis and response to treatment with chenodeoxycholic acid. J Neurol. 2013;260(1):268–74.
21. Berginer VM, Gross B, Morad K, et al. Chronic diarrhea and juvenile cataracts: think cerebrotendinous xanthomatosis and treat. Pediatrics. 2009;123(1):143–7.
22. Mondelli M, Sicurelli F, Scarpini C, Dottit MT, Federico A. Cerebrotendinous xanthomatosis: 11-year treatment with chenodeoxycholic acid in five patients. An electrophysiological study. J Neurol Sci. 2001;190(1–2):29–33.
23. Luyckx E, Eyskens F, Simons A, Beckx K, Van West D, Dhar M. Long-term follow-up on the effect of combined therapy of bile acids and statins in the treatment of cerebrotendinous xanthomatosis: a case report. Clin Neurol Neurosurg. 2014;118:9–11.
24. Bonnot O, Fraidakis MJ, Lucanto R, et al. Cerebrotendinous xanthomatosis presenting with severe externalized disorder: improvement after one year of treatment with chenodeoxycholic acid. CNS Spectr. 2010;15(4):231–6.
25. Berginer VM, Berginer J, Korczyn AD, Tadmor R. Magnetic resonance imaging in cerebrotendinous xanthomatosis: a prospective clinical and neuroradiological study. J Neurol Sci. 1994;122(1):102–8.
26. Zubarioglu T, Kiykim E, Yesil G, et al. Early diagnosed cerebrotendinous xanthomatosis patients: clinical, neuroradiological characteristics and therapy results of a single center from Turkey. Acta Neurol Belg. 2019;119(3):343–50.
27. Nakamura T, Matsuzawa Y, Takemura K, Kubo M, Miki H, Tarui S. Combined treatment with chenodeoxycholic acid and pravastatin improves plasma cholestanol levels associated with marked regression of tendon xanthomas in cerebrotendinous xanthomatosis. Metabolism. 1991;40(7):741–6.
28. Stelten BML, Huidekoper HH, van de Warrenburg BPC, et al. Long-term treatment effect in cerebrotendinous xanthomatosis depends on age at treatment start. Neurology. 2019;92(2):e83–95.
29. Stelten BML, Lycklama À, Nijeholt GJ, et al. Long-term MRI findings in patients with cerebrotendinous xanthomatosis treated with chenodeoxycholic acid. Neurology. 2002;99(13):559–66.
30. Chakraverty S, Griffiths PD, Walls TJ, McAllister VL. Cerebrotendinous xanthomatosis in two sisters: case reports and MR imaging. Clin Radiol. 1995;50(2):117–9.
31. Barkhof F, Verrips A, Wesseling P, et al. Cerebrotendinous xanthomatosis: the spectrum of imaging findings and the correlation with neuropathologic findings. Radiology. 2000;217(3):869–76.
32. Mignarri A, Dotti MT, Federico A, et al. The spectrum of magnetic resonance findings in cerebrotendinous xanthomatosis: redefinition and evidence of new markers of disease progression. J Neurol. 2017;264(5):862–74.
33. Mignarri A, Dotti MT, Del Puppo M, et al. Cerebrotendinous xanthomatosis with progressive cerebellar vacuolation: six-year MRI follow-up. Neuroradiology. 2012;54(6):649–51.
34. Verrips A, Dotti MT, Mignarri A, et al. The safety and effectiveness of chenodeoxycholic acid treatment in patients with cerebrotendinous xanthomatosis: two retrospective cohort studies. Neurol Sci. 2020;41(4):943–9.

18 Lessons Taken from the Israeli Cerebrotendinous Xanthomatosis (CTX) Cohort: Can We Improve Outcomes?

Sharon Hassin-Baer and Hofit Cohen

Introduction

1981–2013

The first international publication on CTX from Israel was that by Berginer and Abeliovich in 1981, where they described six patients (from three families) affected with CTX, which were Sephardic Jews of Moroccan origin. They suspected that this ethnic subgroup of Jews from Jewish North African (NA) descent had a high prevalence of genetic variants in the CTX gene and estimated it to be as common as 1/108 [1]. Furthermore, they recommended that cholestanol levels be determined in cases of undiagnosed cataracts or tendinous xanthomas in childhood or early adolescence and stressed the importance of diagnosis and genetic counseling, in view of possible treatment.

In the following years, variable disease-related features and laboratory findings were described in this population, within several manuscripts, including the identification of three distinct genetic variants in the *CYP27A1* gene in the Jewish NA population [2–8]. In 1984, Berginer and colleagues described the clinical and biochemical outcomes of CDCA treatment in 17 of the Israeli patients that were treated

S. Hassin-Baer (✉)
The Movement Disorders Institute and Department of Neurology, Sheba Medical Center, Ramat Gan, Israel

The Gray Faculty of Health and Medical Studies, Tel Aviv University, Tel Aviv, Israel
e-mail: shassin@tauex.tau.ac.il

H. Cohen
The Gray Faculty of Health and Medical Studies, Tel Aviv University, Tel Aviv, Israel

The Bert W. Strassburger Metabolic Center, Sheba Medical Center, Ramat Gan, Israel

A. Federico et al. (eds.), *Cerebrotendinous Xanthomatosis*,
https://doi.org/10.1007/978-3-031-92526-9_18

at least 1 year, and up to 11 years, concluding that long-term CDCA therapy may correct the biochemical abnormalities and arrest and possibly reverse the progression of CTX [9].

2013–2024

Thirty years later, in 2013, we presented the characteristics and outcomes of 18 Israeli Jewish CTX patients (10 males) representing 11 families (6 of them consanguineous), that were followed up from 2003 to 2012 at the Movement Disorders Institute at Sheba Medical Center (SMDI). Their mean age at evaluation was 35.0 ± 9.2 years, and the mean duration of CDCA treatment was 12.2 ± 6.4 years, up to 23 years. Neurological impairment and ambulation as well as educational and psychosocial outcomes were studied. We found that age at CDCA treatment initiation was the most important factor affecting outcome, and the age of 25 years was determined as a critical age after which patients had a significantly worse neurological and thus outcome. Moreover, we discovered that adherence to therapy was likewise important for a better prognosis [10].

We emphasized the importance of early diagnosis and treatment with CDCA along with patient monitoring and recommended that CTX be included in regular premarital counseling in high-risk populations, focusing on Jews of NA origin. We advised to expand the knowledge of physicians on CTX, through lectures as well as articles in Israeli general medical journals, to increase awareness of the complex of features associated with CTX, including diarrhea, failure to thrive, seizures, intellectual and learning disabilities, cataracts, and tendon xanthomas to be able to reach the diagnosis of a treatable neurometabolic disorder CTX as early as possible.

As of 2024, three patients have died, yet our sample of CTX patients has nearly doubled as several additional patients joined follow-up at the SMDI.

We have become aware of cases of autism spectrum disorders (ASD) associated with CTX, as we have five that have been diagnosed and an additional two suspected. Many of the remaining have been challenged with learning disabilities.

All our patients are treated regularly with CDCA and generally, at present we are impressed by good compliance for most of them; we rarely see further deterioration in the neurological condition, after starting CDCA. This is exclusive to a minority that were diagnosed at a late age, (over 20) some of which continued to slowly deteriorate.

Features of the Metabolic Syndrome and Subclinical atherosclerosis in CTX

There is a well-described high prevalence of vascular changes in CTX [11]; however, the exact mechanism leading to early onset arteriosclerosis is unknown [12]. We evaluated the potential metabolic abnormalities and preclinical vascular changes in Israeli CTX patients in ten young subjects, five males and five females aged

32.7 ± 6.7 years. Risk factors for cardiovascular disease and features of metabolic syndrome were present in all the patients, and in three patients, carotid intima media thickness was higher compared to control subjects. We concluded that assessment for cardiovascular risk factors and premature vascular changes should be implemented with other preventive measures to reduce the risk of atherosclerotic cardiovascular disease in CTX patients [13].

Patients with a recent diagnosis of CTX, delayed despite early and typical presentations

It is worth focusing on three female patients that were recently diagnosed with CTX after presenting with neurological symptoms.

The first was a 24-year-old woman of Soviet Christian origin that had prolonged neonatal jaundice, recovered and developed attention deficit/hyperactivity disorder (ADHD) during childhood, as well as juvenile cataract, and tendon xanthomas. At 20 years, she complained of recurrent dizziness and anxiety and at age 22 years started complaining of walking difficulty and falls. She was found to have mild spastic paraparesis. Brain and spinal MRI were normal. A multi-gene panel including 81 genes recognized as causing hereditary spastic paraplegia (HSP) was negative but whole exome sequencing was positive for two pathogenic *CYP27A1* gene variants, c.1183C > G and c.1184G > A and thus the diagnosis of CTX was confirmed.

Another female patient of Iraqi-Ashkenazi descent presented at the age of 27 years at our clinic. She was reported to have a short phase of neonatal jaundice and normal development throughout childhood, a lifetime history of soft stools and underweight (body mass index of 14 at presentation), severe myopia, and danced as a hobby. At the age of 23 years, she noticed weakness in her legs and stopped dancing and exercising. Two years later, she felt some weakness in her arms. She had no sphincteric complaints. She was first seen by a neurologist at age 26 years who found bilateral pyramidal signs and referred her for general blood tests, and total spinal and brain MRI. She was initially suspected to have a thoracic spinal epidural arteriovenous fistula, which was ruled out by angiography. Her brain MRI was defined as normal. She was then sent for genetic work-up including whole exome sequencing and spastic paraplegia gene panel. She was found to have two nonsense genetic variants in the *CYP27A1* gene, c.446 + 1G > A and c.461G > A. Her plasma cholestanol level was 15.6 mcg/ml. and upon revision of the MRI pathological signals of the dentate nuclei were seen. Ophthalmological examination revealed bilateral cataracts.

The third patient was 25-year-old single woman 10-weeks-pregnant, of Jewish Ashkenazi-Tunisian origin. She had intermittent diarrhea since infancy, which continued all her life. The gastroenterologist work-up turned negative and she was diagnosed with irritable bowel syndrome. Furthermore, she had significant learning difficulties and was diagnosed with ADHD. She underwent two episodes of generalized tonic-clonic seizures, one at age 11 years and one at age 18 years and was diagnosed with photosensitive epilepsy and not treated. At the age of 14 years, following complaining of visual loss, bilateral cataracts were found and bilateral extracapsular cataract extraction (ECCE) was performed. At the age of 24 years, she noticed an action tremor in her right hand. An extramarital pregnancy led to the performance of an expanded carrier screening (ECS) to determine the risk of passing on 150–300 or more genetic diseases. She was found to carry two nonsense genetic variants in the *CYP27A1* gene (c.8451G > A and c.1016C > T), confirming the diagnosis of CTX. Upon examination at our clinic, she had thickened Achilles tendons, but no xanthomas and her neurological examination was unremarkable except for slight right upper limb postural tremor and hypokinesia. Her plasma cholestanol level was 15.95 mcg/ml and subsequent to the consultation, she started CDCA 250 mg TID.

All three women had typical symptoms of CTX but were not suspected clinically to have a bile acid disorder. It was whole exome sequencing that led to the diagnosis of CTX.

Extended Family Presentations

We recently encountered two families, with multiple affected children, that were eventually diagnosed with CTX. The first, of Moroccan Jewish origin, consists of three affected siblings (diagnosed at 13 years, 10 years, and 8 years); all carried a homozygous c.845-1G > A *CYP27A1* genetic variant, and baseline cholestanol levels ranged between 17.4 and 39.7 mcg/ml.

The eldest, who suffered from neonatal jaundice and chronic diarrhea, showed significant developmental delay, and was diagnosed with low-functioning ASD at 1.5 years. He never acquired language and has severe behavioral difficulties. Cataract was diagnosed only at the age of 13 years, after his younger brother (known to have emotional problems) was diagnosed with cataract at 8 years. The third child (female) had high-functioning ASD, mild learning difficulties and epilepsy from the age of 5 years which resolved prior to the CTX diagnosis and treatment. Since diagnosis, all children are treated with CDCA, starting at 5 mg/kg/day TID and continuing dose adjustment with normalization of cholestanol level leading to resolution of diarrhea and no further deterioration.

The second family of Moroccan and Libyan Jewish origin consists of six siblings, with four males diagnosed with CTX at ages 15 years, 12 years, 9 years, and 7 years, all being compound heterozygous to the c.845-1G > A and c.1016C > T genetic variants. Baseline cholestanol levels ranged between 30.9 and 40.6 mcg/ml. The genetic investigation was made 3 years after the diagnosis of cataract in the third affected sibling when the first affected child was 15 years. All affected siblings had cataract (three were operated on) and chronic diarrhea. The eldest affected child also had neonatal jaundice, and over the years, emotional and academic difficulties, later diagnosed with ADHD, anxiety, and had several tendon xanthomas removed. The second affected child was diagnosed at the age of 12 years, had neonatal jaundice, a single episode of febrile convulsions (at the age of 5 years), had tendon xanthomas and was diagnosed with high-functioning ASD. The third affected sibling, the one whose cataract diagnosis led to the genetic investigations, was also diagnosed with ADHD, and suffered from anxiety. The youngest affected sibling also has a diagnosis of high-functioning ASD, anxiety, emotional difficulties, and xanthomas. Since diagnosis, these children have also been treated with CDCA, with similar dose adjustments resulting in normalization of cholestanol levels, resolution of diarrhea, and no further deterioration.

In these two families of Jewish NA descent, with seven siblings manifesting prominent key features of CTX, the diagnostic process was delayed by several years, due to insufficient awareness of CTX by several pediatric medical disciplines. These include general pediatricians, pediatric gastroenterologists, pediatric neurologists, ophthalmologists, and sometimes additional disciplines such as orthopedics and more.

We would like to stress several points regarding these families: Initiation of treatment prior to the onset of clinical symptoms, in the younger asymptomatic siblings of diagnosed patients, may have been effective in preventing the onset of clinical symptoms and irreversible pathology. Genetic screening of juvenile cataract patients, including sequencing of the *CYP27A1* gene, should be performed regularly.

Ignoring or missing the diagnosis in a young adult with a typical medical history, before the degenerative phase of the disease, may result in spinocerebellar degeneration, Parkinsonism, and a cognitive deterioration leading to dementia. Better outcomes for CTX patients depend on the age of diagnosis and initiation of CDCA treatment, the availability of CDCA, adherence to CDCA treatment that is closely related to psychiatric wellbeing, continued patient monitoring, and familial support.

Multidisciplinary CTX Clinic

We recommend the unique model of a specialized multidisciplinary clinic for the best care of patients diagnosed with CTX. The SMDI serves as such a specialty center for CTX. Our clinic consists of combined neurological and a metabolic-endocrine assessment. We invite our patients to an annual follow-up at Sheba Medical Center, for providing support and education, monitoring of the adherence to treatment and laboratory evaluation, and ancillary testing for complications such as those related to enhanced atherosclerosis, osteoporosis, and more.

At the annual visit, a full neurological interview and examination are performed, along with an overview of annual lab testing including cholestanol levels, lipid panel, and bone metabolism assessment.

General Prevention and Early Diagnosis in Israel

We recommend implementing screening for bile acid disorders or CTX in the newborn screening program that is available in Israel, along with premarital genetic counseling and testing in the relevant ethnic groups of NA Jews and the Druze community in Israel.

Summary

We recognize two phases in life for the opportunity to diagnose CTX:

1. Infancy-childhood—those suffering from chronic diarrhea, learning difficulties, intellectual disability, or ASD and possibly seizures and juvenile cataracts.
2. Young adulthood—young adults, with prior history consisting of some or all symptoms above, that develop slowly progressive spastic paraparesis and/or cerebellar ataxia.

Missing the opportunity to diagnose of CTX at an early stage is tragic and results in a range of irreversible intellectual and behavioral impairments. A newborn screening program is the only way to diagnose as early as possible and is justified.

Moreover, the earliest diagnosis of CTX can be achieved by newborn screening programs using dried blood spots and should be applied, if not to all newborns, then to populations in which there is a high carriership of pathogenic *CYP27A1* genetic variants, such as Jews of NA origin and the Druze community.

References

1. Berginer VM, Abeliovich D. Genetics of cerebrotendinous xanthomatosis (CTX): an autosomal recessive trait with high gene frequency in Sephardim of Moroccan origin. Am J Med Genet. 1981;10(2):151–7. https://doi.org/10.1002/ajmg.1320100209.
2. Berginer VM, Foster NL, Sadowsky M, Townsend JA 3rd, Siegel GJ, Salen G. Psychiatric disorders in patients with cerebrotendinous xanthomatosis. Am J Psychiatry. 1988 Mar;145(3):354–7. https://doi.org/10.1176/ajp.145.3.354.
3. Berginer VM, Shany S, Alkalay D, Berginer J, Dekel S, Salen G, Tint GS, Gazit D. Osteoporosis and increased bone fractures in cerebrotendinous xanthomatosis. Metabolism. 1993 Jan;42(1):69–74. https://doi.org/10.1016/0026-0495(93)90174-m.
4. Berginer VM, Berginer J, Korczyn AD, Tadmor R. Magnetic resonance imaging in cerebrotendinous xanthomatosis: a prospective clinical and neuroradiological study. J Neurol Sci. 1994 Mar;122(1):102–8. https://doi.org/10.1016/0022-510x(94)90059-0.
5. Leitersdorf E, Reshef A, Meiner V, Levitzki R, Schwartz SP, Dann EJ, Berkman N, Cali JJ, Klapholz L, Berginer VM. Frameshift and splice-junction mutations in the sterol 27-hydroxylase gene cause cerebrotendinous xanthomatosis in Jews or Moroccan origin. J Clin Invest 1993 Jun;91(6):2488–2496. https://doi.org/10.1172/JCI116484. PMID: 8514861; PMCID: PMC443309.
6. Meiner V, Marais DA, Reshef A, Björkhem I, Leitersdorf E. Premature termination codon at the sterol 27-hydroxylase gene causes cerebrotendinous xanthomatosis in an Afrikaner family. Hum Mol Genet. 1994 Jan;3(1):193–4. https://doi.org/10.1093/hmg/3.1.193.
7. Meiner V, Meiner Z, Reshef A, Björkhem I, Leitersdorf E. Cerebrotendinous xanthomatosis: molecular diagnosis enables presymptomatic detection of a treatable disease. Neurology. 1994 Feb;44(2):288–90. https://doi.org/10.1212/wnl.44.2.288.
8. Reshef A, Meiner V, Berginer VM, Leitersdorf E. Molecular genetics of cerebrotendinous xanthomatosis in Jews of north African origin. J Lipid Res. 1994 Mar;35(3):478–83.
9. Berginer VM, Salen G, Shefer S. Long-term treatment of cerebrotendinous xanthomatosis with chenodeoxycholic acid. N Engl J Med. 1984 Dec 27;311(26):1649–52. https://doi.org/10.1056/NEJM198412273112601.

10. Yahalom G, Tsabari R, Molshatzki N, Ephraty L, Cohen H, Hassin-Baer S. Neurological outcome in cerebrotendinous xanthomatosis treated with chenodeoxycholic acid: early versus late diagnosis. Clin Neuropharmacol. 2013 May-Jun;36(3):78–83. https://doi.org/10.1097/WNF.0b013e318288076a.
11. Kuriyama M, Fujiyama J, Yoshidome H, Takenaga S, Matsumuro K, Kasama T, et al. Cerebrotendinous xanthomatosis: clinical and biochemical evaluation of eight patients and review of the literature. J Neurol Sci. 1991;102:225–32. https://doi.org/10.1016/0022-510x(91)90073-g.
12. Björkhem I, Boberg KM. In: Scriver CR, editor. In inborn errors in bile acid biosynthesis and storage of sterols other than cholesterol. The metabolic basis of inherited disease. 7th ed. New York, NY: McGraw-Hill; 1998. p. 2073–209.
13. Cohen H, Hassin-Baer S, Shaish A. Features of the metabolic syndrome and subclinical atherosclerosis in patients with cerebrotendinous xanthomatosis: an augmented risk for premature cardiovascular disease. Front Genet 2022 Sep 27;13:997069. https://doi.org/10.3389/fgene.2022.997069. PMID: 36238157; PMCID: PMC9550927.

Treatment During Pregnancy in Women with Cerebrotendinous Xanthomatosis (CTX)

19

Aviv Mesika and Tzipora C. Falik-Zaccai

Clinical Presentation of Cerebrotendinous Xanthomatosis (CTX)

Cerebrotendinous xanthomatosis (CTX) is a rare autosomal recessive disorder of bile acid synthesis caused by biallelic pathogenic variants in *CYP27A1* [1]. *CYP27A1* encoding for sterol 27-hydroxylase is one of the crucial enzymes in the cholic acid (CA) and chenodeoxycholic acid (CDCA) synthesis pathways. Impaired production of the sterol 27-hydroxylase enzyme leads to accumulation of cholestanol and C_{27} bile alcohols in the blood and in urine, respectively [2]. Moreover, CTX is associated with abnormally high levels and accumulation of cholestanol and cholesterol in the brain, tendon and bile [3]. The early clinical symptoms of CTX present during infancy and include chronic diarrhea and failure to thrive, followed by childhood or adolescence cataracts and a further progressive disease course with neurological deterioration and potentially debilitation and death [4]. Additional clinical features include learning disabilities and cognitive impairment which become evident in childhood, while premature bilateral cataracts frequently present in childhood or adolescence [5]. Tendon xanthomas and a wide spectrum of neurological symptoms develop in the second and third decades of life [6]. The main neurologic dysfunctions seen in CTX patients are learning impairment, memory loss, cognitive impairment, seizures, dementia, and cerebellar and extrapyramidal dysfunctions which are reported typically in the second and third decades of life, resulting in death in the fifth or sixth decade of life if the condition goes undiagnosed and untreated [4]. CTX is a rare disorder, which is most probably underdiagnosed, as presenting non-specific variable signs and symptoms, and marked phenotype variability with regard to its severity and age of onset, overlap with common pathological conditions [7].

A. Mesika · T. C. Falik-Zaccai (✉)
Azrieli Faculty of Medicine, Bar Ilan University, Safed, Israel

A. Federico et al. (eds.), *Cerebrotendinous Xanthomatosis*,
https://doi.org/10.1007/978-3-031-92526-9_19

The Standard of Care

Chenodeoxycholic acid (CDCA; chenodiol) is the current standard of care in the treatment of CTX [7]. Since CDCA is one of the final metabolites of the bile acid synthesis, routine administration of CDCA helps to restore normal sterols, bile acids, bile alcohols, and cholestanol levels in CTX patients [1]. CDCA also appears to be generally effective in preventing adverse clinical manifestations of the disease from occurring or progressing if administered early enough. Studies have provided supportive evidence for the benefits of long-term therapy with CDCA in order to correct the biochemical abnormalities and arrest or possibly reverse the progression of CTX [8]. Berginer et al. described the long-term effects of CDCA (750 mg per day) in patients with CTX [8]. The CDCA treatment improved the major neurological symptoms in symptomatic patients that included dementia, pyramidal and cerebellar signs, and peripheral neuropathy. Concomitantly, mean plasma cholestanol levels declined threefold, and abnormal bile acid synthesis was suppressed. Moreover, Stelten et al. emphasize the importance of early diagnosis in CTX and provide a rationale to include CTX in newborn screening programs, since treatment started at an early age can reverse and even prevent the development of neurologic symptoms in CTX [9].

CDCA is currently contraindicated for use during pregnancy based on non-CTX animal studies that showed fetal hepatotoxicity and sometimes lethality of healthy baboon, rats, and rhesus monkey fetuses of healthy mothers who were treated with very high doses of CDCA [2]. However, discontinuation of CDCA in pregnancy can be harmful for the mother and potentially the fetus as well [2, 10].

Animal Studies of CDCA Treatment During Pregnancy

Previous animal studies have reported severe warning of possible toxic hazards to human fetuses when the pregnant mother is treated with CDCA. Heywood et al. demonstrated that oral CDCA administration in three dosages of 120 mg/kg/day, reduced to 90 mg/kg/day, and to 60 mg/kg/day, (4–6 times the maximum recommended human dose (MRHD)) to groups of pregnant rhesus monkeys (Macaca mulatta) causes dilatation of the central veins in the hepatic lobules with varying degrees of hepatic-cell necrosis, adrenal extensive hemorrhagic cortical necrosis, and renal interstitial hemorrhage associated with varying degrees of renal vascular dilatation [11]. Additional evidence for the hepatotoxicity of CDCA in primates' pregnant animals was reported by McSherry et al. who showed liver injury induced by CDCA administration in pregnant and neonatal baboons (dosage levels of 0.5 mg/ml CDCA dissolve in ethanol) [12]. In the case of rats, Sprinkle et al. demonstrated that neonates of CDCA fed (0.25% level in the diet from Day 11 of gestation) mothers have a significantly greater pool of CDCA in the bile acids and liver, suggesting maternal-to-fetal transfer of dihydroxy bile acids [13]. Neonatal cholesterol-7α-hydroxylase activity and total tissue bile acid pools were not significantly altered by the increased pool of CDCA, and no hepatotoxic effects on rats maternal, neonatal, and postnatal livers were evident with gestational feeding of CDCA [13].

Regarding teratogenicity, several studies reported that CDCA was not teratogenic or carcinogenic in mice and rats when administered at dosages comparable to those used in humans, although dose-related hepatotoxicity was observed in pregnant rats and lead to embryonic lethality in rats after administration of 120 mg/kg/day CDCA (8 times the MRHD) [14–16]. A possible explanation of hepatotoxicity in the primates' pregnant animals that were fed with CDCA suggests that this phenomenon was likely caused by the inability of the animals to remove excess lithocholic acid, CDCA's primary bacterial metabolite. This issue is not relevant in humans since in humans lithocholic acid is detoxified via formation of sulfate conjugates [17].

Should Women with CTX Continue to Be Treated During Pregnancy?

CDCA is designated by the FDA as pregnancy category X, with a warning that it may cause harm to the fetus [2]. However, as described above this designation is based on non-CTX animal studies with very high-dose CDCA supplementation, which may not be relevant to humans with CTX [2]. The FDA's designation and lack of human data regarding the safety of CDCA treatment for the developing fetus has caused uncertainty for pregnant women with CTX and their health care providers regarding whether CDCA treatment should be continued during pregnancy. We claim that withdrawal of CDCA treatment during pregnancy could not only lead to neurological deterioration of the mother, but it could also lead to the accumulation of cholestanol and C_{27} bile alcohols in the developing fetus [2]. Previous reports of pregnancies of mothers with untreated CTX have shown that complications, including fetal and infant death, appear to be more common [10, 18]. Of ten pregnancies to four untreated mothers with CTX, Yahalom et al. [18], reported two miscarriages in the first trimester and one term stillbirth in untreated mothers and concluded that beginning CDCA treatment as early as possible is crucial to preventing neurological damage and deterioration in CTX all patients and especially in pregnant women. After significant neurological pathology is established, the effect of treatment is limited and deterioration may continue [18]. Further evidence for the importance of continuing CDCA supplementation during pregnancies of CTX affected women is described by Berginer et al. who showed intellectual disability in two of 18 (11%) offspring born to nine untreated mothers with CTX, whereas 11 offspring of seven fathers with CTX showed no abnormalities. This suggests that in untreated CTX women an abnormal intrauterine environment for the developing fetuses might be created [10]. Placental transfer from the mother to fetus of elevated cholestanol and other CTX-associated metabolites, such as C_{27} bile alcohols, may occur which will be harmful to the developing fetus [6, 19]. An abnormal fetal environment from excess maternal cholestanol, bile acid precursors, and bile alcohols may not be alleviated by the immature and reduced sterol 27-hydroxylase activity of the fetus (i.e., an obligatory carrier for one pathogenic *CYP27A1* variant) [20]. A similar situation is seen in mothers with untreated phenylketonuria (PKU), where abnormally high levels of phenylalanine in pregnant women with PKU can affect fetal growth and development, and it is recommended that phenylalanine is monitored and maintained within the normal limits before and throughout the pregnancy [8]. Recently, Falik-Zaccai et al. reported the largest number of CDCA-treated pregnancies in women with CTX [2]. This study suggests that CDCA treatment during pregnancy may be safe for the developing fetus and that the benefits to both mother and fetus far outweigh the risks of CDCA exposure. The study reports 19 pregnancies and long-term offspring outcomes for nine mothers with CTX who were either treated with CDCA or untreated throughout pregnancy. Among 11 pregnancies in mothers who received CDCA treatment, no maternal side effects or complications related to CDCA treatment were reported. One mother was hospitalized with postpartum preeclampsia. However, no hospitalizations or other medical issues, including any related to abnormal liver function, were reported either in mothers or in the newborns. All newborns were born at or near full term, with normal birth weight, and Apgar scores. There was no evidence of hepatotoxicity or teratogenicity from CDCA exposure for the developing fetuses. For eight pregnancies where the mother did not receive CDCA treatment during pregnancy, one woman discontinued treatment at the start of her pregnancy and deteriorated neurologically during the pregnancy (SARA score going from 1.5 to 4 regarding her ataxia). She was not able to recover to her baseline before discontinuing CDCA treatment. Two newborns showed elevated bilirubin days after birth and one showed mixed expressive receptive language developmental disorder at 15 months that required speech and language therapy.

This underlines that discontinuing CDCA treatment during pregnancy may be harmful to the mother and to the developing fetus due to a potentially toxic intrauterine environment. These data support the benefit of continued CDCA treatment in pregnant women with CTX for both the affected women and their offspring.

Furthermore, Duell et al. have reported the experiences and perspectives of two women with CTX from the time of diagnosis through pregnancy and their decisions regarding CDCA treatment during pregnancy. Before becoming pregnant, both women were concerned about potential risks to their newborns if they continued or stopped CDCA treatment during pregnancy. Reassurance from their CTX specialist was the primary factor in their decision to continue treatment during pregnancy. The two pregnancies were complicated by preeclampsia; one gave birth to a healthy infant and the other gave birth to an infant that was later diagnosed with periventricular leukomalacia. Neither experienced CDCA-related complications [21].

Our Suggestion for Treatment of Pregnant Women with CTX

A recent modified Delphi study seeking expert consensus on CTX diagnosis, treatment, and disease management [22] reached 67% agreement with no disagreement with the following statement: research indicates that treating CTX mothers with

CDCA during pregnancy is an important mean of protection against damage to the fetus and miscarriage. This result together with our real-life data as presented in our recent paper [2] provides a basis for standardization of care and highlights key areas where further research is needed to inform best practices for the diagnosis, treatment, and management of patients with CTX [2, 22]. However, despite agreement among most experts, consensus was not reached. This is reflective of the limited data that were available at time of the study, regarding the safety and efficacy of CDCA exposure for the developing fetus. We would like to suggest that our recent publication adds very important information regarding the issues of treating pregnant women with CTX. Although more studies of pregnant women with CTX and their offspring are needed, the real-world data published recently [2, 21] should help physicians and patients make informed decisions about CDCA use during pregnancy in women with CTX and might facilitate revisitation of the category X designation for CDCA in pregnancy as suggested by Falik-Zaccai et al. [2]. Currently, the standard CDCA treatment protocol is 250 mg three times a day, in addition to monitoring the levels of the harmful metabolites in the blood and urine (cholestanol and bile alcohols). Current studies are looking for the identification of new biomarkers that will enable fine-tuning of the treatment regimen and the management of pregnant women with CTX.

Conclusions

Reluctance to administer CDCA to pregnant women with CTX has been present for many years and was based on studies in primate healthy animal models. Although these studies warned from the use of CDCA during pregnancy due to fetal hepatotoxicity and teratogenic effects, it has been shown that animals in these studies were given much higher doses of CDCA compared to the human standard dose of 750 mg per day, and that humans have a different metabolism than the studied animals that allows for the detoxification of the teratogenic metabolite lithocholic acid, which thus reduces the risk for any hepatotoxic and/or teratogenic effects of CDCA in human fetuses unlike what is the case in the studied animals. The real-world data recently published support the benefits of continued CDCA treatment in pregnant women with CTX for both the affected women and their offspring. Future studies need to focus on creating a standard protocol for CDCA treatment in CTX pregnant women. We suggest that Pharma companies should re-evaluate their recommendations according to the new data presented here to enable physicians and patients to make an informed decision regarding continuation of treatment during pregnancy.

References

1. Salen G, Steiner RD. Epidemiology, diagnosis, and treatment of cerebrotendinous xanthomatosis (CTX). J Inherit Metab Dis. 2017;40(6):771–81.
2. Falik-Zaccai TC, Hassin-Baer S, Cohen Kfir N, Duell PB, Neerhof M, Sloma R, et al. Chenodeoxycholic acid (CDCA) treatment during pregnancy in women with cerebrotendinous xanthomatosis (CTX): lessons learned from 19 pregnancies. Genet Med. 2024;26:101086.
3. Leitersdorf E, Safadi R, Meiner V, Reshef A, Björkhem I, Friedlander Y, et al. Cerebrotendinous xanthomatosis in the Israeli druze: molecular genetics and phenotypic characteristics. Am J Hum Genet. 1994;55(5):907–15.
4. Duell PB, Salen G, Eichler FS, DeBarber AE, Connor SL, Casaday L, et al. Diagnosis, treatment, and clinical outcomes in 43 cases with cerebrotendinous xanthomatosis. J Clin Lipidol. 2018;12(5):1169–78. https://doi.org/10.1016/j.jacl.2018.06.008.
5. Reshef A, Meiner V, Berginer VM, Leitersdorf E. Molecular genetics of cerebrotendinous xanthomatosis in Jews of North African origin. J Lipid Res 1994;35(3):478–483. Available from: https://doi.org/10.1016/S0022-2275(20)41198-8.
6. Swartz M, Burman KD, Salen G. Cerebrotendinous xanthomatosis: a cause of cataracts and tendon xanthoma. Am J Med Sci. 1982;283(3):147–52.
7. Mignarri A, Gallus GN, Dotti MT, Federico A. A suspicion index for early diagnosis and treatment of cerebrotendinous xanthomatosis. J Inherit Metab Dis. 2014;37(3):421–9.
8. Berginer VM, Salen G, Shefer S. Long-term treatment of cerebrotendinousxanthomatosis with chenodeoxycholic acid. N Engl J Med. 1984;311:1649–52. https://doi.org/10.1056/NEJM198412273112601 4.
9. Stelten BML, Huidekoper HH, Van De Warrenburg BPC, Brilstra EH, Hollak CEM, Haak HR, et al. Long-term treatment effect in cerebrotendinous xanthomatosis depends on age at treatment start. Neurology. 2019;92(2):E8395.
10. Berginer VM, Carmi R, Salen G. Pregnancy in women with cerebrotendinous xanthomatosis (CTX): high risk condition for fetus and newborn infant? Am J Med Genet. 1988;31(1):11–6.
11. Heywood R, Palmer AK, Foll CV, Lee MR. Letter letter: pathological changesin fetal rhesus monkey induced by oral chenodeoxycholic acid. Lancet. 1973;302:1021. https://doi.org/10.1016/s0140-6736(73)91110-0.
12. McSherry CK, Morrissey KP, Swarm RL, May PS, Niemann WH, Glenn F. Chenodeoxycholic acid induced liver injury in pregnant and neonatal baboons. Ann Surg. 1976;184:490–9. https://doi.org/10.1097/00000658-197610000-00012.
13. Sprinkle DJ, Hassan AS, Subbiah MT. Effect of chenodeoxycholic acid feeding during gestation in the rat on bile acid metabolism and liver morphology. Proc Soc Exp Biol Med. 1984;175:386–97. https://doi.org/10.3181/00379727-175-41811.
14. Celle G, Cavanna M, Bocchini R, et al. Chenodeoxycholic acid (CDCA) versus ursodeoxycholic acid (UDCA): a comparison of their effects in pregnant rats. Arch Int Pharmacodyn Ther. 1980;246:149–58.
15. Kitao T, Kamishita S, Yoshikawa H, Sakaguchi M. Terttogenicity studies of chenodeoxycholic acid in rats – influence in fetuses of rats. Yokuri Chiryo. 1982;10:3887–901.
16. Akohoshi H, Miyashita T, Tazuko K. Effects of chenadeoxycholicacid, administered in the orgonogenetic period, on the pre and post-natal development of rat's and mouse's offsprings. Pharmacometrics. 1978;15(1047–1055):12.
17. Allan RN, Thistle JL, Hofmann AF, Carter JA, Yu PY. Lithocholate metabolism during chenotherapy for gallstone dissolution. 1. Serum levels of sulphated and unsulphated lithocholates. Gut. 1976;17(6):405–12.
18. Yahalom G, Tsabari R, Molshatzki N, Ephraty L, Cohen H, Hassin-Baer S. Neurological outcome in cerebrotendinous xanthomatosis treated with chenodeoxycholic acid: early versus late diagnosis. Clin Neuropharmacol. 2013;36(3):78–83.

19. Clayton PT, Verrips A, Sistermans E, Mann A, Mieli-Vergani G, Wevers R. Mutations in the sterol 27-hydroxylase gene (CYP27A) cause hepatitis of infancy as well as cerebrotendinous xanthomatosis. J Inherit Metab Dis. 2002;25(6):501–13.
20. Skrede S, Björkhem I, Kvittingen EA, East C, Grundy S, Skrede S. Reduced c27-steroid 26-hydroxylase activity in heterozygotes for cerebrotendinous xanthomatosis. Scand J Clin Lab Invest. 1988;48(5):425–9.
21. Duell PB, Dutta R, Wolf A, Rosengrant H. Treatment of cerebrotendinous xanthomatosis in pregnancy: patient and physician perspectives. J Clin Lipidol. 2023;17(5):700–3. https://doi.org/10.1016/j.jacl.2023.07.002.
22. Stelten BML, Dotti MT, Verrips A, Elibol B, Falik-Zaccai TC, Hanman K, et al. Expert opinion on diagnosing, treating and managing patients with cerebrotendinous xanthomatosis (CTX): a modified Delphi study. Orphanet J Rare Dis. 2021;16(1):1–18. https://doi.org/10.1186/s13023-021-01980-5.

20 Cerebrotendinous Xanthomatosis (CTX) Presenting as Neonatal Cholestasis, Its Diagnosis and Treatment with Primary Bile Acids, Cholic and Chenodeoxycholic Acids

Kenneth D. R. Setchell, Wujuan Zhang, and Jian-she Wang

Abbreviations

BASD	Bile acid synthesis disorder(s)
ESI	Electrospray ionization mass spectrometry
FAB-MS	Fast atom bombardment ionization mass spectrometry
GC-MS	Gas chromatography-mass spectrometry
LC-MS/MS	Liquid chromatography-tandem mass spectrometry
m/z	Mass/charge ratio

Introduction

A deficiency in the activity of sterol 27-hydroxylase (CYP27A1) manifests as the rare lipid-storage disease of cerebrotendinous xanthomatosis (CTX; OMIM#213700), first described by Van Bogaert et al. [1]. This autosomal recessive disease has an estimated average prevalence of about 1:70,000, although this may be underestimated [2]. CTX has been well characterized clinically and biochemically [3–12]

K. D. R. Setchell (✉) · W. Zhang
Department of Pathology and Laboratory Medicine, Cincinnati Children's Hospital Medical Center, Cincinnati, OH, USA
e-mail: kenneth.setchell@cchmc.org

J.-s. Wang
Center for Pediatric Liver Diseases, Children's Hospital of Fudan University, Shanghai, China

Department of Pediatrics, Shanghai Medical College of Fudan University, Shanghai, China

A. Federico et al. (eds.), *Cerebrotendinous Xanthomatosis*,
https://doi.org/10.1007/978-3-031-92526-9_20

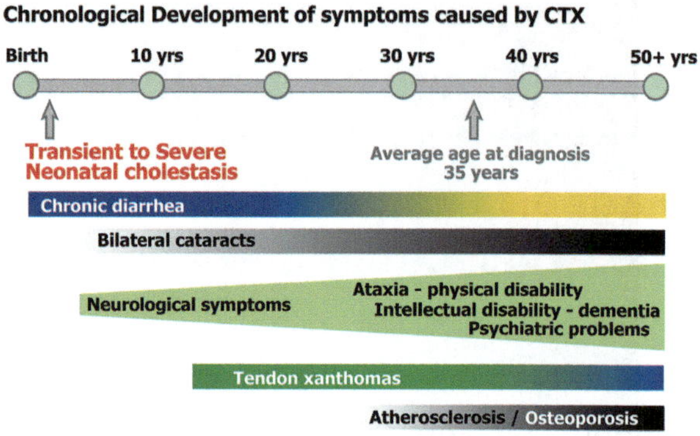

Fig. 20.1 The sequence and typical age of onset of symptoms associated with a deficiency in sterol 27-hydroxylase (CYP27A1) presenting as cerebrotendinous xanthomatosis

and shown to be caused by many different pathogenic variants in the sterol 27-hydroxylase (*CYP27A1*) gene, including insertion, deletion, and point mutations [7, 13–15]. CTX generally becomes symptomatic in the first decades of life and is characterized by a range of neurological abnormalities, xanthomas in the tendons, premature atherosclerosis, dementia, diarrhea, and cataracts. The broad spectra of symptoms overlap and can vary in severity and undiagnosed or untreated are progressive (Fig. 20.1). Biochemically, CTX can be distinguished from other conditions involving xanthomatous deposits by (i) significantly reduced primary bile acid synthesis, specifically chenodeoxycholic acid, (ii) elevations in biliary, urinary, blood, and fecal excretion of bile alcohol glucuronides, (iii) relatively low to normal plasma cholesterol concentration, with deposition of cholesterol and 5α-cholestanol in tissues, and (iv) 10–100-fold elevations in the concentrations of 5α-cholestanol in plasma and cerebrospinal fluid. The symptomatology is most likely the result of chronic lifetime deposition of large amounts of 5α-cholestanol in tissues [3, 6]. Cholestanol is a neurotoxin and may be responsible for neuronal cell death in the cerebellum [16]. Its synthesis and accumulation in the brain may conceivably explain the neurological symptomology in CTX. Early diagnosis of CTX is therefore important because successful therapeutic strategies using oral primary bile acid therapy [17–22] may lead to biochemical and clinical improvements, and evidence suggests the best prognosis occurs with early therapeutic intervention [23, 24]. A Dutch study of 56 CTX patients, with a median follow-up of 8 years, reported a more favorable outcome in terms of reversal or prevention of the development of neurological symptoms when chenodeoxycholic acid (CDCA) treatment was started before the age of 24 years [23].

Historical Perspective Unraveling the Biochemical Basis for CTX

Salen and co-workers [4, 5] first demonstrated the metabolic defect in CTX to be an impairment in oxidation of the cholesterol side chain, and that chenodeoxycholic acid synthesis was reduced to a greater extent than cholic acid synthesis [5, 25]

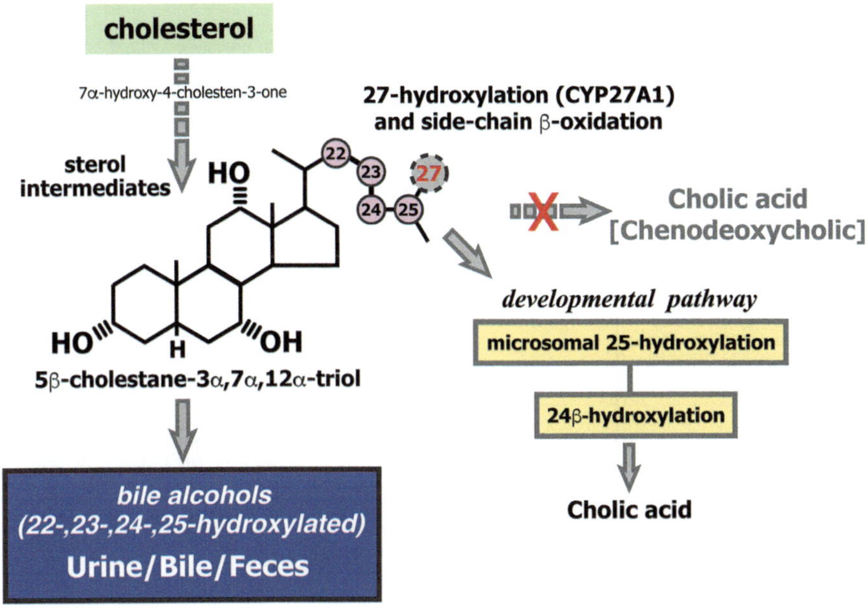

Fig. 20.2 The biochemical defect in the pathway for bile acid synthesis from cholesterol in cerebrotendinous xanthomatosis

(Fig. 20.2). Synthesis rates for chenodeoxycholic acid in adult CTX patients ($n = 3$) were 1.1 ± 0.9 mg/day (normal range 9.3 ± 1.2 mg/day, $n = 7$) compared with 13.7 ± 3.2 mg/day for cholic acid (normal range 10.7 ± 1.4 mg/day) [25]. Initially CTX was thought to be caused by a deficiency in sterol 24-hydroxylase [26], but later studies by Björkhem and co-workers indicated that a deficiency in the mitochondrial sterol-27-hydroxylase (CYP27A1, formerly referred to as C-26 hydroxylase) was the cause [27]. In support of this contention were the observations that (i) the mitochondrial fraction from the liver from a patient with CTX was completely devoid of sterol-27-hydroxylase activity [27]; (ii) the amount of 5β-cholestane-3α,7α,12α-triol, the substrate for this enzyme, in liver homogenates was 50-fold higher than normal [27]; (iii) 27-hydroxycholesterol concentrations in the serum of patients with CTX are markedly reduced or undetectable [28]; (iv) intravenous administration of radiolabeled sterol precursors revealed that only substrates with a C-27 hydroxy group were converted to cholic acid [27]; and (v) the increased amounts of bile alcohol glucuronides synthesized in this defect are polyhydroxylated in the side chain and the steroid rings in many positions [29], except carbon atom C-27. The latter is evident in the example of a typical bile alcohol profile of the feces from an adult with CTX (Fig. 20.3) analyzed by gas chromatography-mass spectrometry (GC-MS) [30]. It is highly probable that the diarrhea seen early in life and reportedly occurring in >50% of adults with CTX [31–33] is caused by the cathartic action of high intraluminal concentrations of these bile alcohols.

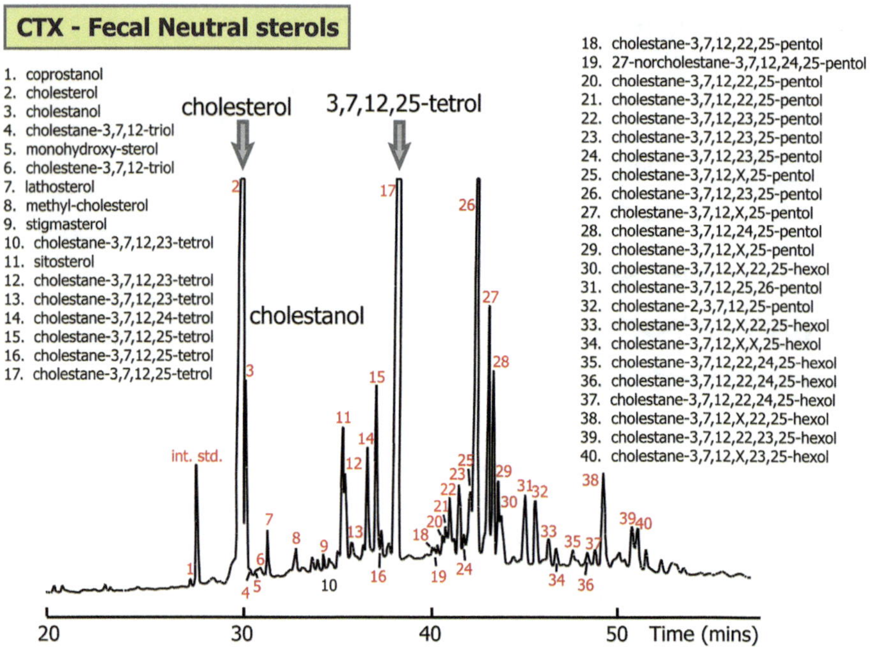

Fig. 20.3 Typical GC profiles for bile alcohols excreted in the feces of an adult patient with cerebrotendinous xanthomatosis (CTX). The trimethylsilyl ether derivatives of bile alcohols were separated on a 25 m DB-1 capillary column, temperature programmed from 225 to 295 °C with a gradient of 2 °C/min after initial and final isothermal periods of 5 min and 20 min, respectively. Neutral steroids were identified by GC-MS based on the electron ionization (70 eV) mass spectrum compared with reference compounds. The stereochemistry of a number of bile alcohols is uncertain, but the position of the assigned hydroxyl groups is accurate and based on fragmentation patterns. X denotes an undetermined assignment of the position of the hydroxyl group [30]

To explain the significantly increased levels of the bile alcohol, 5β-cholestane-3α,7α,12α,25-tetrol in CTX, it was initially proposed to be the result of a deficiency in microsomal 24(S)hydroxylation [6]; this reaction normally yields 5β-cholestane-3α,7α,12α,24,25-pentol. Studies using this radiolabeled cholestanepentol showed it was converted to cholic acid, indicating there was an alternative pathway to that of the classical C-27 hydroxylation pathway for cholic acid synthesis [34]. The quantitative importance of this pathway in health has however been established to be relatively minor in adults [35]. Furthermore, if the primary defect in CTX was a deficiency in 24(S)-hydroxylase, this would not explain the greatly reduced synthesis of chenodeoxycholic acid [36] relative to cholic acid. The reduced CDCA synthesis rate is explained by the fact that in humans it is mainly synthesized via the C-27 hydroxylation pathway. A deficiency in sterol 27-hydroxylase (CYP27A1) also leads to elevations in 5β-cholestane-3α,7α-diol and

7α-hydroxy-4-cholesten-3-one [37], making these sterol intermediates available for 12α-hydroxylation and preferential conversion to cholic acid via the C-25 hydroxylation pathway [27]. Interestingly, microsomal 12α-hydroxylase activity is threefold higher in patients with CTX [25]. So, overall, cholic acid synthesis is not impaired in CTX. Finally, evidence reinforcing a sterol-27-hydroxylase deficiency as the primary enzyme defect in CTX was established following the cloning of the cDNA [14, 38, 39]. Point mutations in the gene located on the long arm of chromosome 2 were identified in CTX and expressed in COS cells, and the resulting sterol 27-hydroxylase enzyme was found to be inactive [39]. Thus, the early controversy over the biochemical basis of CTX was finally settled with molecular studies clearly establishing the primary defect in CTX to be due to a deficiency in the activity of mitochondrial sterol 27-hydroxylase (CYP27A1) (Fig. 20.2).

Significance of 5α-Cholestanol Production in CTX

The elevation in 5α-cholestan-3β-ol (5α-cholestanol) in the nervous system of CTX patients first observed by Menkes et al. and the high plasma concentration of this sterol is a unique biochemical feature of the disease [3, 6]. The origins of the increased 5α-cholestanol may be from elevations in the precursor, 4-cholesten-3-one [40]; hepatic microsomes prepared from CTX patients have been shown to produce three times more 4-cholesten-3-one than similar preparations from healthy controls. By pulse-labeling techniques, 4-cholesten-3-one was shown to yield labeled cholestanol, while the corresponding 7α-hydroxyl intermediate, 7α-hydroxy-4-cholesten-3-one was converted to bile acids and not 5α-cholestanol. An alternative pathway for the formation of cholestanol was proposed implicating hepatic, rather than intestinal 7α-dehydroxylation with the production of a cholest-4,6-dien-3-one intermediate [41, 42]. Evidence to support this pathway was the finding of increased levels of 7α-hydroxy-4-cholesten-3-one and cholest-4,6-diene-3-one in CTX and the observation that cholestyramine treatment, which stimulates cholesterol 7α-hydroxylase activity [43, 44], increases 5α-cholestanol output, whereas the opposite occurs during chenodeoxycholic acid feeding [45]. The neurological dysfunction observed in CTX, while not completely understood, seems to be a consequence of cholestanol and cholesterol deposition in tissues [3, 6]. However, interestingly, reductions in plasma 5α-cholestanol concentrations with primary bile acid therapy are not always associated with neurological improvement. Sterol 27-hydroxylase is found in extrahepatic tissues [46–48], so it is possible that some of the manifestations of the disease may be the result of non-hepatic perturbations in metabolism. Studies in a rat model found that cholestanol induces apoptosis of cerebellar neurons with the suggestion that this could induce cerebellar ataxia in CTX patients [16]. Early diagnosis of CTX, a disease that can be relatively asymptomatic and missed in the early years, is crucial to prevent or limit the progressive accumulation of sterols in tissues over the long term.

Pediatric Presentation of CTX

CTX is usually diagnosed in adulthood with an average age at the time of diagnosis being around 35 years of age. In a review of 54 patients with CTX, the age at diagnosis ranged from 7 to 55 years, and the majority were diagnosed in the third decade of life. Onset of symptoms as early as 1 year of age was noted from clinical histories of some of the adults [7]. The sequelae and timing of the emergence of the clinical manifestations of CTX and onset and severity of the symptoms varies considerably among patients and the symptomologies may overlap (Fig. 20.1). Until recently, CTX was rarely diagnosed in children, only rarely mentioned in childhood [31, 49, 50], and never diagnosed in the neonatal period. Cholestatic liver disease, now a recognized early feature, was never considered a classical feature of CTX [51–56]. This may be explained by the fact that cholic acid synthesis takes place, albeit at sub-optimal rates, by an alternative 25-hydroxylation pathway [34] that results in the production of low but nevertheless sufficient levels of primary bile acids to ultimately facilitate bile flow in adults. However, in healthy infants, there is a natural physiologic cholestasis in the immediate neonatal period [57, 58] because at birth the primary bile acid pool is small and the bile acid transporters are underdeveloped [59–61]. Perhaps not surprising, neonatal cholestasis may be prolonged, or even fatal in newborns with CTX because of the compromised primary bile acid pool size due to the sterol 27-hydroxylase deficiency [52, 53]. It is possible that the jaundice is missed as a signature for CTX in the neonatal period because it may resolve within a few weeks to months with the patient remaining asymptomatic for many years thereafter [51]. This clinical course again underlines the importance of introducing CTX into neonatal screening programs.

We speculate that cholestasis may have conceivably occurred in early life in most adults diagnosed with CTX but that it resolves as the bile acid pool expands by an increase in cholic acid synthesis via the compensatory 25-hydroxylation pathway to levels just sufficient to stimulate and maintain bile flow. In the year 2000, we first described cholestatic liver disease as one of the earliest features of CTX [51]. The patient, a 3-month-old boy born in a first cousin marriage, was being investigated for persistent conjugated hyperbilirubinemia, elevated serum transaminases, and low GGT, but normal cholesterol. There was a history of pale stools, and the patient had hepatomegaly. Diagnosis was based upon markedly elevated urinary bile alcohol glucuronides determined by fast atom bombardment ionization mass spectrometry (FAB-MS) analysis [62]. Subsequent DNA analysis confirmed a homozygous pathogenic variant in *CYP27A1*. Several later reports confirmed that CTX can be associated with hepatobiliary injury in infancy [53, 54]. More recently, we described the largest cohort of infants ($n = 8$) with homozygous or compound heterozygous pathogenic variants in *CYP27A1* that presented with neonatal cholestasis, of which four died from liver failure, and one underwent liver transplantation [52].

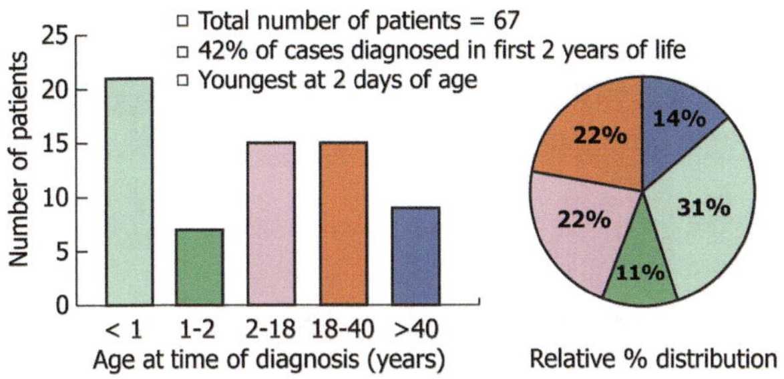

Fig. 20.4 Summary of the numbers of patients diagnosed with cerebrotendinous xanthomatosis from a mass spectrometry screening program at the Cincinnati Children's Hospital Medical Center. Urine samples were analyzed from >19,000 patients, mostly presenting with idiopathic cholestasis, for investigation of possible of bile acid synthesis disorders. The distribution and proportion of CTX cases based on age at the time of diagnosis is shown

Rapid deterioration in liver function leading to liver failure and liver transplantation was reported for a biochemically and genetically confirmed 5-month-old infant with CTX [55], further highlighting that the cholestasis can be severe [52, 53].

Since establishing in 1987 a mass spectrometry-based screening program for the diagnosis of bile acid synthesis disorders (BASD) at the Cincinnati Children's Hospital Medical Center [62] >20,000 urine samples have been screened, most for investigation of underlying causes of idiopathic cholestasis. Two percent of the patients screened were positive for a BASD. A total of 67 cases of CTX were identified (Fig. 20.4). Based on age at the time of diagnosis, 31% of these cases were less than 1 year of life, and 42% were identified in the first 2 years of life. One infant was diagnosed with CTX at 2 days of age. But for the presentation of cholestasis, these cases may have been missed or gone undiagnosed until much later in life. Cholestasis may be either transient [51], or severe enough to be fatal [52, 53] or necessitate liver transplantation [52, 55].

There is a paucity of information on the histological features of cholestasis in CTX because few liver biopsies have been performed or reported [52, 55]. Figure 20.5a shows the liver histology from a 4-month-old infant diagnosed with CTX and neonatal cholestasis before any therapy had begun. This light microscopy reveals a picture of severe neonatal hepatitis with ballooning of hepatocytes, bridging fibrosis, marked inflammation, and giant-cell transformation with periportal fibrosis (Fig. 20.5a). Similar features of marked intralobular cholestasis, hepatocellular disarray, and giant-cell transformation were more recently described for the liver histology of three CTX patients aged 2, 4 and 6 months of age presenting with neonatal cholestasis [52] and for a 4-month-old infant with CTX [55].

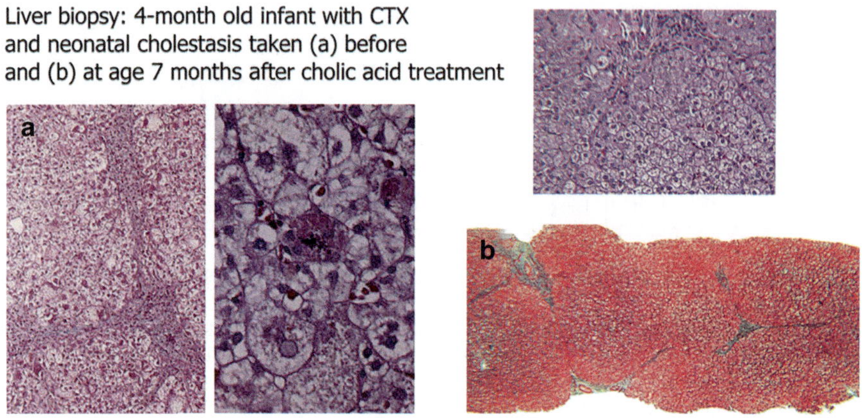

Fig. 20.5 Liver histology from a patient with cerebrotendinous xanthomatosis presenting as neonatal cholestasis before (**a**) and after (**b** and **c**) treatment with cholic acid

Biochemical Diagnostic Approaches to CTX

The biochemical diagnosis of CTX historically relied upon the measures of serum or plasma 5α-cholestanol and cholesterol with gas chromatography, or GC-MS. Cholesterol is usually normal or low in most CTX cases and 5α-cholestanol elevated. Thus, an elevated 5α-cholestanol or 5α-cholestanol/cholesterol ratio was used as a basis for diagnosis [63]. This however is not specific to CTX as 5α-cholestanol can be elevated in other conditions, such as sitosterolemia and cholestatic liver diseases.

Plasma 7α-hydroxy-4-cholesten-3-one (also referred to as C4, 7αC4, or sterol-C4), a surrogate marker for bile acid synthesis rate [64, 65], initially measured by GC-MS [64], and later by LC-MS/MS method that incorporated a derivatization step was shown by DeBarber et al. to be diagnostically more sensitive than 5α-cholestanol for CTX [66]. However, 7α-hydroxy-4-cholesten-3-one has limitations in that it has been shown to be elevated in cases of short bowel syndrome, bile acid malabsorption, and with increased fecal bile acid loss as occurs with chronic diarrhea [67].

DeBarber [68, 69] and others [70] have reported 7α,12α-dihydroxy-4-cholesten-3-one to be a sensitive and specific plasma biomarker for diagnosis of CTX, as well as a useful biomarker for detection of CTX from newborn dried blood spots [68, 69]. In plasma from ten adult CTX patients, concentrations of this oxo-sterol intermediate were reported to be >3862 times that in unaffected adult controls and there was clear delineation between CTX and non-CTX samples. Measurement of 7α,12α-hydroxy-4-cholesten-3-one has limitations in that derivatization and chromatographic resolution is required for sensitivity to perform dried blood spot testing [69, 71] and isobaric interferences may occur for derivatized analyte with approaches that are necessary for high throughput neonatal screening [72]. The most sensitive and specific biochemical diagnostic biomarker for CTX is measurement of bile alcohols in urine, serum/plasma, or blood. Impaired oxidation of the cholesterol side chain results in accelerated cholesterol synthesis and metabolism and greatly increased production and excretion of bile alcohol glucuronides [4, 73–76] which are excreted in high concentrations in urine [62, 76–78]. These bile alcohols have the common 5β-cholestane-3α,7α,12α-triol nucleus with additional hydroxyl groups in the side chain mainly at positions C-22, C-23, C-24, and C-25 (Fig. 20.2). The major bile alcohol secreted in bile and excreted in feces is the 5β-cholestane-3α,7α,12α,25-tetrol, while the more polar 5β-cholestane-3α,7α,12α,23,25-pentol predominates in urine [75, 76, 78, 79]. The difference in these patterns may be due either to more efficient renal excretion of the more polar pentol, or a result of renal C-23 hydroxylation of 5β-cholestane-3α,7α,12α,25-tetrol. These bile alcohols are conjugated to glucuronic and sulfuric acids and found in bile and urine predominantly as conjugates [75, 78] or as double-conjugates [52]. The latter is notable in neonates and infants because sulfation of steroids is major metabolic pathway in early life. Bile alcohol sulfates are also found in more primitive vertebrate species [29]. The position of conjugation of bile alcohols was elucidated from nuclear magnetic resonance (NMR) studies. In the bile alcohol tetrol isolated from bile, the glucuronide moiety was shown to be at carbon atom C-3, and the structure assigned as 5β-cholestane-3α,7α,12α,25-tetrol-3-O-β-glucuronide. For the bile alcohol pentol isolated from urine, it is in the side chain at carbon C-23 and assigned 5β-cholestane-3α,7α,12α, 23S,25-pentol-23-O-β-glucuronide [80, 81].

For more than 4 decades, we have utilized FAB-MS, one of the oldest soft-ionization techniques, for the screening of urine for bile acid synthesis disorders, including CTX [62, 77]. Urine is a concentrated ultrafiltrate of plasma and as such is highly enriched in metabolites of interest. This untargeted "metabolomic" approach is rapid and specific, although not the most quantitatively sensitive. Given that FAB-MS is an obsolescent technique and not generally available to most laboratories, direct loop injection, or flow injection analysis (FIA) electrospray ionization (ESI) tandem mass spectrometry offers an alternative approach [53, 82, 83] and yields similar mass spectra, although in our experience ESI may generate more doubly charged ions than FAB-MS. Definitive identification of CTX is possible from the presence of intense deprotonated molecular ions at *m/z* 611, 627 and 643 (Fig. 20.6) reflective of elevated levels of urinary glucuronide conjugates of tetrahydroxy-, pentahydroxy-, and hexahydroxy-bile alcohols, concomitant with a markedly reduced or total lack of excretion of primary bile acids, most notably chenodeoxycholic acid conjugates [62, 77]. Urinary bile alcohol sulfates are also evident in the mass spectrum from the ions at *m/z* 515, and 531 (Fig. 20.6). Sulfated bile alcohols are a dominant feature of the bile of patients with CTX and evident in neonatal CTX plasma and if present at high levels may be associated with a poor outcome [52]. Sulfated bile alcohols may be useful biomarkers for neonatal dried bloodspot screening and their use should be explored. The possibility of missing CTX should perhaps be considered in neonatal screening where a single bile

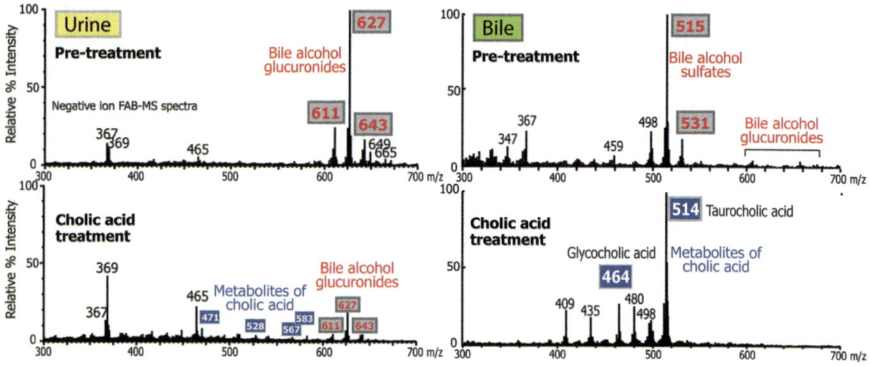

Fig. 20.6 Typical negative ion FAB-MS mass spectra of the urine and bile from a patient with cerebrotendinous xanthomatosis at the time of diagnosis and after treatment with cholic acid (10–15 mg/day). Urine is characterized by dominant ions at m/z 611, 627, and 643 representing excreted glucuronide conjugates of bile alcohol tetrols, pentols, and heptols. In bile, ions at m/z 515 and 531 are prominent that correspond to sulfate conjugates of bile alcohol tetrols and pentols. After cholic acid treatment, ions at m/z 514 and m/z 464 appear that represent taurine and glycine-conjugated cholic acid, confirming uptake, hepatic conjugation, and secretion into bilew

alcohol glucuronide is selected, although there have been no false negative results to date for newborn dried bloodspots from known CTX patients. By 2 years of age, the urinary FAB-MS mass spectrum generally shifts to resemble that observed for adults. Finally, 27-hydroxycholesterol, less commonly measured because it is more analytically challenging, would be another diagnostic biomarker for CTX because the lack of CYP27A1 activity leads to negligible or absence of 27-hydroxycholesterol in most biological matrices [70, 84].

Biochemical Screening Approaches to CTX

Given the importance of early diagnosis, neonatal screening programs based on MS/MS analysis of dried blood spots have begun to be revised to include CTX diagnosis [72, 85, 86]. The most significant and specific biomarker is 5β-cholestane-3α,7α,12α,25-tetrol-3-O-β-glucuronide, which is present in dried blood spots [84]. However, this bile alcohol glucuronide also accumulates in other diseases, including peroxisomal disorders and cholestatic syndromes, so that sole reliance on absolute concentration of 5β-cholestane-3α,7α,12α,25-tetrol-3-O-β-glucuronide may not be sufficiently specific for a neonatal diagnosis of CTX. To overcome this problem, the ratio of 5β-cholestane-3α,7α,12α,25-tetrol glucuronide/taurochenodeoxycholic acid and taurocholic acid was explored and found to be highly specific for neonatal diagnosis [85]. In adults, bile acids are conjugated to glycine and taurine with a ratio of approximately 3:1 [87]. However, in the fetal and neonatal periods, taurine conjugation predominates [88] [89] and since chenodeoxycholic synthesis is impaired in CTX, while cholic acid is not [4], utilizing this ratio was shown to greatly enhance the sensitivity and specificity to diagnose CTX neonatally. In other cholestatic liver diseases, except the previously described BASD [62], both chenodeoxycholic and cholic acid conjugates are elevated in serum/blood. The testing approach involved the use of dried blood spots on paper (Guthrie) cards, solvent extraction of bile acids and bile alcohols, and the addition of a cocktail of stable-labeled internal standards. The extracts were analyzed by flow-injection tandem mass spectrometry, monitoring specific ion transitions for each metabolite and internal standard and from the measured concentrations, the ratios of bile alcohol to bile acids were calculated [85]. In a small pilot study of 217 Guthrie cards from patients with CTX, Zellwegers, and healthy preterm and term infants, definitive separation of these groups was possible based on the ratios of the bile alcohol-tetrol to the taurine-conjugated primary bile acids [85]. A similar approach was applied to the screening of 32,000 dried blood spots from newborns. In this case, 5β-cholestane-3α,7α,12α,25-tetrol-3-O-β-glucuronide was used a first-tier biomarker, with samples then assessed for the ratio of 5β-cholestane-3α,7α,12α,25-tetrol-3-O-β-glucuronide to taurochenodeoxycholic acid. This approach had a zero false positive rate with one newborn from this cohort identified with CTX by these criteria and confirmed from the finding of two pathogenic variants in *CYP27A1* [72]. A two-tier approach comparing flow injection analysis with a chromatographic LC-MS/MS method that included the measurement of the bile alcohol-tetrol and the sterol intermediate, 7α,12α-dihydroxy-4-cholen-3-one by polarity switching was also evaluated for analysis of DBS samples collected prospectively, and from genetically confirmed CTX patients in a high-risk Israeli population. Both tiers proved to be specific for identifying CTX [86].

Biochemical Approaches to Monitor Efficacy of Therapy in CTX

While the utility of the bile alcohol/bile acid ratio has very high specificity and sensitivity for screening for CTX, it may be less useful in monitoring response to bile acid therapies because the bile alcohol/bile acid ratio will be skewed by the presence of the conjugated primary bile acids and their metabolites from oral bile acid therapy. Of more relevance to monitoring therapy are the absolute bile alcohol concentrations and the changes in 5α-cholestanol, which can be measured by specific targeted assays, as the goal of therapy with primary bile acids is to suppress hepatic bile acid synthesis and to reduce bile alcohol and 5α-cholestanol production. Plasma 7α-hydroxy-4-cholesten-3-one, a surrogate marker for bile acid synthesis rate [64, 65], responds more rapidly than 5α-cholestanol to bile acid therapy [66] and has been proposed as the optimal marker for the evaluation of therapy to shut down bile acid synthesis in CTX [90].

Primary Bile Acid Therapy for CTX—Chenodeoxycholic and Cholic Acids

The main therapeutic goal in the treatment in all the genetic defects in bile acid synthesis (BASD), including CTX, is to inhibit endogenous bile acid synthesis through negative feedback inhibition [91] to thereby reduce the levels of atypical disease-causing bile acids and their intermediates [62]. The size of the bile acid pool and its daily synthesis is tightly controlled by negative feedback inhibition from bile acids returning during the enterohepatic circulation to regulate the expression of the rate-limiting enzyme, cholesterol 7α-hydroxylase (CYP7A1) [92], through the nuclear receptor FXR and the protein FGF19 [93–95]. For bile acid synthesis disorders presenting with cholestasis, which is an early feature of CTX in infancy [51–56], the effect of primary bile acid therapy is to facilitate bile flow, because primary bile acids provide the driving force for the maintenance of bile flow [96]. An added benefit is to increase intraluminal bile salt concentrations above the CMC for lipid absorption [97, 98]. Feeding primary bile acids, either cholic or chenodeoxycholic, simply tricks the liver into believing it has normal synthetic function, and through this homoeostatic control, atypical bile acid and sterol production is reduced, concomitant with clinical improvements. This therapeutic approach has been highly successful in treating bile acid synthesis disorders [62].

Chenodeoxycholic acid (CDCA) has been the standard treatment for CTX for about the last four decades [17]. In part, this may have been because of its availability as an approved drug for gallstone dissolution [99, 100] so that it could be used off-label, and until recently, the lack of availability of a pharmaceutical grade cholic acid (Cholbam®), the other primary bile acid. Very recently, the US Food and Drug Administration (FDA) granted chenodeoxycholic acid (Chenodal®) Orphan drug designation for cerebrotendinous xanthomatosis (CTX). In a landmark publication in NEJM, Salen et al. treated 17 adult CTX patients with 250 mg t.i.d of oral chenodeoxycholic acid and showed that plasma 5α-cholestanol and biliary bile alcohol levels could be significantly lowered or normalized, with the added benefit of stabilization or improvement in neurological and neurocognitive symptoms in many of the patients [17, 20, 101]. These studies led to the conclusion that CDCA was a clinically useful therapy for CTX, and it has remained the standard of care ever since. The long-term improvement in neurological status of CTX patients has however proven variable, with a spectrum of improvement, no improvement, or progression of the symptoms among patients [24, 33, 45, 102–105]. However, more recently data have emerged to suggest that the timing of therapeutic intervention with CDCA may be a critical factor in its effectiveness [23, 104]. Data now show that when CDCA treatment is initiated after 24 years of age, patients had worse outcome and were significantly more limited in ambulation, were more cognitively impaired, and showed deterioration of neurologic symptoms, with Parkinsonism as a treatment-resistant feature, despite improvements in biochemistries related to biomarkers. These findings again highlight the importance of early diagnosis and the critical need for inclusion of CTX in neonatal screening programs to afford early therapeutic intervention.

In the case of pediatric CTX patients, some caution is warranted in the use of CDCA. It is a relatively hydrophobic and membrane-damaging bile acid [98], with a risk of hepatotoxicity, despite that it is one of the two major primary bile acids synthesized by the healthy liver. In the large National Cooperative Gallstone study, CDCA was found to elevate serum transaminases in 3% of patients and raise serum LDL-cholesterol in 85% of patients [106]. In an Italian study, 10% of subjects treated with CDCA developed a transaminasemia [107]. It can be speculated that hypertransaminasia is likely to be the consequence of an overload of CDCA, as in adult gallstone patients, CDCA synthesis rates are normal, unlike CTX where CDCA synthesis is markedly reduced. In other words, hepatotoxicity seen in patients with gallstones treated with CDCA does not necessarily mean that adult CTX patients would show the same adverse effects, and indeed, hepatotoxicity is very rarely if ever reported as a complication of CDCA used in adult CTX patients. However, CDCA was reported to be hepatotoxic when administered to a 2-week-old infant with genetically confirmed CTX [108]. At a dose of 15 mg/kg bw/day, the child developed jaundice and hepatomegaly, which resolved after stopping treatment. After lowering the dose to 5 mg/kg bw/day, the serum liver enzymes and cholestanol normalized and remained normal up to 2.8 years of age [108]. Recently, a 4-month-old infant genetically confirmed with CTX was started on CDCA and developed progressive liver disease requiring its discontinuation, and the infant then underwent liver transplantation (Setchell—unpublished). Similar observations of hepatotoxicity from CDCA use in infants with the Δ^4–3-oxosteroid 5β-reductase (AKR1D1) deficiency were reported in our own studies, but after dose adjustment by titrating against the extent of reduction in atypical bile acids, normalization of LFTs was achieved with the optimal dose of CDCA being 4–10 mg/kg bw/day among patients, and the patients became symptom-free over periods ranging 0.5–7.0 years at the lower doses [109]. A further potential concern for CDCA use in neonates and children is the cathartic property of this hydrophobic bile acid, especially as a high proportion of CTX patients present with diarrhea [31, 32]. In a comparative study of CDCA and UDCA for cholesterol gallstone dissolution, diarrhea was a major reason for subject dropout and occurred in up to 30% of the CDCA group (2.8% in the UDCA group) in the first 3 months of treatment, and loose stools persisted beyond 6–12 months [107]. Alternately, diarrhea may not be an issue in CTX patients who have little or no CDCA to begin with and has only extremely rarely been reported as an adverse effect of CDCA treatment of CTX. In a 1987 report of a Dutch study of CTX, one patient was switched from CDCA to cholic acid because of diarrhea, nausea, and abnormal liver function test from CDCA treatment [103]. In our early development of a treatment for BASD, the combined use of cholic and chenodeoxycholic led to severe diarrhea in an infant with AKR1D1 deficiency that resolved after switching to cholic acid monotherapy (unpublished). This ultimately was the rationale for our use of cholic acid monotherapy for the treatment of BASD [62].

Cholic acid is approved by the US Food and Drug Administration (FDA) and the European Medicines Agency (EMA) for the treatment of CTX [110] and leads to a decrease in plasma 5α-cholestanol [19]. It has proven to be life-saving therapy for patients with bile acid synthesis disorders, has no known hepatoxicity, and is well-tolerated by infants and children [18, 19, 62, 111–117]. Cholic acid is more hydrophilic than CDCA (Fig. 20.7) [98] and has an excellent safety profile based on its use for almost 40 years in BASD. For this reason, it should be considered as an alternative treatment option for pediatric CTX patients. The argument against using cholic acid has always been that it does not bind as well as CDCA to the nuclear receptor FXR to suppress CYP7A1 expression [92, 118, 119], the ultimate target of therapy. These comparative binding affinities have largely been derived from in vitro cell systems that lack a bile acid transporter, and as cholic acid is more hydrophilic than CDCA [98] and has different affinities for serum proteins [120], its uptake into the cells will be expectedly lower in the absence of a transporter. However, when a bile acid transporter is introduced into cells, cholic acid is an effective activator of FXR [118]. Furthermore, the in vivo ability of cholic acid to activate FXR is unquestionable based on its clinical effectiveness in suppressing atypical bile acid synthesis in patients with BASD. The safety and clinical efficacy were recognized by the Food and Drug Administration approval of the NDA (NDA 205–270) for the treatment of BASD, with oral cholic acid therapy showing impressive normalization in serum transaminases and improvement in liver histology concomitant with suppression in the urinary excretion of the atypical bile acids. Cholic acid would therefore be expected to be effective on the key biochemical endpoints in CTX, and this has indeed been confirmed [18, 19, 21, 103].

Several studies attest to the effectiveness of cholic acid in pediatric CTX in treating the hepatic and neurological manifestations. Pierre et al. first reported on the effect of cholic acid in stabilizing the progression of cognitive deterioration, suppressing bile alcohol glucuronides, and normalizing serum liver function tests in two affected infants with a confirmed homozygous pathogenic variant in *CYP27A1* [18]. A 3-month-old that presented with jaundice that had resolved by 5-months of age and liver function that had normalized by 8 months of age. He was started on cholic acid (15 mg/kg bw/day) at 14 months of age and showed a good biochemical response concomitant with a marked suppression in urinary bile alcohol excretion. By 8 years of age, he was clinically normal with no xanthomas or cataracts and developmentally stable. A sister, without cholestasis, was started on cholic acid at 5

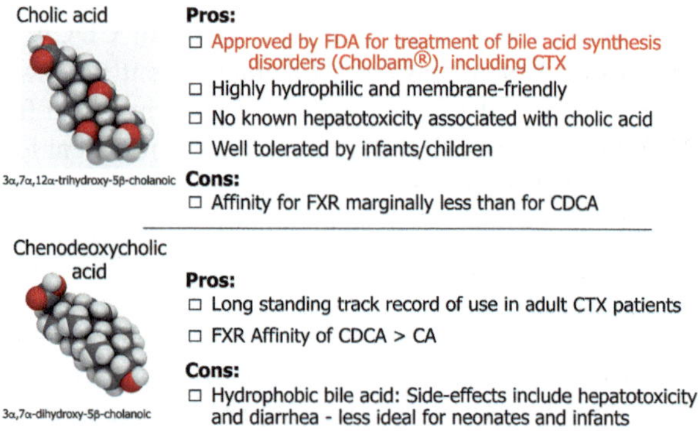

Fig. 20.7 Comparison of structures and properties of cholic acid and chenodeoxycholic (CDCA) acid and the pros and cons of their use in the treatment of CTX patients

months of age. Her delayed verbal skills noted at 3 years had improved by 7 years of age, and a brain MRI was normal [18]. Interestingly, Koopman et al. in 1985 reported positive effects of cholic acid on neurological function and showed that cholic acid and CDCA both suppressed bile alcohol synthesis in CTX patients [21]. It was concluded that either cholic or chenodeoxycholic acid are the therapies of choice for the treatment of CTX, and cholic acid was preferentially recommended [21]. Data to support the efficacy of cholic acid in resolving liver disease in three of four infants with CTX was included in the NDA submitted to the FDA that led to the approval of cholic acid (Cholbam®) for the treatment of BASD. Features of the liver histology of infants with cholestasis caused by BASD have been well documented [117], but liver biopsies are rarely performed for CTX. However, Fig. 20.5 shows the pre- and post-treatment effects of cholic acid therapy (60 mg/day) on the liver histology of an infant with neonatal cholestasis and CTX. By age 7 months, a near normalization in liver histology is evident with a resolution of the inflammatory activity observed pre-treatment (Fig. 20.5b).

In a recent study of the effect of cholic acid therapy in 12 adult CTX patients (five that had prior CDCA treatment and then switched to cholic acid, and seven that were non-treatment naïve) cholic acid (500–750 mg/day) markedly reduced or normalized plasma 5α-cholestanol levels in the latter group [19]. Reportedly, five patients in the non-treatment naïve group showed clinical improvement, one remained stable, and one deteriorated after 830 days treatment, while overall 10/12 patients improved while on cholic acid. The mean age at the time of diagnosis and follow-up was 32.9 years and 798 days, respectively. No adverse effects were observed with cholic acid treatment, whereas elevated transaminases were noted in some patients on CDCA. It was concluded that cholic acid may be a suitable alternative to CDCA for CTX especially in patients with side effects from CDCA [19]. Overall, cholic acid has been shown to be a safe and effective therapy for BASD, is FDA and EMA approved for CTX, and has a superior safety profile to that of CDCA. What is not known is whether long-term cholic acid treatment can consistently or universally arrest or improve the neurological manifestations of CTX because it has not been in clinical use for as long as CDCA. Furthermore, there have been no systematic studies to compare the efficacy of the two primary bile acids. Indirectly, our own data indicate that cholic acid is as effective on the key biochemical parameters in CTX (Setchell & Zhang 2023, unpublished and presented at the Falk XXVII International Congress on Bile Acids: Bile Acids in Health and Disease, Edinburgh 2025). In a study of 26 patients with CTX, who were treated either with cholic acid ($n = 16$) or CDCA ($n = 10$), both bile acids resulted in a clinically meaningful lowering from baseline of the key bile alcohol 5β-cholestan-3α,7α,12α,25-tetrol glucuronide in urine (Fig. 20.8). The average percentage reduction from baseline in urinary bile alcohols was 70% for cholic acid and 90% for CDCA, findings that indicate both bile acids effectively and similarly reduce bile alcohol synthesis with the difference unlikely to be clinically significant.

Other treatment strategies (Fig. 20.9) have been explored for CTX. Ursodeoxycholic acid (UDCA), a highly polar and hypercholeretic bile acid [99, 100, 121], is the mainstay for treating cholestatic liver but is ineffective in terms of suppressing the

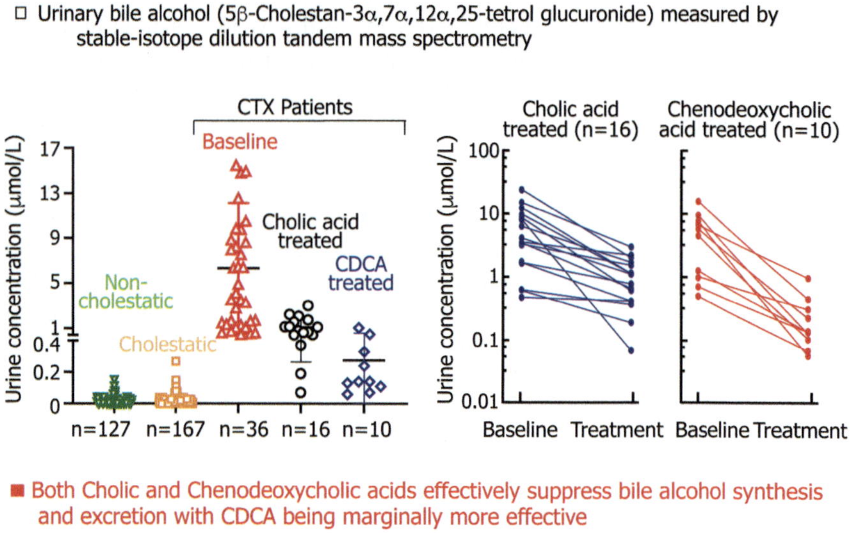

Fig. 20.8 Concentrations of the major bile alcohol glucuronide, 5β-cholestane-3α,7α,12α,25-tetrol-3-O-β-glucuronide in the urine of non-cholestatic pediatric controls (n = 127), pediatric patients with idiopathic cholestasis (n = 167), patients with CTX (adult and pediatric combined (n = 36) at the time of diagnosis and following treatment with cholic (n = 16), or chenodeoxycholic acid (n = 10). Also shown is a comparison of the change from baseline in the urinary excretion of 5β-cholestane-3α,7α,12α,25-tetrol-3-O-β-glucuronide in CTX patients treated with cholic acid (n = 16) or chenodeoxycholic acid (n = 10)

Fig. 20.9 Summary of the treatment options for CTX that have been evaluated showing the effects on the major biochemical targets and endpoints of treatment

Treatment	CYP7A1	HMG-CoA reductase	Bile alcohols	Cholesterol	Cholestanol
CDCA:	⇩	⇩	⇩	⇩/No effect	⇩
Statins:	No effect	⇩	No effect	⇩	No effect
CDCA/Statins:	⇩	⇩⇩	⇩	⇩⇩	⇩
Cholic:	⇩	⇩	⇩	No effect	⇩
UDCA:	slight ⇧	⇩	No effect	No effect	No effect
Clofibrate:	No effect	No effect	-	-	⇩
Cholestyramine:	⇧	⇧	⇧	-	⇧

- No head-to-head comparisons of CDCA vs Cholic acid in CTX
- CDCA is considered to improve neurological symptoms*

*Note: Study of CTX patients (N=25) found neurological symptoms deteriorated in 60% of patients and 20% died while on long-term CDCA therapy (Piro-de-la-Fuente B, et al 2011)

production of bile alcohols in CTX patients [21]. Indeed, it is mildly stimulatory on bile acid synthesis and when used to treat the most common BASD, the 3β-hydroxy-Δ^5-C_{27}-steroid oxidoreductase (HSD3B7) deficiency, it was shown to increase the production of atypical and hepatotoxic 3β-hydroxy-Δ^5 bile acids [122]. It therefore cannot be recommended for CTX. Likewise, the bile acid binding resin, cholestyramine, which stimulates the activity of CYP7A1 to increase bile acid synthesis [43, 123], was shown to increase bile alcohol and cholestanol levels in adult CTX patients. It was used in a challenge test to detect carriers of CTX [124]. Statins, which inhibit HMG-CoA reductase to lower cholesterol levels, were found to have no definitive short-term clinical benefit even though serum cholesterol and 5α-cholestanol levels were reduced [125]. However, primary bile acid therapy may be more effective in CTX if combined with an HMG-CoA reductase inhibitor. A few studies have shown that the combined regimen of CDCA and statin lowers serum cholesterol and cholestanol beyond that of CDCA alone, but it is difficult to know if this translates into any long-term clinical benefit [126–130]. No studies have combined cholic acid with statins and our early experience of combining cholic acid with chenodeoxycholic was discontinued due to the cathartic effects of chenodeoxycholic acid in an infant. Whether combining the two primary bile acids to treat adult CTX would be superior to monotherapy is unknown.

In conclusion, cholic acid, approved in 2015 by the FDA, offers another alternative approach for the treatment of CTX, particularly for neonatal and pediatric patients, with an option to switch to CDCA in the event of non-optimized biochemical, or poor clinical responses. The caveat to this proposal is that there is presently a paucity of data on whether long-term cholic acid monotherapy alters the neurological progression of the disease [18]. Long-term studies to compare clinical outcome on cholic acid versus chenodeoxycholic acid in CTX are therefore needed.

Acknowledgments Acknowledged is the support of the many physicians that have submitted samples to the BASD mass spectrometry screening program since its inception in 1986, to Brian Wolfe for technical support with instrumentation and in performing the mass spectrometry analysis, my superb laboratory support staff including, Stephanie Galandi and Stacey Reed for their support in sample preparation and organizational input to the program. Finally, mention and recognition of my close friend and colleague James Heubi MD, who sadly passed away in 2021, and in whom we formed a superb physician-scientist partnership that led to our development of cholic acid (Cholbam®) monotherapy as an approved treatment for bile acid synthesis disorders. We appreciate the help of our pathologist Kevin Bove MD, who passed away October 25 2024, for help with interpretation of the liver biopsies.

Declarations of Conflict of Interest KDRS holds minor equity as co-founder of Asklepion Pharmaceuticals and is a consultant to Mirum Pharmaceuticals that market both cholic (Cholbam®) and chenodeoxycholic (Chenodal®) acids. None of the other authors have anything to declare.

References

1. Van Bogaert L, Scherer HJ, Epstein E. Une forme cerebrale de la cholesterinose generalisee. Paris: Masson et Cie; 1937.
2. Appadurai V, DeBarber A, Chiang PW, Patel SB, Steiner RD, Tyler C, et al. Apparent underdiagnosis of Cerebrotendinous Xanthomatosis revealed by analysis of ~60,000 human exomes. Mol Genet Metab. 2015;116(4):298–304.
3. Menkes JH, Schimschock JR, Swanson PD. Cerebrotendinous xanthomatosis. The storage of cholestanol within the nervous system. Arch Neurol. 1968;19(1):47–53.
4. Setoguchi T, Salen G, Tint GS, Mosbach EH. A biochemical abnormality in cerebrotendinous xanthomatosis. Impairment of bile acid biosynthesis associated with incomplete degradation of the cholesterol side chain. J Clin Invest. 1974;53(5):1393–401.

5. Salen G, Grundy SM. The metabolism of cholestanol, cholesterol, and bile acids in cerebrotendinous xanthomatosis. J Clin Invest. 1973;52(11):2822–35.
6. Salen G. Cholestanol deposition in cerebrotendinous xanthomatosis. A possible mechanism. Ann Intern Med. 1971;75(6):843–51.
7. Verrips A, Hoefsloot LH, Steenbergen GC, Theelen JP, Wevers RA, Gabreels FJ, et al. Clinical and molecular genetic characteristics of patients with cerebrotendinous xanthomatosis. Brain. 2000;123(Pt 5):908–19.
8. Barkhof F, Verrips A, Wesseling P, van Der Knaap MS, van Engelen BG, Gabreels FJ, et al. Cerebrotendinous xanthomatosis: the spectrum of imaging findings and the correlation with neuropathologic findings. Radiology. 2000;217(3):869–76.
9. Moghadasian MH. Cerebrotendinous xanthomatosis: clinical course, genotypes and metabolic backgrounds. Clin Invest Med. 2004;27(1):42–50.
10. Nie S, Chen G, Cao X, Zhang Y. Cerebrotendinous xanthomatosis: a comprehensive review of pathogenesis, clinical manifestations, diagnosis, and management. Orphanet J Rare Dis. 2014;9:179.
11. Mignarri A, Dotti MT, Federico A, De Stefano N, Battaglini M, Grazzini I, et al. The spectrum of magnetic resonance findings in cerebrotendinous xanthomatosis: redefinition and evidence of new markers of disease progression. J Neurol. 2017;264(5):862–74.
12. Koyama S, Sekijima Y, Ogura M, Hori M, Matsuki K, Miida T, et al. Cerebrotendinous Xanthomatosis: molecular pathogenesis, clinical Spectrum, diagnosis, and disease-modifying treatments. J Atheroscler Thromb. 2021;28(9):905–25.
13. Gallus GN, Dotti MT, Federico A. Clinical and molecular diagnosis of cerebrotendinous xanthomatosis with a review of the mutations in the CYP27A1 gene. Neurol Sci. 2006;27(2):143–9.
14. Cali JJ, Hsieh CL, Francke U, Russell DW. Mutations in the bile acid biosynthetic enzyme sterol 27-hydroxylase underlie cerebrotendinous xanthomatosis. J Biol Chem. 1991;266(12):7779–83.
15. Berginer VM, Abeliovich D. Genetics of cerebrotendinous xanthomatosis (CTX): an autosomal recessive trait with high gene frequency in Sephardim of Moroccan origin. Am J Med Genet. 1981;10(2):151–7.
16. Inoue K, Kubota S, Seyama Y. Cholestanol induces apoptosis of cerebellar neuronal cells. Biochem Biophys Res Commun. 1999;256(1):198–203.
17. Berginer VM, Salen G, Shefer S. Long-term treatment of cerebrotendinous xanthomatosis with chenodeoxycholic acid. N Engl J Med. 1984;311(26):1649–52.
18. Pierre G, Setchell K, Blyth J, Preece MA, Chakrapani A, McKiernan P. Prospective treatment of cerebrotendinous xanthomatosis with cholic acid therapy. J Inherit Metab Dis. 2008;31(Suppl 2):S241–5.
19. Mandia D, Chaussenot A, Besson G, Lamari F, Castelnovo G, Curot J, et al. Cholic acid as a treatment for cerebrotendinous xanthomatosis in adults. J Neurol. 2019;266(8):2043–50.
20. Salen G, Meriwether TW, Nicolau G. Chenodeoxycholic acid inhibits increased cholesterol and cholestanol synthesis in patients with cerebrotendinous xanthomatosis. Biochem Med. 1975;14(1):57–74.
21. Koopman BJ, Wolthers BG, van der Molen JC, Waterreus RJ. Bile acid therapies applied to patients suffering from cerebrotendinous xanthomatosis. Clin Chim Acta. 1985;152(1–2):115–22.
22. Pedley TA, Emerson RG, Warner CL, Rowland LP, Salen G. Treatment of cerebrotendinous xanthomatosis with chenodeoxycholic acid. Ann Neurol. 1985;18(4):517–8.
23. Stelten BML, Huidekoper HH, van de Warrenburg BPC, Brilstra EH, Hollak CEM, Haak HR, et al. Long-term treatment effect in cerebrotendinous xanthomatosis depends on age at treatment start. Neurology. 2019;92(2):e83–95.
24. Yahalom G, Tsabari R, Molshatzki N, Ephraty L, Cohen H, Hassin-Baer S. Neurological outcome in cerebrotendinous xanthomatosis treated with chenodeoxycholic acid: early versus late diagnosis. Clin Neuropharmacol. 2013;36(3):78–83.

25. Salen G, Shefer S, Tint GS, Nicolau G, Dayal B, Batta AK. Biosynthesis of bile acids in cerebrotendinous xanthomatosis. Relationship of bile acid pool sizes and synthesis rates to hydroxylations at C-12, C-25, and C-26. J Clin Invest. 1985;76(2):744–51.
26. Salen G, Shefer S, Cheng FW, Dayal B, Batta AK, Tint GS. Cholic acid biosynthesis: the enzymatic defect in cerebrotendinous xanthomatosis. J Clin Invest. 1979;63(1):38–44.
27. Oftebro H, Bjorkhem I, Skrede S, Schreiner A, Pederson JI. Cerebrotendinous xanthomatosis: a defect in mitochondrial 26-hydroxylation required for normal biosynthesis of cholic acid. J Clin Invest. 1980;65(6):1418–30.
28. Javitt NB, Kok E, Cohen B, Burstein S. Cerebrotendinous xanthomatosis: reduced serum 26-hydroxycholesterol. J Lipid Res. 1982;23(4):627–30.
29. Une M, Hoshita T. Natural occurrence and chemical synthesis of bile alcohols, higher bile acids, and short side chain bile acids. Hiroshima J Med Sci. 1994;43(2):37–67.
30. Setchell KDR, Street JM, Sjovall J. Fecal bile acids. In: Setchell KDR, Kritchevsky D, Nair PP, editors. The bile acids: methods and applications. New York: Plenum Press; 1988. p. 441–570.
31. van Heijst AF, Wevers RA, Tangerman A, Cruysberg JR, Renier WO, Tolboom JJ. Chronic diarrhoea as a dominating symptom in two children with cerebrotendinous xanthomatosis. Acta Paediatr. 1996;85(8):932–6.
32. Verrips A, van Engelen BG, Wevers RA, van Geel BM, Cruysberg JR, van den Heuvel LP, et al. Presence of diarrhea and absence of tendon xanthomas in patients with cerebrotendinous xanthomatosis. Arch Neurol. 2000;57(4):520–4.
33. Duell PB, Salen G, Eichler FS, DeBarber AE, Connor SL, Casaday L, et al. Diagnosis, treatment, and clinical outcomes in 43 cases with cerebrotendinous xanthomatosis. J Clin Lipidol. 2018;12(5):1169–78.
34. Shefer S, Cheng FW, Dayal B, Hauser S, Tint GS, Salen G, et al. A 25-hydroxylation pathway of cholic acid biosynthesis in man and rat. J Clin Invest. 1976;57(4):897–903.
35. Duane WC, Pooler PA, Hamilton JN. Bile acid synthesis in man. In vivo activity of the 25-hydroxylation pathway. J Clin Invest. 1988;82(1):82–5.
36. Salen G, Shefer S, Mosbach EH, Hauser S, Cohen BI, Nicolau G. Metabolism of potential precursors of chenodeoxycholic acid in cerebrotendinous xanthomatosis (CTX). J Lipid Res. 1979;20(1):22–30.
37. Bjorkhem I, Oftebro H, Skrede S, Pedersen JI. Assay of intermediates in bile acid biosynthesis using isotope dilution–mass spectrometry: hepatic levels in the normal state and in cerebrotendinous xanthomatosis. J Lipid Res. 1981;22(2):191–200.
38. Andersson S, Davis DL, Dahlback H, Jornvall H, Russell DW. Cloning, structure, and expression of the mitochondrial cytochrome P-450 sterol 26-hydroxylase, a bile acid biosynthetic enzyme. J Biol Chem. 1989;264(14):8222–9.
39. Cali JJ, Russell DW. Characterization of human sterol 27-hydroxylase. A mitochondrial cytochrome P-450 that catalyzes multiple oxidation reaction in bile acid biosynthesis. J Biol Chem. 1991;266(12):7774–8.
40. Salen G, Shefer S, Tint GS. Transformation of 4-cholesten-3-one and 7 alpha-hydroxy-4-cholesten-3-one into cholestanol and bile acids in cerebrotendinous xanthomatosis. Gastroenterology. 1984;87(2):276–83.
41. Skrede S, Bjorkhem I, Buchmann MS, Hopen G, Fausa O. A novel pathway for biosynthesis of cholestanol with 7 alpha-hydroxylated C27-steroids as intermediates, and its importance for the accumulation of cholestanol in cerebrotendinous xanthomatosis. J Clin Invest. 1985;75(2):448–55.
42. Skrede S, Buchmann MS, Bjorkhem I. Hepatic 7 alpha-dehydroxylation of bile acid intermediates, and its significance for the pathogenesis of cerebrotendinous xanthomatosis. J Lipid Res. 1988;29(2):157–64.
43. Grundy SM, Ahrens EH Jr, Salen G. Interruption of the enterohepatic circulation of bile acids in man: comparative effects of cholestyramine and ileal exclusion on cholesterol metabolism. J Lab Clin Med. 1971;78(1):94–121.

44. Bjorkhem I, Reihner E, Angelin B, Ewerth S, Akerlund JE, Einarsson K. On the possible use of the serum level of 7 alpha-hydroxycholesterol as a marker for increased activity of the cholesterol 7 alpha-hydroxylase in humans. J Lipid Res. 1987;28(8):889–94.
45. Verrips A, Dotti MT, Mignarri A, Stelten BML, Verma S, Federico A. The safety and effectiveness of chenodeoxycholic acid treatment in patients with cerebrotendinous xanthomatosis: two retrospective cohort studies. Neurol Sci. 2020;41(4):943–9.
46. Bjorkhem I, Andersson O, Diczfalusy U, Sevastik B, Xiu RJ, Duan C, et al. Atherosclerosis and sterol 27-hydroxylase: evidence for a role of this enzyme in elimination of cholesterol from human macrophages. Proc Natl Acad Sci USA. 1994;91(18):8592–6.
47. Babiker A, Andersson O, Lindblom D, van der Linden J, Wiklund B, Lutjohann D, et al. Elimination of cholesterol as cholestenoic acid in human lung by sterol 27-hydroxylase: evidence that most of this steroid in the circulation is of pulmonary origin. J Lipid Res. 1999;40(8):1417–25.
48. Crisby M, Nilsson J, Kostulas V, Bjorkhem I, Diczfalusy U. Localization of sterol 27-hydroxylase immuno-reactivity in human atherosclerotic plaques. Biochim Biophys Acta. 1997;1344(3):278–85.
49. Cruysberg JR, Wevers RA, Tolboom JJ. Juvenile cataract associated with chronic diarrhea in pediatric cerebrotendinous xanthomatosis. Am J Ophthalmol. 1991;112(5):606–7.
50. Wevers RA, Cruysberg JR, Van Heijst AF, Janssen-Zijlstra FS, Renier WO, Van Engelen BG, et al. Paediatric cerebrotendinous xanthomatosis. J Inherit Metab Dis. 1992;15(3):374–6.
51. Setchell KDR, O'Connell N, Russell DW, Kelly DA. A unique case of cerebrotendinous xanthomatosis in infancy with cholestatic liver disease further highlights bile acid synthetic defects as an important category of metabolic liver disease (Abstract). XX International Bile Acid Meeting, 13–14 June, Amsterdam, Falk Symposium 165 (Abstract). 2000.
52. Gong JY, Setchell KDR, Zhao J, Zhang W, Wolfe B, Lu Y, et al. Severe neonatal cholestasis in Cerebrotendinous Xanthomatosis: genetics, immunostaining, mass spectrometry. J Pediatr Gastroenterol Nutr. 2017;65(5):561–8.
53. von Bahr S, Bjorkhem I, Van't Hooft F, Alvelius G, Nemeth A, Sjovall J, et al. Mutation in the sterol 27-hydroxylase gene associated with fatal cholestasis in infancy. J Pediatr Gastroenterol Nutr. 2005;40(4):481–6.
54. Clayton PT, Verrips A, Sistermans E, Mann A, Mieli-Vergani G, Wevers R. Mutations in the sterol 27-hydroxylase gene (CYP27A) cause hepatitis of infancy as well as cerebrotendinous xanthomatosis. J Inherit Metab Dis. 2002;25(6):501–13.
55. Pietrobattista A, Spada M, Candusso M, Boenzi S, Dionisi-Vici C, Francalanci P, et al. Liver transplantation in an infant with cerebrotendinous xanthomatosis, cholestasis, and rapid evolution of liver failure. Pediatr Transplant. 2022;26(6):e14318.
56. Degrassi I, Amoruso C, Giordano G, Del Puppo M, Mignarri A, Dotti MT, et al. Case report: early treatment with Chenodeoxycholic acid in Cerebrotendinous Xanthomatosis presenting as neonatal cholestasis. Front Pediatr. 2020;8:382.
57. Balistreri WF, Suchy FJ, Farrell MK, Heubi JE. Pathologic versus physiologic cholestasis: elevated serum concentration of a secondary bile acid in the presence of hepatobiliary disease. J Pediatr. 1981;98(3):399–402.
58. Suchy FJ, Balistreri WF, Heubi JE, Searcy JE, Levin RS. Physiologic cholestasis: elevation of the primary serum bile acid concentrations in normal infants. Gastroenterology. 1981;80(5 pt 1):1037–41.
59. Watkins JB, Ingall D, Szczepanik P, Klein PD, Lester R. Bile-salt metabolism in the newborn. Measurement of pool size and synthesis by stable isotope technic. N Engl J Med. 1973;288(9):431–4.
60. Watkins JB, Szczepanik P, Gould JB, Klein P, Lester R. Bile salt metabolism in the human premature infant. Preliminary observations of pool size and synthesis rate following prenatal administration of dexamethasone and phenobarbital. Gastroenterology. 1975;69(3):706–13.
61. Heubi JE, Balistreri WF, Suchy FJ. Bile salt metabolism in the first year of life. J Lab Clin Med. 1982;100(1):127–36.

62. Setchell KD, Heubi JE. Defects in bile acid biosynthesis–diagnosis and treatment. J Pediatr Gastroenterol Nutr. 2006;43(Suppl 1):S17–22.
63. Koopman BJ, van der Molen JC, Wolthers BG, de Jager AE, Waterreus RJ, Gips CH. Capillary gas chromatographic determination of cholestanol/cholesterol ratio in biological fluids. Its potential usefulness for the follow-up of some liver diseases and its lack of specificity in diagnosing CTX (cerebrotendinous xanthomatosis). Clin Chim Acta. 1984;137(3):305–15.
64. Axelson M, Sjovall J. Potential bile acid precursors in plasma–possible indicators of biosynthetic pathways to cholic and chenodeoxycholic acids in man. J Steroid Biochem. 1990;36(6):631–40.
65. Galman C, Arvidsson I, Angelin B, Rudling M. Monitoring hepatic cholesterol 7alpha-hydroxylase activity by assay of the stable bile acid intermediate 7alpha-hydroxy-4-cholesten-3-one in peripheral blood. J Lipid Res. 2003;44(4):859–66.
66. DeBarber AE, Connor WE, Pappu AS, Merkens LS, Steiner RD. ESI-MS/MS quantification of 7alpha-hydroxy-4-cholesten-3-one facilitates rapid, convenient diagnostic testing for cerebrotendinous xanthomatosis. Clin Chim Acta. 2010;411(1–2):43–8.
67. Freudenberg F, Gothe F, Beigel F, Rust C, Koletzko S. Serum 7-alpha-hydroxy-4-cholesten-3-one as a marker for bile acid loss in children. J Pediatr. 2013;163(5):1367–71 e1.
68. DeBarber AE, Luo J, Giugliani R, Souza CF, Chiang JP, Merkens LS, et al. A useful multi-analyte blood test for cerebrotendinous xanthomatosis. Clin Biochem. 2014;47(9):860–3.
69. DeBarber AE, Luo J, Star-Weinstock M, Purkayastha S, Geraghty MT, Chiang JP, et al. A blood test for cerebrotendinous xanthomatosis with potential for disease detection in newborns. J Lipid Res. 2014;55(1):146–54.
70. Hoflinger P, Hauser S, Yutuc E, Hengel H, Griffiths L, Radelfahr F, et al. Metabolic profiling in serum, cerebrospinal fluid, and brain of patients with cerebrotendinous xanthomatosis. J Lipid Res. 2021;62:100078.
71. Bleyle L, Huidekoper HH, Vaz FM, Singh R, Steiner RD, DeBarber AE. Update on newborn dried bloodspot testing for cerebrotendinous xanthomatosis: an available high-throughput liquid-chromatography tandem mass spectrometry method. Mol Genet Metab Rep. 2016;7:11–5.
72. Hong X, Daiker J, Sadilek M, DeBarber AE, Chiang J, Duan J, et al. Toward newborn screening of cerebrotendinous xanthomatosis: results of a biomarker research study using 32,000 newborn dried blood spots. Genet Med. 2020;22(10):1606–12.
73. Shefer S, Dayal B, Tint GS, Salen G, Mosbach EH. Identification of pentahydroxy bile alcohols in cerebrotendinous xanthomatosis: characterization of 5beta-cholestane-3alpha, 7alpha, 12alpha, 24xi, 25-pentol and 5beta-cholestane-3alpha, 7alpha, 12alpha, 23xi, 25-pentol. J Lipid Res. 1975;16(4):280–6.
74. Hoshita T, Yasuhara M, Kihira K, Kuramoto T. Identification of (23S)-5beta-cholestane-3alpha, 7alpha, 12alpha, 23, 25-pentol in cerebrotendinous xanthomatosis. Steroids. 1976;27(5):657–64.
75. Hoshita T, Yasuhara M, Une M, Kibe A, Itoga E, Kito S, et al. Occurrence of bile alcohol glucuronides in bile of patients with cerebrotendinous xanthomatosis. J Lipid Res. 1980;21(8):1015–21.
76. Wolthers BG, Volmer M, van der Molen J, Koopman BJ, de Jager AE, Waterreus RJ. Diagnosis of cerebrotendinous xanthomatosis (CTX) and effect of chenodeoxycholic acid therapy by analysis of urine using capillary gas chromatography. Clin Chim Acta. 1983;131(1–2):53–65.
77. Egestad B, Pettersson P, Skrede S, Sjovall J. Fast atom bombardment mass spectrometry in the diagnosis of cerebrotendinous xanthomatosis. Scand J Clin Lab Invest. 1985;45(5):443–6.
78. Shimazu K, Kuwabara M, Yoshii M, Kihira K, Takeuchi H, Nakano I, et al. Bile alcohol profiles in bile, urine, and feces of a patient with cerebrotendinous xanthomatosis. J Biochem. 1986;99(2):477–83.
79. Yasuhara M, Kuramoto T, Hoshita T, Itoga E, Kito S. Identifications of 5 beta-cholestane-3 alpha, 7 alpha, 12 alpha, 23 beta-tetrol, 5 beta-cholestane-3 alpha, 7 alpha, 12 alpha, 24 alpha-tetrol, and 5 beta-cholestane-3 alpha, 7 alpha, 12 alpha, 24 beta-tetrol in cerebrotendinous xanthomatosis. Steroids. 1978;31(3):333–45.

80. Kuramoto T, Fukuda K, Ohshima A, Kihira K, Hoshita T. Determination of the glucurono-conjugated position in bile alcohol glucuronides excreted in urine of a patient with cerebrotendinous xanthomatosis by a nuclear magnetic resonance study. J Biochem. 1994;115(4):655–8.
81. Kuramoto T, Suemura Y, Kihira K, Hiraoka T, Hoshita T. Determination of the glucurono-conjugated position in bile alcohol glucuronides present in a patient with cerebrotendinous xanthomatosis. Steroids. 1995;60(10):709–12.
82. Haas D, Gan-Schreier H, Langhans CD, Rohrer T, Engelmann G, Heverin M, et al. Differential diagnosis in patients with suspected bile acid synthesis defects. World J Gastroenterol. 2012;18(10):1067–76.
83. Mills KA, Mushtaq I, Johnson AW, Whitfield PD, Clayton PT. A method for the quantitation of conjugated bile acids in dried blood spots using electrospray ionization-mass spectrometry. Pediatr Res. 1998;43(3):361–8.
84. Mignarri A, Magni A, Del Puppo M, Gallus GN, Bjorkhem I, Federico A, et al. Evaluation of cholesterol metabolism in cerebrotendinous xanthomatosis. J Inherit Metab Dis. 2016;39(1):75–83.
85. Vaz FM, Bootsma AH, Kulik W, Verrips A, Wevers RA, Schielen PC, et al. A newborn screening method for cerebrotendinous xanthomatosis using bile alcohol glucuronides and metabolite ratios. J Lipid Res. 2017;58(5):1002–7.
86. DeBarber AE, Kalfon L, Fedida A, Fleisher Sheffer V, Ben Haroush S, Chasnyk N, et al. Newborn screening for cerebrotendinous xanthomatosis is the solution for early identification and treatment. J Lipid Res. 2018;59(11):2214–22.
87. Sjovall J. Dietary glycine and taurine on bile acid conjugation in man; bile acids and steroids 75. Proc Soc Exp Biol Med. 1959;100(4):676–8.
88. Encrantz JC, Sjovall J. On the bile acids in duodenal contents of infants and children. Bile acids and steroids 72. Clin Chim Acta. 1959;4:793–9.
89. Setchell KD, Dumaswala R, Colombo C, Ronchi M. Hepatic bile acid metabolism during early development revealed from the analysis of human fetal gallbladder bile. J Biol Chem. 1988;263(32):16637–44.
90. Lutjohann D, Stellaard F, Bjorkhem I. Levels of 7alpha-hydroxycholesterol and/or 7alpha-hydroxy-4-cholest-3-one are the optimal biochemical markers for the evaluation of treatment of cerebrotendinous xanthomatosis. J Neurol. 2020;267(2):572–3.
91. Einarsson K, Hellstrom K, Kallner M. Feedback regulation of bile acid formation in man. Metabolism. 1973;22(12):1477–83.
92. Jelinek DF, Andersson S, Slaughter CA, Russell DW. Cloning and regulation of cholesterol 7 alpha-hydroxylase, the rate-limiting enzyme in bile acid biosynthesis. J Biol Chem. 1990;265(14):8190–7.
93. Hofmann AF. The enterohepatic circulation of bile acids in man. Clin Gastroenterol. 1977;6(1):3–24.
94. Chiang JY. Regulation of bile acid synthesis. Front Biosci. 1998;3:d176–93.
95. Makishima M, Okamoto AY, Repa JJ, Tu H, Learned RM, Luk A, et al. Identification of a nuclear receptor for bile acids. Science. 1999;284(5418):1362–5.
96. Boyer JL. New concepts of mechanisms of hepatocyte bile formation. Physiol Rev. 1980;60(2):303–26.
97. Roda A, Hofmann AF, Mysels KJ. The influence of bile salt structure on self-association in aqueous solutions. J Biol Chem. 1983;258(10):6362–70.
98. Roda A, Minutello A, Angellotti MA, Fini A. Bile acid structure-activity relationship: evaluation of bile acid lipophilicity using 1-octanol/water partition coefficient and reverse phase HPLC. J Lipid Res. 1990;31(8):1433–43.
99. Bachrach WH, Hofmann AF. Ursodeoxycholic acid in the treatment of cholesterol cholelithiasis. Part II Dig Dis Sci. 1982;27(9):833–56.
100. Bachrach WH, Hofmann AF. Ursodeoxycholic acid in the treatment of cholesterol cholelithiasis. Part I. Dig Dis Sci. 1982;27(8):737–61.

101. Salen G, Berginer V, Shore V, Horak I, Horak E, Tint GS, et al. Increased concentrations of cholestanol and apolipoprotein B in the cerebrospinal fluid of patients with cerebrotendinous xanthomatosis. Effect of chenodeoxycholic acid. N Engl J Med. 1987;316(20):1233–8.
102. Pilo de la Fuente B, Ruiz I, Lopez de Munain A, Jimenez-Escrig A. Cerebrotendinous xanthomatosis: neuropathological findings. J Neurol. 2008;255(6):839–42.
103. Waterreus RJ, Koopman BJ, Wolthers BG, Oosterhuis HJ. Cerebrotendinous xanthomatosis (CTX): a clinical survey of the patient population in The Netherlands. Clin Neurol Neurosurg. 1987;89(3):169–75.
104. Stelten BML, Lycklama ANGJ, Hendriks E, Kluijtmans LAJ, Wevers RA, Verrips A. Long-term MRI findings in patients with Cerebrotendinous Xanthomatosis treated with Chenodeoxycholic acid. Neurology. 2022;99(13):559–66.
105. Zubarioglu T, Kiykim E, Yesil G, Demircioglu D, Cansever MS, Yalcinkaya C, et al. Early diagnosed cerebrotendinous xanthomatosis patients: clinical, neuroradiological characteristics and therapy results of a single center from Turkey. Acta Neurol Belg. 2019;119(3):343–50.
106. Schoenfield LJ, Lachin JM. Chenodiol (chenodeoxycholic acid) for dissolution of gallstones: the National Cooperative Gallstone Study. A controlled trial of efficacy and safety. Ann Intern Med. 1981;95(3):257–82.
107. Roda E, Bazzoli F, Labate AM, Mazzella G, Roda A, Sama C, et al. Ursodeoxycholic acid vs. chenodeoxycholic acid as cholesterol gallstone-dissolving agents: a comparative randomized study. Hepatology. 1982;2(6):804–10.
108. Huidekoper HH, Vaz FM, Verrips A, Bosch AM. Hepatotoxicity due to chenodeoxycholic acid supplementation in an infant with cerebrotendinous xanthomatosis: implications for treatment. Eur J Pediatr. 2016;175(1):143–6.
109. Zhang MH, Setchell KD, Zhao J, Gong JY, Lu Y, Wang JS. Delta4-3-oxosteroid-5beta-reductase deficiency: responses to oral bile acid therapy and long-term outcomes. World J Gastroenterol. 2019;25(7):859–69.
110. Cholbam to treat rare bile acid synthesis disorders [press release]. 2015.
111. Gonzales E, Gerhardt MF, Fabre M, Setchell KD, Davit-Spraul A, Vincent I, et al. Oral cholic acid for hereditary defects of primary bile acid synthesis: a safe and effective long-term therapy. Gastroenterology. 2009;137(4):1310–20e1-3.
112. Heubi JE, Bove KE, Setchell KDR. Oral Cholic acid is efficacious and well tolerated in patients with bile acid synthesis and Zellweger Spectrum disorders. J Pediatr Gastroenterol Nutr. 2017;65(3):321–6.
113. Setchell KD, Bragetti P, Zimmer-Nechemias L, Daugherty C, Pelli MA, Vaccaro R, et al. Oral bile acid treatment and the patient with Zellweger syndrome. Hepatology. 1992;15(2):198–207.
114. Daugherty CC, Setchell KD, Heubi JE, Balistreri WF. Resolution of liver biopsy alterations in three siblings with bile acid treatment of an inborn error of bile acid metabolism (delta 4-3-oxosteroid 5 beta-reductase deficiency). Hepatology. 1993;18(5):1096–101.
115. Berendse K, Klouwer FC, Koot BG, Kemper EM, Ferdinandusse S, Koelfat KV, et al. Cholic acid therapy in Zellweger spectrum disorders. J Inherit Metab Dis. 2016;39(6):859–68.
116. Elias ER, Orth LE, Li A, Xu L, Jones SM, Rizzo WB. Cholic acid increases plasma cholesterol in smith-Lemli-Opitz syndrome: a pilot study. Mol Genet Metab Rep. 2024;38:101030.
117. Bove KE, Heubi JE, Balistreri WF, Setchell KD. Bile acid synthetic defects and liver disease: a comprehensive review. Pediatr Dev Pathol. 2004;7(4):315–34.
118. Wang H, Chen J, Hollister K, Sowers LC, Forman BM. Endogenous bile acids are ligands for the nuclear receptor FXR/BAR. Mol Cell. 1999;3(5):543–53.
119. Fujino T, Une M, Imanaka T, Inoue K, Nishimaki-Mogami T. Structure-activity relationship of bile acids and bile acid analogs in regard to FXR activation. J Lipid Res. 2004;45(1):132–8.
120. Roda A, Cappelleri G, Aldini R, Roda E, Barbara L. Quantitative aspects of the interaction of bile acids with human serum albumin. J Lipid Res. 1982;23(3):490–5.
121. Crosignani A, Setchell KD, Invernizzi P, Larghi A, Rodrigues CM, Podda M. Clinical pharmacokinetics of therapeutic bile acids. Clin Pharmacokinet. 1996;30(5):333–58.

122. Zhang W, Jha P, Wolfe B, Gioiello A, Pellicciari R, Wang J, et al. Tandem mass spectrometric determination of atypical 3beta-hydroxy-Delta5-bile acids in patients with 3beta-hydroxy-Delta5-C27-steroid oxidoreductase deficiency: application to diagnosis and monitoring of bile acid therapeutic response. Clin Chem. 2015;61(7):955–63.
123. Kuroki S, Naito T, Okamoto S, Sakai H, Yamashita H, Chijiiwa K, et al. Cholestyramine loading test to assess hepatic reserve for bile acid synthesis in patients with chronic liver diseases. Gastroenterology. 1997;112(4):1277–83.
124. Koopman BJ, Waterreus RJ, Van den Brekel HW, Wolthers BG. Detection of carriers of cerebrotendinous xanthomatosis. Clin Chim Acta. 1986;158(2):179–85.
125. Lewis B, Mitchell WD, Marenah CB, Cortese C, Reynolds EH, Shakir R. Cerebrotendinous xanthomatosis: biochemical response to inhibition of cholesterol synthesis. Br Med J (Clin Res Ed). 1983;287(6384):21–2.
126. Verrips A, Wevers RA, Van Engelen BG, Keyser A, Wolthers BG, Barkhof F, et al. Effect of simvastatin in addition to chenodeoxycholic acid in patients with cerebrotendinous xanthomatosis. Metabolism. 1999;48(2):233–8.
127. Nakamura T, Matsuzawa Y, Takemura K, Kubo M, Miki H, Tarui S. Combined treatment with chenodeoxycholic acid and pravastatin improves plasma cholestanol levels associated with marked regression of tendon xanthomas in cerebrotendinous xanthomatosis. Metabolism. 1991;40(7):741–6.
128. Kuriyama M, Tokimura Y, Fujiyama J, Utatsu Y, Osame M. Treatment of cerebrotendinous xanthomatosis: effects of chenodeoxycholic acid, pravastatin, and combined use. J Neurol Sci. 1994;125(1):22–8.
129. Dotti MT, Lutjohann D, von Bergmann K, Federico A. Normalisation of serum cholestanol concentration in a patient with cerebrotendinous xanthomatosis by combined treatment with chenodeoxycholic acid, simvastatin and LDL apheresis. Neurol Sci. 2004;25(4):185–91.
130. Batta AK, Salen G, Tint GS. Hydrophilic 7 beta-hydroxy bile acids, lovastatin, and cholestyramine are ineffective in the treatment of cerebrotendinous xanthomatosis. Metabolism. 2004;53(5):556–62.

Cholic Acid Treatment in Adults with Cerebrotendinous Xanthomatosis (CTX)

21

Yann Nadjar

Cerebrotendinous xanthomatosis (CTX) is a genetic recessive disease associated with bi-allelic pathogenic genetic variants of *CYP27A1* gene, resulting in decreased 27-hydroxylase enzymatic activity [1] (see corresponding chapters). 27-hydroxylase is a mitochondrial enzyme involved in the normal liver biosynthesis of bile acids from cholesterol. As a consequence of this enzymatic block, several biochemical abnormalities were observed in CTX patients, including strongly increased cholestanol synthesis. Cholestanol accumulation in different organs is thought to be the cause of CTX clinical manifestations, and it is widely used as a blood diagnostic biomarker for CTX although its sensitivity was recently questioned [2] (see corresponding chapters).

Cholic acid (CA) is one of the two primary bile acids synthesized by the human liver, along with chenodeoxycholic acid (CDCA). CDCA is a widely used treatment of CTX [3], and many papers reported the beneficial effect of CDCA treatment in CTX patients since several decades (see corresponding chapters), whereas literature about use of CA is scarce [4].

The main reason explaining that CDCA is widely used as CTX treatment is probably that one of the first observation in CTX that helped to understand the pathophysiology of the disease was the strongly decreased CDCA concentration in bile [5]. CDCA treatment was then shown to be efficient to drastically decrease blood cholestanol [6]. The explanation for these findings are the following (see also corresponding chapters): in CTX, due to the enzymatic block, CDCA is almost not synthesized, whereas physiologically CDCA inhibits the 7α-hydroxylase activity, which is the rate limiting enzyme of bile acids synthesis from cholesterol, through the activation of the nuclear farnesoid X receptor (FXR), a nuclear receptor that

Y. Nadjar (✉)
Neurology Department, Neuro-Metabolism Unit, Reference Center for Metabolic and Lysosomal Neurological Diseases, Hopital Pitié-Salpétrière, AP-HP, Paris, France
e-mail: yann.nadjar@aphp.fr

A. Federico et al. (eds.), *Cerebrotendinous Xanthomatosis*,
https://doi.org/10.1007/978-3-031-92526-9_21

regulates the metabolism of bile acids [7]; therefore, due to the absence of CDCA, 7α-hydroxylase activity is strongly increased in CTX [8]. This increased activity, combined with the enzymatic block, leads to accumulation of bile acids intermediates, and notably the 7α-hydroxy-4-cholesten-3-one, which is the precursor of cholestanol, and bile alcohols that accumulates in CTX. When CDCA is given to treat CTX patients, it reverses the upregulation of the 7α-hydroxylase activity which significantly decreases, and consequently bile acid intermediates like cholestanol stop to accumulate. CDCA treatment acts as a suppressor of the endogenous bile acid synthesis.

CA was less studied than CDCA, probably because CA was found at almost normal concentration in bile from CTX patients. This is due to two combined phenomena: (i) the fact that the enzymatic block in CTX is not part of an accessory biosynthetic pathway leading only to CA synthesis and not CDCA (the B sub-pathway of the classical pathway, physiologically involved in 1% of CA synthesis; see Fig. 21.1, [9]; and (ii) the strongly increased 7α-hydroxylase activity (discussed above). However, CA, as CDCA, can also inhibit 7α-hydroxylase activity through FXR activation, despite it was shown that CA is a less potent activator [10].

Only three articles in the literature report the use of CA in adults diagnosed with CTX, with similar and coherent findings. Koopman and colleagues [11] reported the use of CA in CTX patients for the first time only 1 year after the first report of CDCA use was published and compared the two bile acids effects. They conclude that although both therapies are efficient, CA should be especially recommended. Indeed, Koopman and al showed similar levels of reduction of urinary bile alcohols

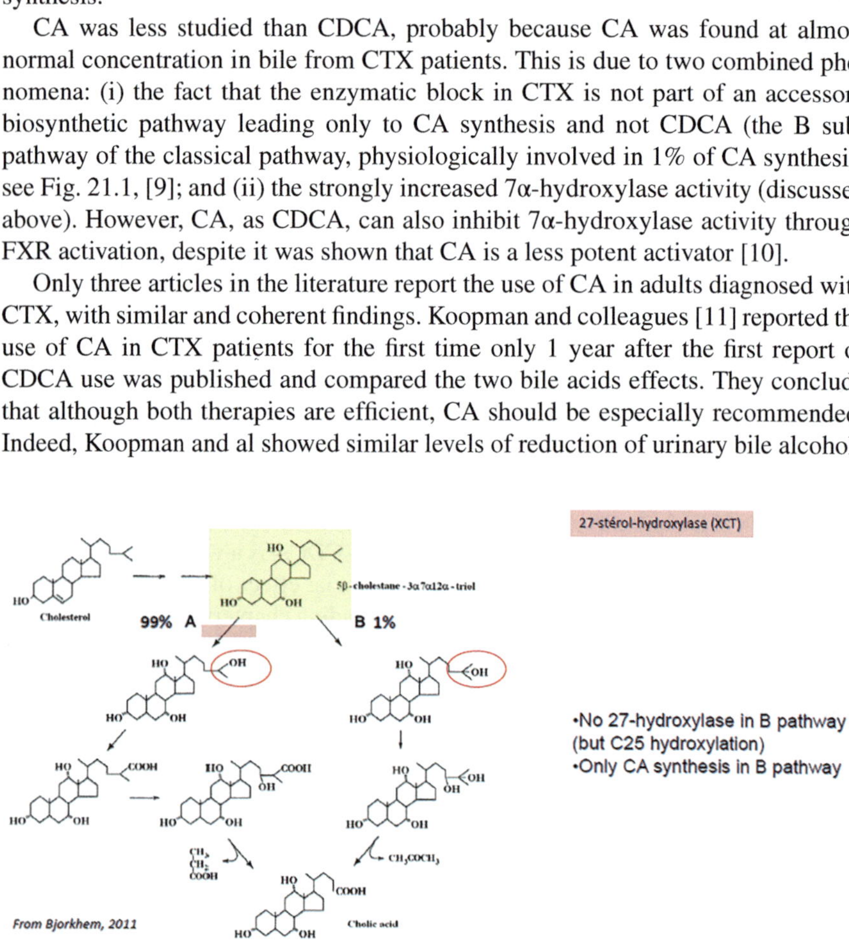

Fig 21.1 Classic pathway of bile acid synthesis from cholesterol is in fact composed of two different sub-pathways, the main one A (corresponding to 99% of the classic pathway activity physiologically and leading to CDCA and CA synthesis), and the accessory one B (corresponding to 1% of the classic pathway activity physiologically, leading only to CA synthesis, and that does not need 27-hydroxylase to function, as opposed to sub-pathway A). Adapted from Björkhem et al, 2010, Cerebrotendinous xanthomatosis: An inborn error in bile acid synthesis with defined mutations but still a challenge. Biochem Biophys Res Commun 396:46–9

in four adult patients (and even better reduction by CA for one patient) and similar clinical evolution with symptoms stabilization, and no adverse reactions with CA, compared to known CDCA adverse events reported when used for gallstone indication (diarrhea, nausea, pruritus, and abnormal liver function tests). Waterreus and colleagues [12] showed a similar biochemical efficiency of CA compared to CDCA (13 analyzed patients) in eight patients, with both monitoring of plasma cholestanol and urinary bile alcohols. Among these eight patients, two had CA treatment only, and six had been also given (previously to CA) ursodeoxycholic treatment or CDCA treatment. One patient with previous CDCA treatment switched because of CDCA related adverse events (severe diarrhea, nausea, and abnormal liver function tests). No patient showed a clear clinical improvement either treated by CDCA or CA in this study (Waterreus et al). Finally, Mandia and colleagues [4] reported findings from 12 CA treated patients, including five previously treated by CDCA (non-naive) who switched from CDCA to CA due to supply issue. All non-naive patients had similar plasma cholestanol levels after switching from CDCA to CA, and all naive patients (i.e., who were only treated by CA) achieved a drastic decrease of plasma cholestanol level under CA compared to baseline cholestanol (and normalization for 4/7, see Fig. 21.2). Two patients clinically deteriorated while treated by CA with progression of the gait disorder; one was naive, switched to CDCA due to disease progression, that continued despite the switch; the other was non-naive and was also deteriorating while treated by CDCA before switching to CA. Interestingly these two patients had vacuolated dentate nucleus in brain MRI, a previously described finding which is associated with a negative prognosis [13]. Both CA and CDCA were well tolerated. Of note, one patient who had repetitive mild elevation of liver enzymes AST (2 N) and ALT (4.7 N) while treated by CDCA, had complete normalization of liver enzymes' levels in repeated blood samples after the switch to treatment with CA.

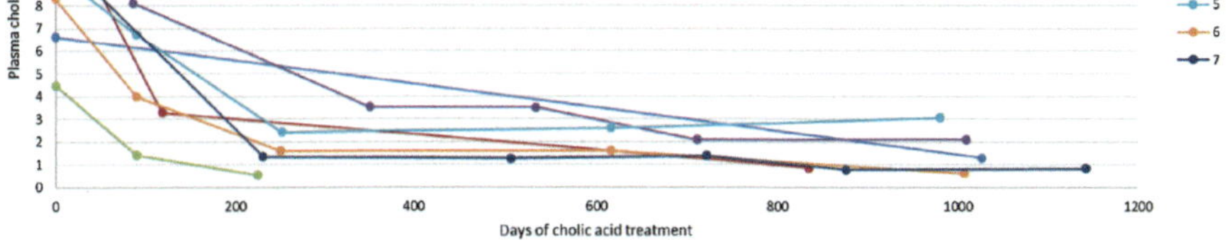

Fig 21.2 Plasma cholestanol levels over time from CA introduction, in seven naive (i.e., not previously treated by CDCA) adult patients. (Adapted from Mandia D et al, 2019, Cholic acid as a treatment for cerebrotendinous xanthomatosis in adults. J Neurol 266:2043–2050)

The adverse events that seem to be more frequent in CDCA compared to CA may be due to its increased detergent capacity that could have a cytotoxic effect through plasmatic membrane lysis [14, 15]. This cytotoxic effect could also be due to the production of lithocolic acid from CDCA by digestive tract flora, as litocholic acid also has a higher detergent capacity than CA.

In conclusion, CA treatment in CTX patients seems as efficient as CDCA in adult patients. However, there are much more studies related to the efficiency of CDCA compared to CA. CDCA and CA have never been directly compared prospectively in a study with high methodological standards. CA could be an interesting therapeutic option in CTX patients treated by CDCA who suffer from disabling adverse events and/or hepatotoxicity. CA might not be an interesting therapeutic option in CTX patients treated by CDCA whose symptoms are progressing despite expected biochemical efficiency of CDCA, as CA and CDCA share the same mechanism of action.

References

1. Nóbrega PR, Bernardes AM, Ribeiro RM, et al. Cerebrotendinous Xanthomatosis: a practice review of pathophysiology, diagnosis, and treatment. Front Neurol. 2022;13:1049850. https://doi.org/10.3389/fneur.2022.1049850.
2. Debarber AE, Duell PB. Update on cerebrotendinous xanthomatosis. Curr Opin Lipidol. 2021;32:123–31.
3. Verrips A, Dotti MT, Mignarri A, Stelten BML, Verma S, Federico A. The safety and effectiveness of chenodeoxycholic acid treatment in patients with cerebrotendinous xanthomatosis: two retrospective cohort studies. Neurol Sci. 2020;41:943–9.
4. Mandia D, Chaussenot A, Besson G, et al. Cholic acid as a treatment for cerebrotendinous xanthomatosis in adults. J Neurol. 2019;266:2043–50.
5. Salen G. Cholestanol deposition in cerebrotendinous xanthomatosis. A possible mechanism. Ann Intern Med. 1971;75:843–51.
6. Berginer VM, Salen G, Shefer S. Long-term treatment of cerebrotendinous xanthomatosis with chenodeoxycholic acid. N Engl J Med. 1984;311:1649–52.
7. Eloranta JJ, Kullak-Ublick GA. The role of FXR in disorders of bile acid homeostasis. Physiology. 2008;23:286–95.
8. Björkhem I. Cerebrotendinous xanthomatosis. Curr Opin Lipidol. 2013;24:283–7.
9. Björkhem I, Hansson M. Cerebrotendinous xanthomatosis: an inborn error in bile acid synthesis with defined mutations but still a challenge. Biochem Biophys Res Commun. 2010;396:46–9.
10. Makishima M, Okamoto AY, Repa JJ, Tu H, Learned RM, Luk A, Hull MV, Lustig KD, Mangelsdorf DJ, Shan B. Identification of a nuclear receptor for bite acids. Science. 1999;284(80):1362–5.
11. Koopman BJ, Wolthers BG, van der Molen JC, Waterreus RJ. Bile acid therapies applied to patients suffering from cerebrotendinous xanthomatosis. Clin Chim Acta. 1985;152:115–22.
12. Waterreus RJ, Koopman BJ, Wolthers BG, Oosterhuis HJ. Cerebrotendinous xanthomatosis (CTX): a clinical survey of the patient population in The Netherlands. Clin Neurol Neurosurg. 1987;89:169–75.
13. Mignarri A, Dotti MT, Federico A, De Stefano N, Battaglini M, Grazzini I, Galluzzi P, Monti L. The spectrum of magnetic resonance findings in cerebrotendinous xanthomatosis: redefinition and evidence of new markers of disease progression. J Neurol. 2017;264:862–74.

14. Di Gregorio MC, Cautela J, Galantini L. Physiology and physical chemistry of bile acids. Int J Mol Sci. 2021;22:1–23.
15. Yasuhara H, Tonooka M, Kamei K, Sakamoto K. Membrane effects of various drugs on isolated rat hepatocytes and erythrocytes. Toxicol Appl Pharmacol. 1985;79:453–60.

Gene Therapy for Cerebrotendinous Xanthomatosis (CTX)

22

Rubén Hernández-Alcoceba, Angie Molina, and Gloria Gonzalez-Aseguinolaza

Gene Therapy: Definition, Modalities, and Tools

The broad definition of gene therapy is the transfer of genetic material to the cells of an organism with a therapeutic purpose. The nucleic acid can be protein-coding double-stranded DNA, messenger RNA (mRNA), small single-stranded DNA or RNA oligonucleotides, interfering RNAs, or other RNA molecules with diverse functions.

A more restrictive definition considers gene therapy to be only those procedures involving the modification of the genetic material in the cells, either by gene addition (supplementation) or gene editing. It excludes the use of small nucleic acids for modulation of gene expression. These latter approaches are similar to conventional drugs in terms of clinical implementation, since the effect is transient requiring periodic administrations, and they allow standard dose adjustments.

All nucleic acids are negatively charged molecules and most of them present high molecular weights. This determines the need of specific vehicles (vectors) capable of delivering their genetic cargo into the cells, or physical methods to increase the plasma membrane permeability. Only small oligonucleotides are active upon direct administration in vivo. Vectors can be derived from viruses (adenoviruses, retroviruses, herpes simplex viruses, adeno-associated viruses, etc.) [1], or they can be chemical formulations such as polyplexes or lipid nanoparticles (LNPs)

R. Hernández-Alcoceba (✉) · A. Molina
University of Navarra, CIMA, Gene Therapy and Regulation of Gene Expression Program, Pamplona, Spain
e-mail: rubenh@unav.es

G. Gonzalez-Aseguinolaza
University of Navarra, CIMA, Gene Therapy and Regulation of Gene Expression Program, Pamplona, Spain

Vivet Therapeutics S.L., Pamplona, Spain

A. Federico et al. (eds.), *Cerebrotendinous Xanthomatosis*,
https://doi.org/10.1007/978-3-031-92526-9_22

[2]. In general, viral vectors are more efficient for the delivery of DNA because they co-opt the active mechanisms for nuclear delivery of their genetic cargo. In contrast, non-viral vectors are gaining popularity for RNA delivery because they are generally safer, less immunogenic, and can be administered multiple times without losing efficacy. The choice of the viral vector depends on the specificities of the indication and the size of the genetic material to be delivered. For maintaining long-term transgene expression in rapidly dividing cells, integrative vectors such as retro/lentiviruses are needed. In contrast, episomal vectors are suitable if the target cell has a low turnover, such as neurons, muscle cells, or hepatocytes. In this case, the current gold standard is adeno-associated viral vectors (AAVs), due to their low pathogenicity and immunogenicity [3]. The main limitation of AAVs is the relatively low cloning capacity (4.7 Kb).

Gene delivery can be achieved using ex vivo or in vivo approaches. When the transfer of genetic material is performed in isolated cells that are then administered to the subject, this modality is called ex vivo gene therapy. In contrast, in vivo gene therapy approaches introduce the vectors directly into the organism. The ex vivo approach allows the use of higher vectors doses or aggressive physical methods without compromising the safety of the therapy, and the modified cells can be characterized prior to infusion. This modality has been successfully used in the clinic for adoptive cancer therapy and gene supplementation for hematopoietic diseases. However, the high cost of the procedure and the need for patient pre-conditioning are stimulating the development of in vivo approaches for these indications. The same applies for the majority of monogenic diseases, in which migration and engraftment of corrected cells in the target organs are not feasible.

Another gene therapy modality showing remarkable progress is gene editing. The versatility of the Clustered Regularly Interspaced Short Palindromic Repeats (CRISPR)-Cas9 technology is allowing a rapid evolution of tools to modify the cellular genome [4]. In this ribonucleoprotein complex, sequence specificity is determined by an RNA guide and cleavage is performed by Cas9 nuclease. In its original format, the CRISPR-Cas9 introduces double-strand DNA breaks, which are rapidly repaired by the cellular machinery by non-homologous end joining (NHEJ), giving rise to insertion or deletions (indels) [5]. In the presence of a DNA template with homology arms for the 5′ and 3′ segments of the broken genome, the homology-directed repair (HDR) program can introduce exogenous DNA material [6]. Further evolution of the technology resulted in Cas9 proteins with the ability to cut only one DNA strand (nickase activity), which increases the safety of this approach [7]. In addition, proteins devoid of nuclease activity (dCas9 or equivalent) can be employed as DNA targeting domains for the development of sequence-specific base editors, thus allowing the correction of mutations without DNA cleavage [8]. Fusion of dCas9 with reverse transcriptases is able to insert small DNA sequences (prime editing), whereas association with recombinases or transposases can direct the insertion of larger fragments [8–11]. In principle, this would allow the incorporation of entire coding sequences of faulty genes in their endogenous chromosomal locations, ensuring nearly physiological transcriptional control and avoiding the need to design specific therapeutic cassettes for individual mutations. Finally, the fusion of dCas9 with artificial transcriptional activators or repressors can be used to modulate transgene expression [12]. However, the caveats of these approaches are the immunogenicity of CRISPR proteins and the potential off-target activity, which become a hurdle for clinical translation.

Application of Gene Therapy for the Treatment of Metabolic Diseases

Metabolic diseases comprise a wide range of disorders that affect a particular metabolic pathway. A report from 2021 described over 1450 inherited metabolic disorders (IMD) mostly resulting from pathogenic variants in specific genes leading to the accumulation of toxic metabolites or the strong reduction of some essential ones [13]. Given the genetic component of these IMD, gene therapy emerges as a promising tool to achieve safe, stable, and efficient correction of a wide range of these diseases.

As mentioned before, AAVs are the leading technology for in vivo gene therapy, with several products approved in the USA and/or other countries for retinal dystrophy (Luxturna), spinal muscular atrophy (Zolgensma), aromatic amino acid decarboxylase deficiency (Upstaza) [14], and hemophilia A and B (Roctavian and Hemgenix, respectively) [15, 16]. The latter applications involve intravenous administration of the vectors for secretion of coagulation factors from transduced hepatocytes.

Given the liver's essential role in the metabolism and its capacity to be transduced by AAV vectors, it is a key gene therapy target for treating IMD. It has been described that mostly all AAV serotypes have a tropism for hepatocytes when injected into the systemic circulation [17]. This fact, combined with the tolerogenic nature of this organ, makes the liver an ideal target for rAAV-based gene therapies. The first liver-directed AAV gene therapy in humans was described in 2006 by Manno et al. when an AAV2 vector expressing the human FIX was administered into hemophilia B patients, achieving therapeutic levels for 2 months with no related toxicity [18]. Subsequent improvements trying to increase vector transduction and FIX expression have led to the approval of a hemophilia B AAV5 gene therapy, Hemgenix [19].

From this experience, a large number of liver-directed AAV gene therapy clinical trials are in progress aiming to treat different metabolic diseases (ClinicalTrials.gov). Depending on the deficiency, the objective of the gene therapy and the threshold of corrected cells needed to achieve a therapeutic effect can vary. According to this, the aim could be (1) to restore the secretion of a defective protein, as in the case of hemophilia or alpha 1-antitrypsin (AAT) deficiency; (2) to reestablish cell autonomous defects within the hepatocytes (as observed for Wilson's disease, acute intermittent porphyria, ornithine transcarbamilase deficiency, among others; or (3) to treat multiorgan metabolic disorders such as lysosomal storage diseases. All these finished and ongoing clinical trials encourage patients diagnosed with liver IMD in which no targeted and effective treatment is currently available and with the advantage that no ongoing therapy adherence is needed.

Current Status of Gene Therapy for CTX

Many factors make CTX a good candidate for gene therapy (Fig. 22.1). First, it is a monogenic disease caused in all cases by homozygous or compound heterozygous biallelic pathogenic variants in the *CYP27A1* gene, encoding the cytochrome P450 sterol 27-hydroxylase enzyme [20]. The pathophysiology of the disease is relatively well understood, at least at the biochemical level [21], and there is no evidence that missense variants exert a dominant negative effect. The length of the coding sequence (1.593 bp) is compatible with the use of AAV vectors as described above. Restoration of *CYP27A1* function in the liver is relevant, considering the role of the sterol 27-hydroxylase enzyme in the bile acid metabolism. Of note, the enzyme is located in the mitochondria, but the gene is transcribed from chromosome 2.

All these considerations sustained the development of a well-established gene supplementation method based on intravenous administration of AAVs for liver transduction [22]. The vectors were evaluated in a mouse model for CTX, carrying

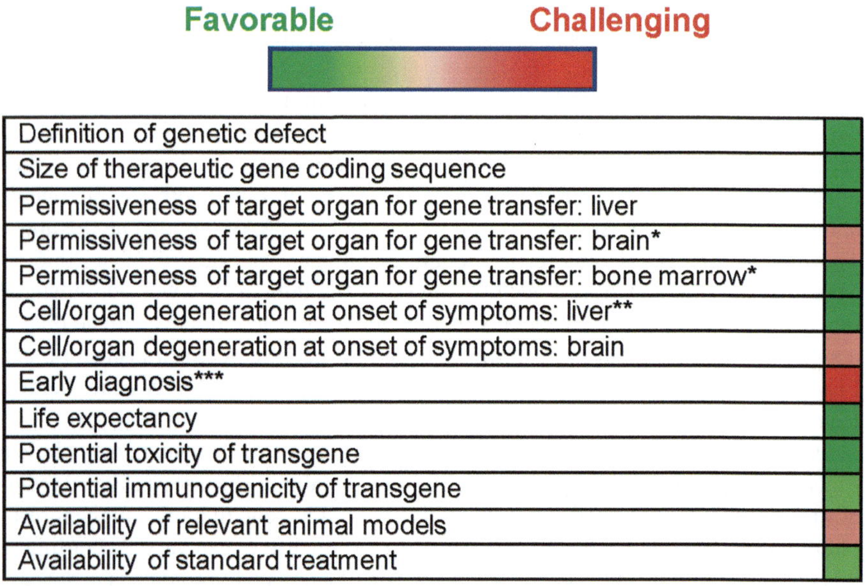

Fig. 22.1 *CYP27A1* gene supplementation for CTX patients: advantages and challenges. Color code indicates the characteristics that favor gene therapy implementation for CTX (dark green) vs. those that do not (dark red). Light colors indicate intermediate situations. *Currently there is no evidence that other organs apart from the liver require gene transfer to address CTX manifestations. **Some patients experience severe neonatal cholestasis, but liver function is not compromised in childhood and adulthood. ***Newborn screening initiatives and increasing awareness about the disease could allow early diagnosis in the future

22a homozygous truncation of *Cyp27a1* exon 8 [23]. These mice recapitulate important metabolic features of CTX, such as elevation of bile acid precursors (cholestanol and 7α-hydroxy-4-cholesten-3-one (7αC4)), reduction of CDCA, and induction of the rate-limiting enzyme cholesterol 7α-hydroxylase (*Cyp7a1*) in the liver. However, the increase in cholestanol is mild (only twofold compared with wild type mice), probably due to the potent detoxifying mechanisms (induction of Cyp3a11 and Cyp46a1) present in mouse liver [24, 25]. As a result, *Cyp27a1*-knockout mice do not develop xanthomas, and neurological manifestations have not been consistently reported.

The therapeutic efficacy of two AAV vectors were compared, differing only in the regulatory sequence used to control *CYP27A1* expression: a strong liver-specific promoter (albumin enhancer fused with the α1 antitrypsin promoter, EAAT) [26] and a portion of the human *CYP27A1* 5′ UTR known to possess promoter activity [27, 28]. In principle, the endogenous promoter would allow expression at physiological levels in all transduced cells. This feature would be relevant if high levels of the sterol 27-hydroxylase were toxic for cells, or if gene supplementation was needed in different cell types such as neurons, macrophages, etc. However, experiments performed in cell lines and in mice indicated that the *CYP27A1* 5′UTR sequence had weak promoter activity compared with EAAT. This proved to be an important limitation for the therapeutic effect of this vector. Only at high doses (5×10^{13} vg/kg), a partial reduction of 7αC4 was observed in the mouse model. In contrast, the liver-specific AAV8-EAAT-CYP27A1 vector achieved complete metabolic correction at 1.5×10^{12} vg/Kg, which is well below the doses of AAV that have been associated with the development of severe adverse effects in clinical trials [29]. This vector dose transduces less than 20% of hepatocytes in mice, but the EAAT promoter sustains the production of the sterol 27-hydroxylase at high levels. This over-expression was well tolerated and may convert the hepatocytes into a metabolic sink for the toxic bile acid intermediates produced in non-transduced cells (Fig. 22.2).

Importantly, *CYP27A1* gene supplementation normalized not only cholestanol and 7αC4 levels in plasma but also the expression of *Cyp7a1* in the liver. Induction of the xenobiotic-responsive cytochrome Cyp3a11 was avoided, suggesting that any other potential toxic metabolites were also likely eliminated. Analysis of the bile acid profile in plasma showed nearly complete normalization of CDCA, cholic acid (CA), and secondary species. The mechanism of action was clearly different from the standard treatment based on oral CDCA administration. In this case, the predominant bile acids were CDCA and derivatives, whereas CA levels remained low in treated animals.

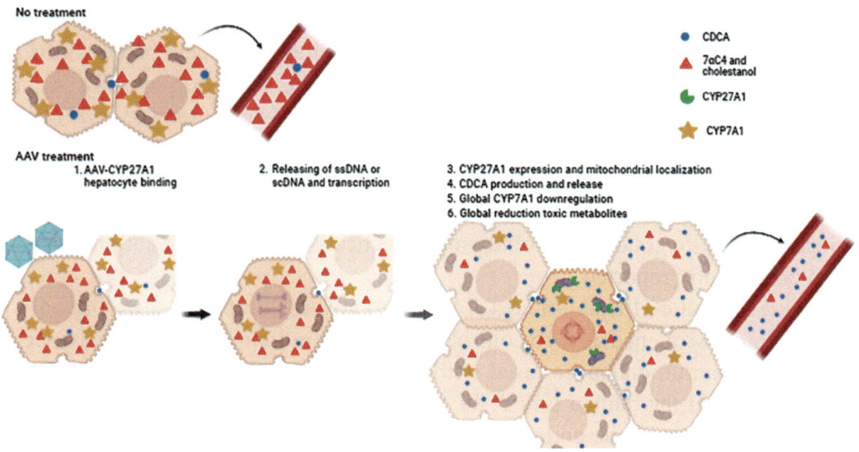

Fig. 22.2 Proposed mechanism of action of gene therapy for CTX. The lack of functional CYP27A1 enzyme in hepatocytes of CTX patients causes a reduction of CDCA. The activation of bile acid biosynthetic pathway by induction of the CYP7A1 enzyme causes accumulation of toxic metabolites. Only cholestanol and 7αC4 are represented for simplicity (red triangles, upper panel). The lower panel represents the different steps of gene supplementation performed by AAV vectors encoding *CYP27A1*. At moderate doses, the vectors can only transduce a subset of hepatocytes in the liver. Once the vector genomes reach the nucleus and acquire a functional conformation, *CYP27A1* is expressed at high levels and the enzyme is localized in the mitochondria. CDCA produced by these cells normalizes its levels systemically, as well as other bile acids, avoiding the induction of CYP7A1 in the whole liver. The accumulation of toxic intermediates is halted, as they are metabolized by transduced hepatocytes. (Created in BioRender.com)

Overview of Alternative Gene Therapy Approaches for CTX

The safety and feasibility of gene supplementation using AAVs in humans are supported by a growing number of clinical trials and approved products [30]. To the best of our knowledge, this is the only gene therapy approach being developed for the treatment of CTX. However, the field is rapidly evolving and provides interesting alternatives. It is worth considering the potential advantages and limitations of these approaches in the context of CTX.

One common limitation of all viral vectors designed for long-term gene supplementation is the immunogenicity of capsids. Neutralizing antibodies (NAbs) and T cell responses may be present in some patients before the treatment, and they will certainly be developed after vector administration. This reduces the eligibility of patients and precludes vector redosing [31]. In addition, inflammatory responses limit the dose of vector that can be safely administered. Although different approaches are being developed to tackle these issues, the use of non-viral vectors carrying therapeutic DNA or RNA is an attractive alternative [32]. They could also reduce the production cost and facilitate the standardization of vectors. The main drawback of non-viral vectors is their low efficacy for delivery of DNA into the nucleus. Although the liver is one of the most accessible organs for non-viral vectors such as LNPs [33], it is not clear if they could reach the threshold needed for metabolic normalization in CTX. To tackle this limitation, one possibility would be to establish a protocol of repeated dosing and monitoring of biochemical markers in blood, with the hope of obtaining incremental liver transduction. Another option is to deliver *CYP27A1* mRNA in the LNP. This could achieve higher expression after each administration, but the need for lifelong maintenance makes this approach less attractive.

The most advanced in vivo gene editing methods employ LNPs to deliver the CRISPR-Cas9 in the form of protein or mRNA, together with the guide RNA [34]. The short exposure to the protein reduces the risk of immune responses and off-target events. The versatility of non-viral vectors allows the incorporation of a DNA template if needed. In the context of CTX, the efficacy of this approach is favored by the permissiveness of the liver. However, the experience gained with the AAV-mediated supplementation of *CYP27A1* indicates that efficient metabolic restoration requires either over-expression in a subset of hepatocytes or low level of expression in the majority of them [22]. With the current gene editing technology, this is difficult to achieve because no selective advantage of corrected hepatocytes is expected. Since strategies based exclusively on gene disruption are not applicable to CTX, current options include base editors, prime editing, or integration of DNA templates [35]. Some *CYP27A1* pathogenic variants are over-represented in particular geographical areas [36] in part due to founder effects [37], and missense variants tend to accumulate in exons 6–8 [38]. However, there is not a precise hotspot for CTX, which means that addressing individual point mutations is not realistic from a healthcare standpoint. These considerations point to site-specific integration of the full *CYP27A1* cDNA as the most attractive gene editing approach for CTX. A common integration site in the transcription start site or exon 1 could be designed for all patients. However, the technologies allowing this process are still in early stages of development [8–11]. In the case of CTX, it is not clear if the potential advantage of endogenous *CYP27A1* regulation in the corrected hepatocytes outweighs the expected reduction of efficacy compared with the AAV-mediated gene supplementation.

Perspectives for Clinical Implementation of Gene Therapy in CTX

Based on the previous experience from other IMD clinical trials, some of the challenges to be addressed to translate the approaches made in the CTX animal model into the clinic, will include (1) strategies to obtain efficient expression with low vector doses, such as the improvement of expression cassettes, vector genomes, and capsids and (2) the management of the patient immune response.

Regarding the design of expression cassettes, different strategies have been used in FDA-approved vectors, including ubiquitous or tissue-specific promoters, enhancers, sequence modification, or addition of regulatory domains. In Luxturna, the human *RPE65* coding sequence was expressed under control of a hybrid chicken β-actin promoter with a cytomegalovirus (CMV) enhancer. The cassette contained a modified Kozak sequence and an artificial poly-adenylation sequence [39]. Similar modifications were included in Zolgensma in which a codon-optimized sequence of the *SMN1* gene was delivered by an AAV9 vector with a self-complementary (sc) structure [40]. The use of scAAV circumvents the conversion of single-stranded DNA (ssDNA) into double-stranded DNA (dsDNA), making gene expression more efficient compared to the natural ssDNA AAV conformation [41].

A drawback of scAAV vectors is the limitation of their cloning capacity to 2.2 Kb. Although this does not prevent the application of this conformation for the delivery of *CYP27A1*, an accurate optimization of transcriptional and post-transcriptional regulatory elements should be performed to guarantee optimal transgene expression without exceeding this size.

It has been reported that AAV induces little innate immunity, as opposed to adenoviruses or other viral vectors [42]. However, unmethylated CpG motifs can be found in AAV preparations and could trigger innate immunity via the stimulation of TLR9 expressed on vertebrate immune cells (such as B cells, natural killer cells, macrophages, and monocytes) [43]. According to this, methylation of those CpGs or their elimination by codon-optimization could decrease the innate inflammatory response.

As mentioned previously, NAbs against AAV capsids is a major concern when thinking about clinical translation [44]. Different strategies to overcome this issue have been used, including (1) AAV capsid modification, (2) removal of patients' antibodies from serum, or (3) depletion of total IgG. All these options could be combined with immunosuppressants to prevent B-cell activation.

As vector-dependent factors contribute to immunogenicity, the use of capsids with low seroprevalence and the design of new capsids are key points. Efforts have been performed to engineer new AAV capsids that cannot be recognized by preexisting NAbs and minimizing the effect on vector production, tissue tropism, or transduction efficiency [45].

Different strategies to remove anti-AAV antibodies from the bloodstream have been described and include plasmapheresis, hemapheresis, and immunoabsorption, in which the removal of antibodies resulted in an increase in gene expression comparable to sero-negative subjects [46–48]. Moreover, the addition of modified empty capsid to the final vector formulation that will act as a bait to bind to NAbs without entering to the target cell has been proposed [49].

More recently, depletion of total IgG using *Streptococcus* sp. immunoglobulin-degrading enzymes (IdeS, IdeZ, and IgdE) has been reported to reduce anti-AAV antibodies in animal models and human sera, and consequently rescuing AAV transduction [50, 51]. Additionally, in a Phase I study, it was shown that IdeS presented a safe profile with no serious adverse events when administered to humans [52].

Even if the removal of antibodies will allow inclusion of sero-positive patients in clinical trials and the re-administration of AAV if needed (especially in children in which organs are still growing), it has the limitation of the transient non-specific removal of all circulating IgG. Attempts have been performed to selectively eliminate anti-AAV antibodies [47, 48], but further studies are still needed to address this hurdle.

Concluding Remarks

As a monogenic disease affecting the liver, CTX fits within the scope of current gene therapy technology targets. The most straightforward and clinically feasible approach is based on gene supplementation using AAV vectors. Although other modalities could be available in the future, the pre-clinical results obtained with this strategy support translation efforts to offer a novel therapeutic alternative to the patients as soon as possible. The availability of validated biochemical markers in blood and urine will facilitate the evaluation of treatment efficacy in clinical trials. Of note, this will make it possible to combine gene therapy with conventional CDCA treatment in initial clinical trials, until the effect of the vector allows reduction or eventually safe withdrawal of the drug. A Phase 3 clinical trial in patients treated with CDCA (ClinicalTrials.gov, NCT04270682) improved the understanding of metabolite behavior after the withdrawal of CDCA. This information will be useful for the design of a gene therapy trial for CTX if the final objective is to obtain metabolic correction after a single dose of the vector.

In summary, additional preclinical studies are still needed to improve the efficacy and safety of vectors for gene supplementation in CTX and to determine the best way to wean patients off the standard treatment.

It is early to speculate about the advantages of gene therapy versus CDCA in the general CTX patient population. The most obvious candidates to be included in a gene therapy clinical trial are those who show partial effect of the drug. Definition of partial response at the biochemical level could involve measurement of other metabolites apart from cholestanol, such as 7αC4; 7α,12α-dihydroxy-4-cholesten-3-one; and cholestane-3β,5α,6β-triol [21, 53]. Problems associated with adherence to the treatment are eliminated with gene therapy, because a single intravenous administration should provide protection for several years. The maximum duration of liver-directed transgene expression after AAV treatment in humans is not known, but it is expected to last more than 10 years according to the experience with hemophilia patients [29, 54]. In the meantime, new approaches are being developed to preserve the efficacy of AAV redosing [31].

Regarding protection from neurological deterioration, the CTX mouse model cannot provide meaningful information. Considering the complete restoration of bile acid metabolism and the efficacy in reducing 7αC4 in blood [22], it is expected that gene therapy will avoid neurological deterioration at least as efficiently as CDCA. Follow-up of infantile CTX patients subjected to liver transplantation will provide valuable information, but the experience is still very scarce [55, 56]. Early treatment will be crucial to increase the chances of success, but the long-term stability of transgene expression can be compromised in a developing liver. In addition, severe cholestasis or any other hepatic dysfunction should be excluded before AAV administration. The need for *CYP27A1* restoration in neurons cannot be completely ruled out, although accumulation of cholestanol in the brain is supposed to depend mainly on the influx of 7αC4 from systemic circulation [57]. If simultaneous expression was needed in liver and brain, it could be addressed using ubiquitous or bifunctional promoters together with modified AAV capsids with the ability to cross the blood-brain barrier.

Apart from the liver, *CYP27A1* is expressed in macrophages and to a lesser extent in other organs such as lung, spinal cord, peripheral nerves, and small intestine (https://www.proteinatlas.org/ENSG00000135929-CYP27A1). The importance of enzyme restoration in these structures is not known. Global expression would be difficult to achieve with a single vector, and it is not expected to play a major role in preventing the most clinically relevant manifestations of the disease. For instance, the sterol 27-hydroxylase expressed in macrophages plays a role in the removal of cholesterol and other atherogenic oxysterols from peripheral tissues [58]. If the defect in this mechanism was responsible for the increase in cardiovascular risk observed in CTX patients, it could be addressed by hematopoietic stem cell-directed gene transfer. However, it has been postulated that CDCA treatment is able to wash out the cholestanol accumulated in the plasma membranes [59]. Therefore, liver-directed gene therapy could be equally protective by reducing toxic metabolites and restoring CDCA in blood.

In summary, gene therapy could be an attractive alternative for CTX in the near future. Coupled with early diagnosis preferably by implementing newborn screening programs, it offers the opportunity to normalize the life of patients and their families.

References

1. Bulcha JT, Wang Y, Ma H, Tai PWL. Viral vector platforms within the gene therapy landscape. Signal Transduct Target Ther [Internet]. 2021; https://doi.org/10.1038/s41392-021-00487-6.
2. Shtykalova S, Deviatkin D, Freund S, Egorova A, Kiselev A. Non-viral carriers for nucleic acids delivery: fundamentals and current applications. Life. 2023;13(4):903.
3. Li C, Samulski RJ. Engineering adeno-associated virus vectors for gene therapy. Nat Rev Genet [Internet]. 2020;21(4):255–72. https://doi.org/10.1038/s41576-019-0205-4.
4. Summary R. CRISPR technology: a decade of genome editing is only the beginning. Science. 2023;379:eadd8643.
5. Cong L, Ran FA, Cox D, Lin S, Barretto R, Habib N, et al. Multiplex genome engineering using CRISPR/Cas systems. Science. 2013;339(6121):819–23.
6. Paquet D, Kwart D, Chen A, Sproul A, Jacob S, Teo S, et al. Efficient introduction of specific homozygous and heterozygous mutations using CRISPR/Cas9. Nature. 2016;533:125.
7. Ran FA, Hsu PD, Lin C-Y, Gootenberg JS, Konermann S, Trevino AE, et al. Double nicking by RNA-guided CRISPR Cas9 for enhanced genome editing specificity. Cell [Internet]. 2013;154(6):1380–9. https://doi.org/10.1016/j.cell.2013.08.021.
8. Newby GA, Liu DR. In vivo somatic cell base editing and prime editing. Mol Ther [Internet]. 2021;29(11):3107–24. https://doi.org/10.1016/j.ymthe.2021.09.002.
9. Pallarès-masmitjà M, Ivan D, Mir-pedrol J, Jaraba-wallace J, Tagliani T, Oliva B, et al. Find and cut-and-transfer (FiCAT) mammalian genome engineering. Nat Comm. 2021;12:1–9.
10. Anzalone AV, Gao XD, Podracky CJ, Nelson AT, Koblan LW, Raguram A, et al. Programmable deletion, replacement, integration and inversion of large DNA sequences with twin prime editing. Nat Biotechnol. 2022;40(5):731–40.
11. Yarnall MTN, Ioannidi EI, Schmitt-ulms C, Krajeski RN, Lim J, Villiger L, et al. Drag-and-drop genome insertion of large sequences without double-strand DNA cleavage using CRISPR-directed integrases. Nat Biotechnol. 2023;41(4):500–12.

12. Bendixen L, Jensen TI, Bak RO. CRISPR-Cas-mediated transcriptional modulation: the therapeutic promises of CRISPRa and CRISPRi. Mol Ther [Internet]. 2023;31(7):1–18. https://doi.org/10.1016/j.ymthe.2023.03.024.
13. Ferreira CR, Zschocke J. An international classification of inherited metabolic disorders (ICIMD). J Inherit Metab Dis. 2021;44:164–77.
14. Kang L, Jin S, Wang J, Lv Z, Xin C, Tan C, et al. Review article AAV vectors applied to the treatment of CNS disorders: clinical status and challenges. J Control Release [Internet]. 2023;355(February):458–73. https://doi.org/10.1016/j.jconrel.2023.01.067.
15. Chuecos MA. Liver directed adeno-associated viral vectors to treat metabolic disease. J Inherit Metab Dis. 2024;47(1):22–40.
16. Nathwani AC, McIntosh J, Sheridan R. Liver gene therapy. Hum Gene Ther. 2022;33(17–18):879–88.
17. Issa SS, Shaimardanova AA, Solovyeva VV. Various AAV serotypes and their applications in gene therapy: an overview. Cells. 2023;12:785.
18. Manno CS, Pierce GF, Arruda VR, Glader B, Ragni M, Rasko JJE, et al. Successful transduction of liver in hemophilia by AAV-Factor IX and limitations imposed by the host immune response. Nat Med. 2006;12(3):342–8.
19. Mullard A. FDA approves first haemophilia B gene therapy. Nat Rev Drug Discov. 2023;22(7):714.
20. Cali JJ, Russell DW. Characterization of human sterol 27-hydroxylase. Mol Biol. 1991;266(12):7774–8.
21. Mignarri A, Magni A, Del Puppo M, Gallus GN, Björkhem I, Federico A, et al. Evaluation of cholesterol metabolism in cerebrotendinous xanthomatosis. J Inherit Metab Dis. 2016;39(1):75–83.
22. Lumbreras S, Ricobaraza A, Baila-rueda L, Gonzalez-aparicio M, Mora-jimenez L, Uriarte I, et al. Gene supplementation of CYP27A1 in the liver restores bile acid metabolism in a mouse model of cerebrotendinous xanthomatosis. Mol Ther Methods Clin Dev [Internet]. 2021;22(September):210–21. https://doi.org/10.1016/j.omtm.2021.07.002.
23. Rosen H, Reshef A, Maeda N, Lippoldt A, Shpizen S, Triger L, et al. Markedly reduced bile acid synthesis but maintained levels of cholesterol and vitamin D metabolites in mice with disrupted sterol 27- hydroxylase gene. J Biol Chem. 1998;273(24):14805–12.
24. Honda A, Salen G, Matsuzaki Y, Batta AK, Xu G, Leitersdorf E, et al. Side chain hydroxylations in bile acid biosynthesis catalyzed by CYP3A are markedly up-regulated in Cyp27−/− mice but not in cerebrotendinous xanthomatosis. J Biol Chem. 2001;276(37):34579–85.
25. Mast N, Li Y, Linger M, Clark M, Wiseman J, Pikuleva IA. Pharmacologic stimulation of cytochrome P450 46A1 and cerebral cholesterol turnover in mice. J Biol Chem. 2014;289(6):3529–38.
26. Kramer MG, Barajas M, Razquin N, Berraondo P, Rodrigo M, Wu C, et al. In vitro and in vivo comparative study of chimeric liver-specific promoters. Mol Ther. 2003 Mar;7(3):375–85.
27. Araya Z, Tang W, Wikvall K. Hormonal regulation of the human sterol 27-hydroxylase gene CYP27A1. Biochem J. 2003;372(2):529–34.
28. Chen W, Chiang JYL. Regulation of human sterol 27-hydroxylase gene (CYP27A1) by bile acids and hepatocyte nuclear factor 4α (HNF4α). Gene. 2003;313(1–2):71–82.
29. George LA, Monahan PE, Eyster ME, Sullivan SK, Ragni MV, Croteau SE, et al. Multiyear factor VIII expression after AAV gene transfer for hemophilia A. N Engl J Med. 2021;385:1961–73.
30. Sayed N, Allawadhi P, Khurana A, Singh V, Navik U, Kumar S, et al. Gene therapy: comprehensive overview and therapeutic applications. Life Sci [Internet]. 2022;294(January):120375. https://doi.org/10.1016/j.lfs.2022.120375.
31. Schulz M, Levy DI, Petropoulos CJ, Bashirians G, Winburn I, Mahn M, et al. Binding and neutralizing anti-AAV antibodies: detection and implications for rAAV-mediated gene therapy. Mol Ther [Internet]. 2023;31(3):616–30. https://doi.org/10.1016/j.ymthe.2023.01.010.
32. Mendes BB, Conniot J, Avital A, Yao D, Jiang X, Zhou X, et al. Nanodelivery of nucleic acids. Nat Rev Methods Primers. 2022;2:24.

33. Kularatne RN, Crist RM, Stern ST. The future of tissue-targeted lipid nanoparticle-mediated nucleic acid delivery. Pharmaceuticals. 2022;15(7):897.
34. Taha EA, Lee J, Hotta A. Delivery of CRISPR-Cas tools for in vivo genome editing therapy: trends and challenges. J Control Release [Internet]. 2022;(342):345–61. https://doi.org/10.1016/j.jconrel.2022.01.013.
35. Doudna JA. The promise and challenge of therapeutic genome editing. Nature. 2022;578(7794):229–36.
36. Leitersdorf E, Safadi R, Meiner V, Reshef A, Bjorkhem I, Friedlander Y, et al. Cerebrotendinous xanthomatosis in the Israeli Druze: molecular genetics and phenotypic characteristics. Am J Hum Genet. 1994;55:907–15.
37. Pilo-de-la-Fuente B, Jimenez-Escrig A, Lorenzo JR, Pardo J, Arias M, Ares-Luque A, et al. Cerebrotendinous xanthomatosis in Spain: clinical, prognostic, and genetic survey. Eur J Neurol. 2011;18(10):1203–11.
38. Verrips A, Hoefsloot LH, Steenbergen GCH, Theelen JP, Wevers RA, Gabreëls FJM, et al. Clinical and molecular genetic characteristics of patients with cerebrotendinous xanthomatosis. Brain. 2000;123(5):908–19.
39. Russell S, Bennett J, Wellman JA, Chung DC, Yu Z, Tillman A, et al. Articles efficacy and safety of voretigene neparvovec (AAV2-hRPE65v2) in patients with RPE65 -mediated inherited retinal dystrophy: a randomised, controlled, open-label, phase 3 trial. Lancet [Internet]. 2017;390(10097):849–60. https://doi.org/10.1016/S0140-6736(17)31868-8.
40. Mendell JR, Al-Zaidy S, Shell R, Arnold WD, Rodino-Klapac LR, Prior TW, et al. Single-dose gene-replacement therapy for spinal muscular atrophy. N Engl J Med [Internet]. 2017;377(18):1713–22. Available from: http://www.nejm.org/doi/10.1056/NEJMoa1706198.
41. Mccarty DM. Self-complementary AAV vectors; advances and applications. Mol Ther. 2008;16(10):1648–56. https://doi.org/10.1038/mt.2008.171.
42. Zaiss A, Liu Q, Bowen GP, Wong NCW, Bartlett JS, Muruve DA. Differential activation of innate immune responses by adenovirus and adeno-associated virus vectors. J Virol. 2002;76(9):4580–90.
43. Bessis N, Garciacozar FJ, Boissier M. Immune responses to gene therapy vectors: influence on vector function and effector mechanisms. Gene Ther. 2004;11:10–7.
44. Boutin S, Monteilhet V, Veron P, Leborgne C, Benveniste O, Montus M, et al. Prevalence of serum IgG and neutralizing factors against adeno-associated virus (AAV) types 1, 2, 5, 6, 8, and 9 in the healthy population: implications for gene therapy using AAV vectors. Hum Gene Ther. 2010;21(6):704–12.
45. Victor L, Klinc KA, Madigan VJ, Castellanos RM, Wells LF. Structure-guided evolution of antigenically distinct adeno-associated virus variants for immune evasion. Proc Natl Acad Sci USA. 2017;114(24):E4812–21.
46. Monteilhet V, Saheb S, Boutin S, Leborgne C, Veron P, Montus M, et al. A 10 patient case report on the impact of plasmapheresis upon neutralizing factors against adeno-associated Virus (AAV) types 1, 2, 6, and 8. Mol Ther. 2011;19(11):2084–91.
47. Bertin B, Veron P, Leborgne C, Deschamps J, Moullec S, Fromes Y, et al. Capsid-specific removal of circulating antibodies to adeno- associated virus vectors. Sci Rep. 2020;10:864.
48. Orlowski A, Katz MG, Gubara SM, Fargnoli AS, Fish KM, Weber T. Successful transduction with AAV vectors after selective depletion of anti-AAV antibodies by immunoadsorption. Mol Ther Methods Clin Dev [Internet]. 2020;16(March):192–203. https://doi.org/10.1016/j.omtm.2020.01.004.
49. Mingozzi F, Anguela XM, Pavani G, Chen Y, Davidson RJ, Hui DJ, et al. Overcoming pre-existing humoral immunity to AAV using capsid decoys. Sci Transl Med. 2014;5(61):1–20.
50. Leborgne C, Barbon E, Alexander JM, Hanby H, Delignat S, Cohen DM, et al. IgG-cleaving endopeptidase enables in vivo gene therapy in the presence of anti-AAV neutralizing antibodies. Nat Med [Internet]. 2020;26(July) https://doi.org/10.1038/s41591-020-0911-7.
51. Ros-Gañan I, Hommel M, Trigueros-motos L, Tamarit B, Ros-ga I, Douar A, et al. Optimising the IgG-degrading enzyme treatment regimen for enhanced adeno-associated virus transduction in the presence of neutralising antibodies. Clin Transl Immunol. 2022;11:1–14.

52. Windstedt L, Jarsum S, Andersson Nordahl E, Olsson A, Runström A, Bockermann R, et al. Complete removal of extracellular IgG antibodies in a randomized dose-escalation phase I study with the bacterial enzyme IdeS – a novel therapeutic opportunity. PLoS One. 2015;10:e0132011.
53. Pajares S, Arias A, García-villoria J, Macías-vidal J, Ros E, Heras JD, et al. Cholestane-3 b, 5 a, 6 b -triol: high levels in Niemann-Pick type C, cerebrotendinous xanthomatosis, and lysosomal acid lipase deficiency. J Lipid Res. 2015;56:1926–35.
54. Shah J, Kim H, Sivamurthy K, Monahan PE, Kim H, Sivamurthy K, et al. Comprehensive analysis and prediction of long- term durability of factor IX activity following etranacogene dezaparvovec gene therapy in the treatment of hemophilia B. Curr Med Res Opin [Internet]. 2023;39(2):235–45. https://doi.org/10.1080/03007995.2022.2133492.
55. Shen CH, Wang ZX. Liver transplantation due to cerebrotendinous xanthomatosis end-stage liver disease. World J Pediatr. 2018;14(4):414–5.
56. Pietrobattista A, Spada M, Candusso M, Boenzi S, Vici CD, Francalanci P, et al. Liver transplantation in an infant with cerebrotendinous xanthomatosis, cholestasis, and rapid evolution of liver failure. Pediatr Transplant. 2022;26(6):1–6.
57. Båvner A, Shafaati M, Hansson M, Olin M, Shpitzen S, Meiner V, et al. On the mechanism of accumulation of cholestanol in the brain of mice with a disruption of sterol 27-hydroxylase. J Lipid Res. 2010;51:2722–30.
58. Babiker A, Andersson O, Lund E, Xiu R, Deeb S, Reshef A, et al. Elimination of cholesterol in macrophages and endothelial cells by the sterol 27-hydroxylase mechanism. J Biol Chem. 1997;272(42):26253–61.
59. Seyama Y. Cholestanol metabolism, molecular pathology, and nutritional implications. J Med Food. 2003;6(March):217–24.

Part VII

Cerebrotendinous Xanthomatosis (CTX): Presentation in Infants and Children and Ophthalmic Involvement

Cerebrotendinous Xanthomatosis (CTX) Pediatric Presentation

23

Tanyel Zubarioglu, Ertugrul Kıykım, and Cigdem Aktuglu-Zeybek

Introduction

Cerebrotendinous xanthomatosis (CTX) was first described by Van Bogaert et al. in 1937. They observed lipid-like deposits in postmortem brain tissue samples, particularly in cerebellar white matter and in the cerebral peduncles of a patient with cerebellar and pyramidal signs, myoclonus of the soft palate, mental retardation, cataract, and tendon xanthomas. The clinical findings first appeared at the age of 12 years, whereas the diagnosis was not made until the third decade of life [1].

After the reporting of the first cases, research studies on CTX focused on different topics. In 1984, chenodeoxycholic acid (CDCA) was introduced as a long-term treatment option, and improvement with CDCA therapy was reported [2]. After methodological studies on diagnostic and prognostic biomarkers, a suspicion index was developed in 2014 by Mignarri et al. to promote early diagnosis and treatment [3].

CTX diagnosis is via biochemical measurement of cholestanol and/or characteristic bile alcohols, and the gold standard for confirmation of diagnosis is by genetic testing for biallelic pathogenic variants in *CYP27A1* [4]. In 2021, the first expert consensus review was published. All experts involved in the collaboration agreed that age at diagnosis and early initiation of treatment had the greatest impact on treatment outcomes, and CDCA was considered a lifelong replacement therapy that, if started early, could significantly improve prognosis because it might be able to reverse the pathophysiological process in CTX [4]. Because CTX patients are usually diagnosed in adulthood, knowledge of the pediatric presentations of the disease plays a critical role in early diagnosis and treatment. In this chapter, we discuss the clinical spectrum of CTX in a pediatric cohort.

T. Zubarioglu (✉) · E. Kıykım · C. Aktuglu-Zeybek
Istanbul University-Cerrahpaşa, Cerrahpaşa Faculty of Medicine, Division of Pediatric Nutrition and Metabolism, Istanbul, Turkey
e-mail: tanyel.zubarioglu@iuc.edu.tr

A. Federico et al. (eds.), *Cerebrotendinous Xanthomatosis*,
https://doi.org/10.1007/978-3-031-92526-9_23

Natural History of Cerebrotendinous Xanthomatosis: Review of the Literature

The clinical phenotype of CTX includes both neurologic and extra-neurologic findings. Developmental delay, intellectual disability, cerebellar, pyramidal and extra-pyramidal signs, dementia, psychiatric manifestations, peripheral neuropathy, parkinsonism, seizures, and spinal involvement have all been listed as neurologic findings of the disease. Juvenile cataract, tendon xanthomas, cholestatic jaundice, infantile hepatitis, and chronic diarrhea are the most reported extra-neurologic findings, along with skeletal and cardiovascular findings and pulmonary system involvement [5, 6]. Juvenile cataract, osteoporosis with bone fractures and tooth loss, atherosclerosis, and neurologic disorders with dementia and/or parkinsonism suggest a general premature aging process in CTX [7]. Cerebrotendinous xanthomatosis may be considered a pediatric disease, usually diagnosed in adulthood. The majority of reported patients are diagnosed in the third decade of life, as the diagnostic delay is more than 20 years in some cases [3, 8–11]. Given this striking delay, the natural history of the disease and pediatric case reports should be focused on to increase clinician awareness of early diagnosis and intervention.

Studies on the natural history of the disease were mainly conducted in adult CTX patients. In a study of 54 CTX patients, Verrips et al. mentioned chronic diarrhea as the earliest clinical finding of CTX. Neurological symptoms, including pyramidal and cerebellar involvement, appeared after the second decade of life. Cataract and tendon xanthomas contributed to the clinical phenotype after late adolescence. Electromyogram (EMG) studies confirmed that polyneuropathy was reported as a late finding of the disease [9]. In another study with a large sample size, Mignarri et al. [3] pointed to neonatal jaundice as an early clinical manifestation of CTX in infancy. Neurological manifestations in childhood included intellectual disability and seizures, while psychiatric changes usually occurred after the second decade of life, in addition to cerebellar and pyramidal involvement. In addition to polyneuropathy, osteoporosis and parkinsonism have also been reported as later findings [3]. The natural history of the CTX cohort of Degos et al. [12] showed that chronic diarrhea was one of the most common signs, often starting within the first year of life. Cataract and school difficulties usually followed between the ages of 5 and 15 years. Motor dysfunction leading to difficulty walking and/or psychiatric symptoms were not observed until the second decade of life [12]. Similar to the findings mentioned above, data from CTX studies in adults indicate that clinical symptomatology in children was dominated by extra-neurological findings, while neurological findings were present in adults. Osteoporosis and tendon xanthomas were also reported as symptoms in adults [13–15]. Data on the natural history of CTX patients from different cohorts are summarized in Table 23.1.

Table 23.1 Data on the natural history of CTX patients from different cohorts

	Verrips [9]	Lee [13]	Pilo de la Fuente [11]	Mignarri [3]	Degos [12]	Duell [10]	Yunisova [14]	Badura-Stronka [8]
Number of patients	54	19	25	55	13	43	7	6
Age of onset (years)	14 ± 11.6	26%: onset in childhood 26%: onset in adolescence 48%: onset in adulthood	19.2 ± 11.2	9.5 ± 9	4.2 ± 3.3	N/A	12.4 ± 10.6	5.41 ± 3.29
Age of diagnosis (years)	33.5 ± 10.9	42 ± 9.8	38.0 ± 10.7	35.5 ± 11.8	30.4 ± 14.9	31.76 ± 10.61	38.7 ± 9.6	25.5 ± 11.76
Tendon xanthomas (years)	50% (27/54) 24.7 ± 11.3	100% (19/19)	56% (14/25)	78% (43/55) 25.6 ± 9.6	23% (3/13)	77% (33/43)	100% (7/7) 28.4 ± 10.1	33% (2/6)
Cataract (years)	96% (52/54) 19.7 ± 11.2	74% (14/19)	92% (23/25)	89% (49/55) 17.0 ± 14.5	85% (11/13) 15.4 ± 13.8	70% (30/43)	85% (6/7) 13.1 ± 7.2	100% (6/6)
Chronic diarrhea (years)	35% (19/54) 9.8 ± 9.9	N/A	92% (23/25)	40% (22/55) 3.7 ± 6.8	77% (10/13) neonatal	53% (23/43)	42% (3/7) 4.0 ± 1.0	83% (5/6)
Neonatal jaundice (years)	N/A	N/A	N/A	15% (8/55)	None		N/A	N/A
Osteoporosis (years)	N/A	21% (4/19)	N/A	67% (20/30) 38.6 ± 10.1	31% (4/13)	N/A	42% (3/7)	50% (3/6)

(continued)

Table 23.1 (continued)

	Verrips [9]	Lee [13]	Pilo de la Fuente [11]	Mignarri [3]	Degos [12]	Duell [10]	Yunisova [14]	Badura-Stronka [8]
Cerebellar signs (years)	65% (35/54) 27.8 ± 10.5	89% (17/19)	83% (20/24)	36% (20/55) 28.7 ± 9.3	54% (7/13) 33 ± 13.8	81% (35/43)[a]	100% (7/7) 25.2 ± 7.3	67% (4/6)
Pyramidal signs (years)	72% (39/54) 27.6 ± 8.9	89% (17/19)	92% (23/25)	64% (35/55) 27.4 ± 10.1	69% (9/13) 33 ± 13.8		100% (7/7) 31.8 ± 6.9	50% (3/6)
Intellectual disability (years)	61% (33/54)	N/A	48% (12/25)	60% (33/55) 6.5 ± 3.1	85% (11/13) 9.9 ± 3.2	74% (32/43)	100% (7/7) 10.4 ± 1.9	100% (6/6)
Psychiatric disturbances (years)	N/A	N/A	61% (14/23)	44% (24/55) 23.4 ± 13.3	46% (6/13) 21.2 ± 11.7	N/A	42% (3/7) 25.6 ± 9.2	67% (4/6)
Seizures (years)	26% (14/54) 24.0 ± 15.5	N/A	32% (8/25)	33% (18/55) 10.3 ± 9.9	7% (1/13)	N/A	42% (3/7) 4.0 ± 1.0	33% (2/6)
EMG-confirmed polyneuropathy (years)	79% (19/24) 28.3 ± 6.6	N/A	67% (12/18)	70% (21/30) 35.4 ± 9.2	77% (10/13)	N/A	28% (2/7)	50% (3/6)
Parkinsonism (years)	N/A	N/A	N/A	9% (5/55) 38.4 ± 16.2 years	N/A	N/A	14% (1/7) 30 years	N/A

[a]Data reflects overall neurological involvement; cerebellar and pyramidal involvement was not reported separately

Pediatric Cerebrotendinous Xanthomatosis Cohort in the Literature

Considering the age of the first symptom and the corresponding age at diagnosis of CTX patients, it becomes clear that there is a diagnostic delay that is often of at least two decades. The therapeutic effect of CDCA can be dramatic if initiated before the onset of disabling motor and psychiatric symptoms. Therefore, the focus should be on pediatric case reports and clinical trials to raise clinicians' awareness of early diagnosis and symptoms during the optimal therapeutic window of childhood.

Highlighting the pediatric patients in the adult CTX studies mentioned above, it is notable that Duell [10] reported neurological findings in four of the five pediatric patients among the 43 CTX patients reported. Speech delay and limited vocabulary were a remarkable feature of these pediatric patients [10]. Pilo-de-la-Fuente observed pyramidal signs, ataxia, and neuropathy in a 14-year-old patient [11]. Badura-Stronka reported behavioral disturbances and rapid, unclear speech in a 13-year-old patient [8]. When evaluating pediatric CTX studies, it becomes clearer that the neuropsychiatric involvement of CTX observed in individual case reports can begin early in the course of the disease, even in early childhood.

In a pediatric CTX study involving six patients, three patients were found to have cataracts, two had chronic diarrhea, and one had persistent neonatal jaundice. Four patients had developmental delay and five had cognitive impairment. None of the patients showed pyramidal and extrapyramidal signs. However, all patients had at least one of the cerebellar signs, in particular intention tremor. Peripheral neuropathy was confirmed by EMG in five of the six patients. Psychiatric manifestations were observed in three patients. Regarding the effects on the skeletal system, severe osteoporosis with a history of fractures with mild trauma was noted in two patients [16]. The results of another pediatric CTX study from Turkey were consistent with the previous study. Of the seven pediatric patients, six had ataxia and four had polyneuropathy. Two patients were found to have early osteoporosis and one of them had a history of bone fractures [17].

According to data from both pediatric CTX studies mentioned above and individual case reports, cerebellar signs, peripheral neuropathy, psychiatric findings, and early osteoporosis should be cited as warning signs in addition to other known findings such as cataract, chronic diarrhea, developmental delay, and cognitive decline for the early diagnosis of CTX.

At-Risk Population Screening in Cerebrotendinous Xanthomatosis

To serve the purpose of early diagnosis, in addition to knowledge of clinical findings, screening of at-risk populations could potentially be a good method, as CTX is not part of any national screening programs although accurate newborn screening assays have been developed [18, 19]. In the literature, screening studies on CTX mainly focus on cataract. In different studies, the prevalence of CTX varies from

0.9% to 3.3% in patients with juvenile onset bilateral idiopathic cataract, and it has been mentioned that ophthalmologists play an important role in facilitating early diagnosis of the disease [20–23].

Recently, it's become clear that psychiatric involvement may occur before the development of neurological findings. In addition, autism spectrum disorder has been recently identified as a common feature of children with CTX. In a Dutch CTX cohort, autism spectrum disorder (ASD) was described in 10 of the 77 patients, and ASD was highlighted as an early and probably underestimated common feature in CTX [24]. Plasma cholestanol testing for CTX has been recommended as a diagnostic strategy in patients with atypical psychosis as part of investigations for inborn errors of metabolism [25]. Behavioral/personality disorders, mood/affective disorders, psychosis, catatonia, anxiety, and dementia have been included among the psychiatric manifestations of the disease. Fraidakis et al. reported that psychiatric manifestations in CTX follow a bimodal/bitemporal pattern. In the advanced stages of the disease, dementia and various neuropsychiatric findings, including behavioral/personality disorders, affective/mood disorders, or psychotic disorders, were mentioned. In childhood and adolescence, however, neuropsychiatric manifestations associated with learning difficulties or intellectual disability predominate [26].

Involvement of the skeletal system is an important and debilitating finding in CTX patients. In advanced stages of the disease, severe osteoporosis leads to pathologic fractures, exacerbated by ataxia. The assessment of osteoporosis and changes in bone density during CDCA therapy has been widely reported in adult CTX patients [27–29]. However, recent studies in pediatric CTX patients have shown that osteoporosis is also part of the clinical spectrum in childhood and can even lead to fractures [16, 17, 30]. In this context, it should be recommended to include osteoporosis as a clinical feature of CTX and for CTX to be considered a diagnostic possibility especially in children who also have intellectual disability.

Finally, chronic diarrhea is considered one of the earliest and cardinal symptoms of the disease [4, 5, 31]. However, no screening study for CTX has yet been published in a cohort with diarrhea analogous to the studies of cataracts. There may be several reasons for this situation. Diarrhea in CTX patients is nonspecific, and children may not identify changes in defecation patterns or bring them to parents' attention. In addition, childhood diarrhea has a multifactorial course, so selecting the right individuals to consider for a CTX diagnosis can be challenging. Additional research evaluating children with chronic diarrhea for CTX in order to determine the prevalence in such groups is indicated. It seems likely that CTX may be diagnosed early in selected children with chronic diarrhea in the future.

High-Risk Populations in Cerebrotendinous Xanthomatosis and Newborn Screening

Estimates derived from the frequency of disease-causing mutations in the *CYP27A1* gene suggest that the incidence of CTX in Europeans is between 1:134,970 and 1:416,358, in Africans between 1:263,222 and 1:468,624, in Latinos between 1:71,677 and 1:148,914, in East Asians between 1:64,267 and 1:64,712, and in South Asians between 1:36,072 and 1:75,601 [32]. In certain groups in Israel, such as Moroccan Jews and a specific Druze community in Galilee, the prevalence of CTX is much higher [33–35]. Remarkably, in this Druze population, the frequency of carriers of the pathogenic founder variant c.355delC in the *CYP27A*1 gene was 1:11 [36].

Measurement of the elevated levels of cholestanetetrol glucuronide (GlcA-tetrol) concentration and its ratio to tauro-chenodeoxycholic acid (t-CDCA) proved to be an informative, sensitive, and reliable method of newborn screening in CTX. The ratio of tauro-trihydroxycholestanoic acid (t-THCA)/GlcA-tetrol has also been used to avoid false-positive results due to other cholestatic diseases such as Zellweger spectrum disorders [18, 19].

In a prospective pilot study targeting the Druze population, 366 dried blood spot (DBS) samples from newborns were examined using a two-tier screening approach for CTX newborn screening. All positive samples underwent further analysis for the c.355delC variant of the *CYP27A1* gene, which resulted in a carrier frequency of 1:30, giving an estimated disease prevalence of 1:3600 in this population [37].

Based on the advances in methods for CTX newborn screening and the detection of increased carrier rates in high-risk populations, it is anticipated that prenatal and postnatal screening will be critical, particularly in areas with a high estimated prevalence. It is crucial that early detection and intervention play a major role in preventing progressive neurodegeneration. Initiating treatment from the time of birth, facilitated by early detection through newborn screening, can significantly improve outcomes for patients with this treatable metabolic disorder.

Conclusions

It is of great importance to improve the awareness and knowledge of clinicians from different disciplines such as gastroenterology, pediatrics, ophthalmology, dermatology, neurology, and psychiatry about CTX disease, as age at diagnosis and early initiation of treatment are considered to have the biggest positive impact on treatment outcomes. It is recommended to include CTX in the differential diagnosis of children with chronic diarrhea, xanthoma, bilateral juvenile cataract, intellectual disability, cerebellar signs, psychiatric disorders, autism, early osteoporosis, and polyneuropathy. The delays in diagnosis and treatment in CTX will only be obviated with a two-pronged approach of widespread screening and increased suspicion for the condition in the appropriate clinical setting.

References

1. Van Bogaert L, Scherer HJ, Epstein E. Une forme cerebrale de la cholesterinose generalisee. Paris: Masson et Cie; 1937.
2. Berginer VM, Salen G, Shefer S. Long-term treatment of cerebrotendinous xanthomatosis with chenodeoxycholic acid. N Engl J Med. 1984;311(26):1649–52.
3. Mignarri A, Gallus GN, Dotti MT, Federico A. A suspicion index for early diagnosis and treatment of cerebrotendinous xanthomatosis. J Inherit Metab Dis. 2014;37(3):421–9.
4. Stelten BML, Dotti MT, Verrips A, Elibol B, Falik-Zaccai TC, Hanman K, et al. Expert opinion on diagnosing, treating and managing patients with cerebrotendinous xanthomatosis (CTX): a modified Delphi study. Orphanet J Rare Dis. 2021;16(1):353–70.
5. Federico A, Gallus GN. Cerebrotendinous xanthomatosis. In: Adam MP, Mirzaa GM, Pagon RA, Wallace SE, Bean LJH, Gripp KW, Amemiya A, editors. GeneReviews® [Internet]. 2003 [updated 2022 Mar 17]. Seattle: University of Washington; 1993–2023.
6. Nie S, Chen G, Cao X, Zhang Y. Cerebrotendinous xanthomatosis: a comprehensive review of pathogenesis, clinical manifestations, diagnosis, and management. Orphanet J Rare Dis. 2014;9:179–89.
7. Dotti MT, Salen G, Federico A. Cerebrotendinous xanthomatosis as a multisystem disease mimicking premature ageing. Dev Neurosci. 1991;13(4–5):371–6.
8. Badura-Stronka M, Hirschfeld AS, Winczewska-Wiktor A, Budzyńska E, Jakubiuk-Tomaszuk A, Piontek A, et al. First case series of Polish patients with cerebrotendinous xanthomatosis and systematic review of cases from the 21st century. Clin Genet. 2021;101(2):190–207.
9. Verrips A, Hoefsloot LH, Steenbergen GC, Theelen JP, Wevers RA, Gabreëls FJ, et al. Clinical and molecular genetic characteristics of patients with cerebrotendinous xanthomatosis. Brain. 2000;123(5):908–19.
10. Duell PB, Salen G, Eichler FS, DeBarber AE, Connor SL, Casaday L, et al. Diagnosis, treatment, and clinical outcomes in 43 cases with cerebrotendinous xanthomatosis. J Clin Lipidol. 2018;12(5):1169–78.
11. Pilo-de-la-Fuente B, Jimenez-Escrig A, Lorenzo JE, Pardo JR, Arias Ares-Luque A, et al. Cerebrotendinous xanthomatosis in Spain: clinical, prognostic, and genetic survey. Eur J Neurol. 2011;18(10):1203–11.
12. Degos B, Nadjar Y, Amador Mdel M, Lamari F, Sedel F, Roze E, et al. Natural history of cerebrotendinous xanthomatosis: a paediatric disease diagnosed in adulthood. Orphanet J Rare Dis. 2016;11:41–4.
13. Lee MH, Hazard S, Carpten JD, Yi S, Cohen J, Gerhardt GT, Salen G, Patel SB. Fine-mapping, mutation analyses, and structural mapping of cerebrotendinous xanthomatosis in U.S. pedigrees. J Lipid Res. 2001;42(2):159–69.
14. Yunisova G, Tufekcioglu Z, Dogu O, Bilgic B, Kaleagasi H, Akca Kalem S, Lohmann E, Gurvit HI, Emre M, Hanagasi HA. Patients with lately diagnosed cerebrotendinous xanthomatosis. Neurodegener Dis. 2019;19(5–6):218–24.
15. Wong JC, Walsh K, Hayden D, Eichler FS. Natural history of neurological abnormalities in cerebrotendinous xanthomatosis. J Inherit Metab Dis. 2018;41(4):647–56.
16. Zubarioglu T, Kiykim E, Yesil G, Demircioglu D, Cansever MS, Yalcinkaya C, Aktuglu-Zeybek C. Early diagnosed cerebrotendinous xanthomatosis patients: clinical, neuroradiological characteristics and therapy results of a single center from Turkey. Acta Neurol Belg. 2017;119(3):343–50.
17. Kısa PT, Yildirim GK, Hismi BO, Dorum S, Kusbeci OY, Topak A, et al. Patients with cerebrotendinous xanthomatosis diagnosed with diverse multisystem involvement. Metab Brain Dis. 2021;36(6):1201–11.
18. Vaz FM, Jamal Y, Barto R, Gelb MH, DeBarber AE, Wevers RA, et al. Newborn screening for cerebrotendinous xanthomatosis: a retrospective biomarker study using both flow-injection and UPLC-MS/MS analysis in 20,000 newborns. Clin Chim Acta. 2023;539:170–4.

19. Vaz FM, Bootsma AH, Kulik W, Verrips A, Wevers RA, Schielen PC, et al. A newborn screening method for cerebrotendinous xanthomatosis using bile alcohol glucuronides and metabolite ratios. J Lipid Res. 2017;58(5):1002–7.
20. Freedman SF, Del Monte MA, Diva U, Donahue SP, Drack AV, Dutta R, et al. Prevalence of cerebrotendinous xanthomatosis among patients diagnosed with early-onset idiopathic bilateral cataracts: final analysis. J AAPOS. 2023;27(4):208–11.
21. Fernández-Eulate G, Martin GC, Dureau P, Speeg-Spatz C, Brassier A, Gillard P, et al. Prospective cholestanol screening of cerebrotendinous xanthomatosis among patients with juvenile-onset unexplained bilateral cataracts. Orphanet J Rare Dis. 2022;17(1):434–9.
22. Atilla H, Coskun T, Elibol B, Kadayifcilar S, Altinel S, GEN-EYE-I Working Group. Prevalence of cerebrotendinous xanthomatosis in cases with idiopathic bilateral juvenile cataract in ophthalmology clinics in Turkey. J AAPOS. 2021;25(5):269.e1–6.
23. Freedman SF, Brennand C, Chiang J, DeBarber A, Del Monte MA, Duell PB, Fiorito J, Marshall R. Prevalence of cerebrotendinous xanthomatosis among patients diagnosed with acquired juvenile-onset idiopathic bilateral cataracts. JAMA Ophthalmol. 2019;137(11):1312–6.
24. Stelten BML, Bonnot O, Huidekoper HH, van Spronsen FJ, van Hasselt PM, Kluijtmans LAJ, Wevers RA, Verrips A. Autism spectrum disorder: an early and frequent feature in cerebrotendinous xanthomatosis. J Inherit Metab Dis. 2017;41(4):641–6.
25. Sedel F, Baumann N, Turpin JC, Lyon-Caen O, Saudubray JM, Cohen D. Psychiatric manifestations revealing inborn errors of metabolism in adolescents and adults. J Inherit Metab Dis. 2007;30(5):631–41.
26. Fraidakis MJ. Psychiatric manifestations in cerebrotendinous xanthomatosis. Transl Psychiatry. 2013;3(9):e302.
27. Wejjakul W, Chatmaitri S, Wattanarojanaporn T, Pongkunakorn A, Ittiwut C, Shotelersuk V. Bilateral femoral neck fractures in cerebrotendinous xanthomatosis treated by hip arthroplasties: the first case report and literature review. J Orthop Case Rep. 2017;7(5):54–8.
28. Berginer VM, Shany S, Alkalay D, Berginer J, Dekel S, Salen G, Tint GS, Gazit D. Osteoporosis and increased bone fractures in cerebrotendinous xanthomatosis. Metabolism. 1993;42(1):69–74.
29. Martini G, Mignarri A, Ruvio M, Valenti R, Franci B, Del Puppo M, Federico A, Nuti R, Dotti MT. Long-term bone density evaluation in cerebrotendinous xanthomatosis: evidence of improvement after chenodeoxycholic acid treatment. Calcif Tissue Int. 2012;92(3):282–6.
30. Zübarioğlu T, Bilen İP, Kıykım E, Doğan BB, Enver EÖ, Cansever MŞ, Zeybek AÇA. Evaluation of the effect of chenodeoxycholic acid treatment on skeletal system findings in patients with cerebrotendinous xanthomatosis. Turk Pediatri Ars. 2019;54(2):113–8.
31. Brass EP, Stelten BML, Verrips A. Cerebrotendinous xanthomatosis-associated diarrhea and response to chenodeoxycholic acid treatment. JIMD Rep. 2020;56(1):105–11.
32. Appadurai V, DeBarber AE, Chiang PW, Patel SB, Steiner RD, Tyler C, et al. Apparent underdiagnosis of cerebrotendinous xanthomatosis revealed by analysis of ~60,000 human exomes. Mol Genet Metab. 2015;116(4):298–304.
33. Reshef A, Meiner V, Berginer VM, Leitersdorf E. Molecular genetics of cerebrotendinous xanthomatosis in Jews of north African origin. J Lipid Res. 1994;35(3):478–83.
34. Leitersdorf E, Reshef A, Meiner V, Levitzki R, Schwartz SP, Dann EJ, et al. Frameshift and splice-junction mutations in the sterol 27-hydroxylase gene cause cerebrotendinous xanthomatosis in Jews or Moroccan origin. J Clin Invest. 1993;91(6):2488–96.
35. Leitersdorf E, Safadi R, Meiner V, Reshef A, Björkhem I, Friedlander Y, et al. Cerebrotendinous xanthomatosis in the Israeli Druze: molecular genetics and phenotypic characteristics. Am J Hum Genet. 1994;55(5):907–15.
36. Falik-Zaccai TC, Kfir N, Frenkel P, Cohen C, Tanus M, Mandel H, et al. Population screening in a Druze community: the challenge and the reward. Genet Med. 2008;10(12):903–9.
37. DeBarber AE, Kalfon L, Fedida A, Fleisher Sheffer V, Ben Haroush S, et al. Newborn screening for cerebrotendinous xanthomatosis is the solution for early identification and treatment. J Lipid Res. 2018;59(11):2214–22.

Ophthalmic Manifestations in Cerebrotendinous Xanthomatosis (CTX)

24

Z. I. Segal

Introduction

Cerebrotendinous xanthomatosis (CTX) is a rare autosomal recessive metabolic disease. It has been reported in people worldwide. Genetic studies revealed biallelic pathogenic variants in the sterol 27-hydroxylase gene, result in markedly diminished activity of the enzyme in CTX patients. This genetic defect is associated with elevated plasma cholestanol levels and consequently its accumulation in the brain, lens, tendons, and other tissues [1, 2]. Prevalence between genders change among studies [3, 4]. The age of CTX onset is variable, although most clinical presentations appear in the first or second decade of life. Clinical features are insidious and unpredictable. Cataracts and diarrhea are the most often presenting symptoms in childhood but are not always present [5]. Except for bilateral cataract, some authors described additional ophthalmic involvement, including retinal and optic nerve disorders. Tendon xanthomas may be present at the time of diagnosis or years later, while neurological symptoms, leading to significant motor, cognitive, and behavioral disability, develop later in life [6]. Between the fourth and sixth decades, death usually occurs as a consequence of progressive neurologic deterioration, pseudobulbar paralysis, or acute myocardial infarction [7].

Treatment with chenodeoxycholic acid (CDCA) can limit or even reverse the progression of neurologic deficits if treatment is started at an early age, whereas failure to diagnose this disease will inevitably result in severe and irreversible neurological disability [1, 8]. Hence, early clinical and genetic diagnoses have an important role in preventing the morbidity and mortality of the disease. Therefore, even in the absence of cataract, a diagnosis of CTX should be considered in the presence of other suggestive symptoms [9].

Z. I. Segal (✉)
Ophthalmology Department, Galilee Medical Center, Nahariya, Israel

The Azrieli Faculty of Medicine, Bar-Ilan University, Safed, Israel

A. Federico et al. (eds.), *Cerebrotendinous Xanthomatosis*,
https://doi.org/10.1007/978-3-031-92526-9_24

Ophthalmic Involvement in CTX

(a) *Bilateral Cataract*

General Consideration

Cataract is a cloudy area in the lens within the eye which is typically clear (Fig. 24.1). Cataracts are very common as people get older. In fact, more than half of all Americans age 80 or older either have cataracts or have had surgery to get rid of cataracts [10]. Most cataracts develop slowly and don't disturb eyesight early on. But with time, cataracts will eventually affect vision causing blurry, hazy, or less colorful vision.

Many etiologies may cause cataracts which include age (old age and congenital), genetic syndromes, systemic diseases (skin, endocrine, renal etc.), medication, trauma, radiation, inadequate nutrition, previous eye surgery, and hyperbaric oxygen therapy [11].

Cataracts can be classified as congenital, infantile, juvenile, presenile, and senile. Congenital or infantile cataracts present within the first year of life, a juvenile cataract presents within the first decade of life, a presenile cataract presents before the age of about 45 years, and senile or age-related cataract presents after that [12].

In CTX, childhood-onset cataracts are a common early symptom, described in 92% of patients. Cataracts precede neurological signs and tendon xanthomas, and if present, are considered useful for early diagnosis [5].

Lipid Metabolism in Cataract

The concept suggesting a possible involvement of lipids in human cataract is based on the early description of lipoidal material in the crystalline lens reported by Berzelius in 1825 [13]. In 1965, cataractous human lens showed higher amounts of cholesterol, cephalins, lecithin, and sphingomyelin when compared to normal lens which carried already large amounts of cholesterol [14]. Cholesterol represents about 40% of the total lipids of human lens fibers which is unique in its high cholesterol content, and increases, over time, to a level that is incomparable with other tissue/organ cells [15].

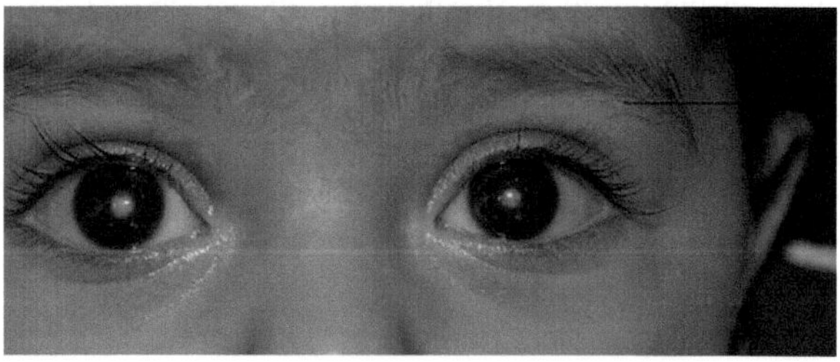

Fig. 24.1 Child with bilateral mature cataracts

Generally, the cholesterol sources in the human body come either from the diet (exogenous cholesterol) or is synthesized de novo (endogenous cholesterol). Dietary cholesterol accounts for approximately 30% of the total cholesterol in the human body, whereas about 70% of cholesterol is derived from cholesterol biosynthesis [16].

In contrast to other tissues, the uptake of dietary cholesterol by the lens is minimal. The human aqueous humor supplies nutrients to the avascular lens maintaining lens transparency. Yet, due to anterior and equatorial lens epithelium barrier, the lens depends less on the diet cholesterol and synthesizes cholesterol de novo or remodels its own lipids for fiber cell membrane formation [17–19]. Thus, any disorders that alter cholesterol synthesis may cause unfavorable consequences in the lens lipid membrane structure and disturbance of the lens fiber cell membrane homeostasis [20].

Knowledge of the spatial distribution of lipids in the intraocular lens is important for understanding the physiology and biochemistry of this unique tissue and for gaining a better insight into the mechanisms underlying diseases of the lens. About 172 lipid species were identified mainly as sphingomyelins, phosphatidyl-cholines, and phosphatidylethanolamines. In addition, 20 phosphatidylcholines, 6 phosphatidylethanolamines, and 4 phosphatidic acids were also detected [21]. The lens transmit light through thousands of cellular membranes rich in phospholipids especially dihydrosphingomyelin. Most of the lipids are associated with proteins. Sphingolipids represent 60% of human lens and contributes the main integral part in its transparency [22]. When proteins lose their stability due to conformational changes, the protein–lipid interaction gets weaker resulting in protein aggregation and cataractous lens formation [23]. The change in the lipid to lipid and lipid to protein-lipid interactions damages the lenticular fiber membranes arrangement by forming widespread of vacuoles and clusters of undulating membranes which scatter the light and impairs the vision.

Oxidative stress is considered to have an important pathogenic role in degenerative eye diseases [24]. Oxidative stress can damage tissues, leading to changes in tissue structure and function, increased vascular permeability, microvascular abnormalities, and neovascularization, such as lens crystallin denaturation and retina degeneration [25, 26]. Therefore, oxidative stress is considered as another mechanism of cataract formation.

Cataracts form when the crystallin protein inside the lens gradually aggregates after an injury or misfolds to form an insoluble turbid protein that scatters light. The mechanisms responsible for this protein change include oxidative stress, osmotic pressure changes, and phase separation between protein and water [27]. The oxidative stress mechanism causes decrease in the antioxidant capacity of the lens resulting in an increase in oxidative pressure within the lens or a decrease in the ability to remove reactive oxidative species (ROS) leading to lens opacification [28].

Studies have shown that cholesterol contributes to the impermeability of oxygen across the lens membranes. Maintaining low levels of oxygen is important to the lens to prevent oxidation and cataract formation. One of the main functions of the mitochondria, present in the epithelium and outer cortical fibers [29], is to degrade oxygen [30]. The cholesterol-related impermeability of the membranes to oxygen may help to keep oxygen in the outer regions of the lens long enough for the mitochondria to degrade it.

Lipid peroxidation caused by free radicals is the initial mechanism leading to the occurrence of cataracts. It includes increased concentrations of primary molecular lipid peroxidaion products, such as diene conjugates, lipid hydroperoxides, oxy-derivatives of phospholipid fatty acids [31]. This mechanism increases the cell membrane permeability resulting in protein function loss and formation of cataract [32, 33]. In addition, lens epithelial cells that act to maintain the stability and transparency of the environment inside the lens are damaged by ROS. The apoptotic cells produce additional amount of ROS, causing degeneration and loss of function of the lens [34]. The Na+/K+-ATPase on the membrane of lens epithelial cells is also influenced by ROS, resulting in sodium and water accumulation within the cells and formation of lens opacification [35, 36].

Bile acids (BA) eliminate cholesterol, aid in lipid transport, and stimulate bile flow and biliary phospholipid secretion [37]. BAs are produced in hepatocytes and are transported to the gallbladder through bile canaliculi. There are two major pathways for BA synthesis: the classical and alternative pathways [38]. The classical pathway is initiated by cholesterol 7α-hydroxylase (CYP7A1) and regulated by farnesoid X receptor (FXR) [39, 40]. CYP7A1 is the only rate-limited enzyme in BA synthesis and leads to the production of the two primary BAs: cholic acid (CA) and chenodeoxycholic acid (CDCA). The alternate pathway is initiated by sterol 27-hydroxylase (CYP27A1), a mitochondrial cytochrome P450 enzyme that is widely distributed in macrophages and most tissues [39, 41]. Studies have shown that the alternative pathway contributes to around 9% of total BA synthesis in human hepatocytes [37]. Initiation by CYP27A1, followed by CYP7B1 (25-hydroxycholesterol 7-alpha-hydroxylase), leads to the synthesis of CA and CDCA in the liver and extrahepatic tissues [37, 41]. A deficiency of sterol 27-hydroxylase leads to reduced production of CDCA and subsequently to upregulation of cholesterol 7α-hydroxylase. Upregulation of the rate-limiting enzyme in the classic bile acid pathway results in elevated levels of 7α-hydroxy-4-cholesten-3-one, an efficient precursor to cholestanol [42]. In patients with CTX, most of the cholestanol accumulation is derived from 7α-hydroxylated metabolites of cholesterol, 7α-hydroxy-4-cholesten-3-one being the most important [42, 43]. Development and progression of CTX are secondary to the further efficient conversion of 7α-hydroxy-4-cholesten-3-one into cholestanol and bile alcohols by two different pathways [42, 44, 45]. Consequently, increased cholesterol metabolites, such as cholestanol, accumulate mainly in the brain, lenses, and tendons, leading to the characteristic clinical manifestations of CTX. Elevated serum cholestanol and urine bile alcohols are the biochemical diagnostic hallmarks in CTX [45]. The increased content of cholestanol in cataract patients with CTX was found when they compared with the senile lens nuclei used as a control [46]. Moreover, some studies showed cataract stabilization in patients treated with CDCA [47], whereas others did not experience complete resolution and they had to undergo surgery [48].

Clinical Presentation

Juvenile bilateral cataract is considered to be one of the clinical hallmarks of CTX (76–88% of patients based on a review of selected international case series) [49, 50]. Childhood-onset bilateral cataracts are a common presentation in patients with CTX [51]. However, patients with juvenile-onset unexplained bilateral cataract should benefit from a plasma cholestanol analysis for suspected CTX, even in the absence of other CTX clinical manifestations [52]. Within the bilateral juvenile cataract, CTX prevalence is relatively high (2% to approximately 4%) [53–55] when comparing the estimated bilateral childhood cataracts in the general population as 3–68 per 100,000 [56]. The lens opacities usually develop within the first 3 decades of life, often between the ages of 4 and 18 years. These patients develop irregular cortical opacities, anterior polar cataracts, or dense posterior subscapular cataracts. Fleck lenticular deposits may be an early sign of CTX [11, 52]. Screening using the Mignarri suspicion index and cholestanol blood levels can be helpful in identifying suspected cases of CTX [57].

Posterior subcapsular cataracts (PSC) form in the back of the lens, aside the capsule which holds the lens in place. As the cataract develops, it will increasingly obstruct the path of light and cause glare. This type of cataract is commonly found in children and even infants. The progression of a PSC cataract is typically more rapid than other forms of cataract. PSC cataracts can compromise one's reading vision, cause glare or halos around lights during the night, and may result in worsened vision in bright-light settings. If left untreated, posterior subcapsular cataracts may result in significant impairment of vision and can progress to the point of blindness (Fig. 24.2).

Although descriptions of the cataract types in CTX are largely lacking, some reports show the presence of posterior subcapsular cataracts with particular fleck-like opacities in patients with CTX [48, 57, 58]. Anterior sutural cataract near the anterior capsule was also described in CTX patient [58].

Congenital/juvenile/pediatric cataract may appear in many multiorgan disorders associated with dysmorphism, metabolic errors, and some neurological involvement. Two examples for such disorders are myotonic dystrophy type 1 (DM1) or Steinert's disease and galactokinase deficiency or galactosemia type II. Juvenile cataract with neurologic disorders in DM1 shows a "Christmas tree" morphology [59], which differs in appearance from the fleck-like opacities found in CTX

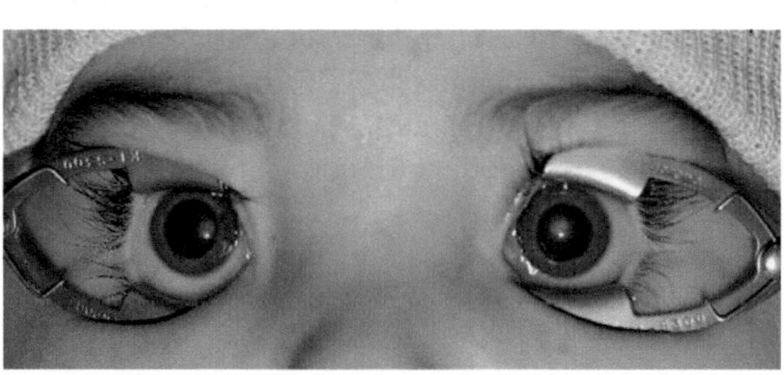

Fig. 24.2 Bilateral posterior subcapsular polar cataract

patients. In galactokinase deficiency, as in CTX, bilateral cataract is the most common manifestation [60]. Galactokinase deficiency is a rare inborn error of galactose metabolism that frequently results in the formation of nuclear cataracts [61]. In this genetic disorder, cataract develops due to accumulation of galactitol in the lens, causing osmotic swelling of lens fibers, rupture of the cell membrane, and protein denaturation that opacies the lens. Cataract changes are reversible only if galactose is withdrawn from food before the rupture of the cell membrane [62].

Treatment of cataract depends on the time of discovery. When the lens opacities are mild and no visual disturbances occur, the patients should be followed up until the time when cataract surgery is needed. Removal of the cataract is performed when the eye sight and general proper functioning (reading, driving, watching television, etc.) are reduced. Because of underdiagnosis of CTX, most of the patients when diagnosed suffer already from bilateral as it appears early in life, and they need cataract surgery immediately after discovery. Others reach genetic counseling when they are already pseudophakic as the cataract surgery was performed previously. The prognosis of cataract surgery depends on the age of diagnosis, time of surgery, surgical complications, and postoperative treatment. One of the most common complications in infantile/juvenile cataract is deprivational amblyopia. For this reason, cataract lens removal should be considered early in life with proper postoperative strict follow-up.

Early medical treatment is based on recognition of CTX based on genetic testing and a positive family history for the disease. Treatment with chenodeoxycholic acid (CDCA) may prevent or reduce the appearance of lens opacities in those patients [47].

(b) *Retinal Involvement*

General Consideration

Knowledge of the clinical phenotype of completely lacking sterol 27-hydroxylase activity may provide some insight into the ocular significance of cholesterol 27-oxygenation. Among several clinical manifestations of CTX, CYP27A1 deficiency leads to ocular diverse symptoms that include involvement of the eye's posterior segment. Presence of optic disc pallor, cholesterol-like crystals in the vitreous, retinal vessel sclerosis, cholesterol-like deposits along the vascular arcades, RPE defects on fluorescein angiography (FA) were described (Fig. 24.3) [63, 64].

Fundus examinations are difficult in patients with cataracts, which limit visualization of the retina. Therefore, for a number of years, cataracts were thought to be the only ocular symptom of CTX. However, it has become clear that ocular involvement in CTX is more widespread than previously described [65], suggesting that CYP27A1 is as important for normal retinal function as it is for general health.

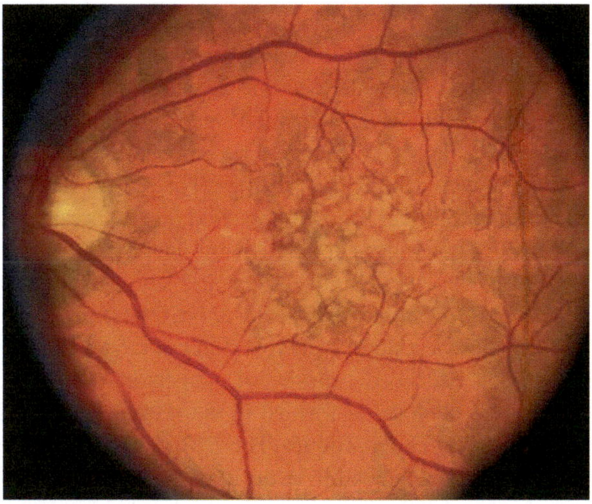

Fig. 24.3 Lipid deposits (drusen) beneath the retina

Retinal Lipid Metabolism

Proper functioning of the human retina depends on cholesterol, which is utilized in multiple physiological processes. Similar to other organs in the human body, the retina obtains cholesterol from two distinct sources: de nova synthesis of cholesterol and import of cholesterol from extraretinal sources. Unlike the blood-brain barrier, the blood-retina barrier allows uptake of cholesterol from the circulation via a lipoprotein-based/receptor-mediated mechanism into the RPE and all layers of the neural retina [65]. On the hand, correlative in situ hybridization studies have supported the hypothesis that (rod) photoreceptor cells, Müller cells, and RPE cells have the capacity to synthesize isoprenoids, such as cholesterol. However, there is no evidence to unambiguously determine whether or not de novo cholesterol synthesis can account for the steady-state levels of cholesterol found in the retina or whether de novo synthesis is both necessary and sufficient to meet the multiple needs of the retina for cholesterol [66].

Under normal conditions, cholesterol homeostasis is tightly regulated. Also, cholesterol exists in the neural retina overwhelmingly in unesterified form, and sterol intermediates are present in minimal to negligible quantities. However, under certain pathological conditions, either due to an inborn error in cholesterol biosynthesis or as a consequence of exposure to selective inhibitors of enzymes in the cholesterol pathway, the ratio of sterol intermediates to cholesterol in the retina can rise dramatically and persist, in some cases resulting in progressive degeneration that significantly compromises the structure and function of the retina.

Quantification of the oxysterols in the human retina revealed that 27-COOH is the most abundant enzymatic product of cholesterol oxidation in this organ, significantly exceeding the levels of Preg and 24-OH cholesterol. 27S-hydroxylase that hydroxylates cholesterol at the C27 position has been detected by immunohistochemistry in monkey's retina, localized primarily in photoreceptor inner segments (cell bodies), with minimal expression in Müller cells, RPE cells, ganglion cells, the nerve fiber layer, and the endothelial cells of the choriocapillaris [67]. Based upon these results, one would expect to detect appreciable levels of 27-hydroxycholesterol in the retina. However, when the steady-state levels of 27-hydroxycholesterol were quantified, they were found to be below the detection limit in bovine and human retinas as well as in RPE cells [68]. The reason for that is CYP27A1 localization in photoreceptor inner segments showed faint expression throughout the retina, including Müller cells, ganglion cells, and nerve fibers [65]. Faint CYP27A1 expression was also observed in the RPE and choriocapillaris [67]. On the other hand, 3β-hydroxy-5-cholestenoic acid (27-COOH), an oxidation product derived from 27-hydroxycholesterol, was found in human and bovine retina and RPE in amounts that far exceeded those of 24-hydroxycholesterol. This suggests that 27-hydroxycholesterol formed in the retina is immediately converted to the corresponding 27-COOH product. The 27-COOH level is higher in human retina than in the RPE and undetectable in the choroid. By way of comparison, the levels of oxysterols are >1000-fold lower than the levels of cholesterol in retina and RPE cells. If CYP27A1 is highly abundant in photoreceptor inner segments and this site is the major source of retinal 27-COOH, then the 27-oxygenated cholesterol metabolite has to leave the photoreceptor inner segments and be transported within the retina to the site(s) where it can enter systemic circulation. In total, these findings not only exclude the choroid as a source of contamination for the 27-COOH found in the retina but also are consistent with reverse cholesterol transport from the retina to the RPE and into the choroidal circulation.

Studies with cultured human macrophages showed that the nature of the acceptor outside the cell affects the intracellular cholesterol to be metabolized to 27-OH or 27-COOH [69]. Consequently, cholesterol has to be transported from the outer to the inner membrane to be metabolized by CYP27A1, but the nature of this process in photoreceptor inner segments is unknown. CYP27A1 activity depends on the phospholipid content of the membranes in which this enzyme is embedded [70]. Cholesterol removal from the retina likely varies, depending on cell type. Multiple oxysterols (Preg and 24-OH) are produced in the retinal neurons, and one predominant oxysterol, 27-COOH, is probably generated in the photoreceptor inner segments and RPE [69]. Overall, oxidation to 27-COOH seems to be the predominant mechanism for cholesterol elimination from the retina and RPE [68].

As mentioned previously, the bile acid pathway plays an important role in cholesterol metabolism. In the retina as well as in the brain, bile acid biosynthesis relies mainly on the alternate pathway. The first step in the alternate pathway is initiated by the conversion of cholesterol into 27-hydroxycholesterol via CYP27A1. Subsequently, oxysterol 7α-hydroxylase (CYP7B1), through subsequent hydroxylation, leads to the formation of primary bile acids: cholic acid and chenodeoxycholic acid [71].

Cholesterol involvement is implicated in several retinal pathologies, such as in age-related macular degeneration, where large cholesterol-rich deposits are a hallmark feature [39]. CYP27A1 and CYP46A1 are two enzymes that are important for ocular function in humans. In the retina, CYP27A1 is the principal hydroxylase that catalyzes the hydroxylation of cholesterol for BA synthesis to account for the majority of enzymatic cholesterol elimination in the retina [70]. Deficiency in CYP27A1 as seen in *CTX* may cause premature retinal degeneration [39]. Combined deficiency in CYP27A1 and CYP46A1 results in neovascularization and lipid accumulation in the mouse retina [72].

Study using Cyp27a1$^{-/-}$ mice model showed dysregulation of retinal cholesterol homeostasis, including unexpected upregulation of retinal cholesterol biosynthesis [72]. The major findings of the study are that dysregulated retinal cholesterol homeostasis leads to focal depositions of cholesterol along Bruchs membrane (BrM; the inner choroidal layer) and the development of retinal choroidal anastomosis (RCA) in the involved areas. In addition, Müller cells, the predominant glial cell type of the retina, are reported to play a role in neovascularization (NV) [73]. Near the injured area, healthy Müller cells expressed general activation in response to hypoxia, while other Müller cell bodies were disorganized and gliotic [39]. The presence of an abnormal vascular process demonstrated blood vessel patency in vivo and revealed that the permeability of the blood vessels is increased. Leakage from these vessels was later observed as lipid deposits in the areas of abnormal vascularization and thus support a model for AMD wherein lipid lesions in BrM elicit choroidal NV [74, 75].

(c) *Optic Nerve Involvement*

Optic nerve involvement in CTX has been reported previously; therefore, medical caretakers should examine the optic nerve very thoroughly. Optic neuropathy with optic disc paleness is a common finding in patients with CTX (Fig. 24.4) [63, 64]. About 50–80% of affected patients exhibit a prolonged or diminished visual-evoked potential (VEP) latency in the presence or absence of an abnormal fundus [63, 76]. Considering the pathophysiology of CTX, which involves the accumulation of cholesterol and cholestanol in virtually all tissues, nonarthritic ischemic optic neuropathy (NAION) is considered in the differential diagnosis of a patients with optic neuropathy. However, the presence of contrast-enhanced optic nerves on

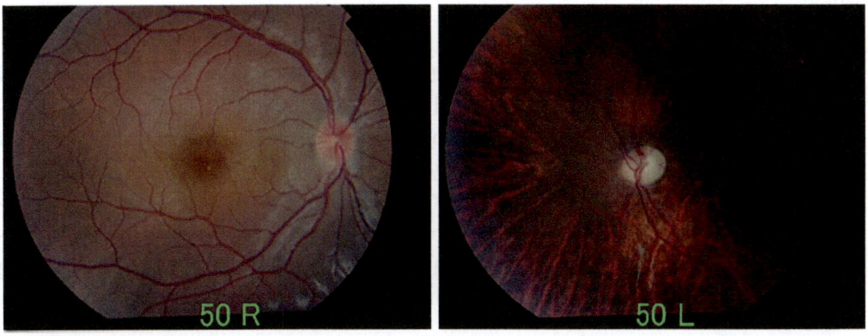

Fig. 24.4 Optic atrophy in the left eye

MRI and spontaneous recovery of visual acuity turns NAION a less likely diagnosis [77].

A different consideration for optic neuropathy in CTX may be related to the myelin membrane of the optic nerve. One of the prominent biochemical characteristics that distinguishes myelin from other membranes is its high lipid-to-protein ratio; lipids account for at least 70% of the dry weight of myelin membranes [78]. The lipid-rich composition of myelin is likely to contribute to the frequent occurrence of myelin defects in lipid metabolism disorders, including hypomyelination (decreased myelin production), dysmyelination (abnormally formed myelin), and demyelination (degenerative loss of myelin). Inherited forms of these diseases are particularly informative and provide direct insight into the underlying molecular mechanisms. These include defects in the metabolism of all myelin-enriched lipids, as seen in Smith-Lemli-Opitz syndrome (SLOS), cerebrotendinous xanthomatosis (CTX), and Tangier disease (TD). The defects of these disorders may result in accumulation of various metabolic precursors from lipid biosynthesis to levels that are toxic to the myelinating glial cells or at least interfere with normal myelin membrane structure [79, 80]. CTX and TD lead to accumulation of 7α-hydroxy-4-cholesten-3-one and cholestanol (in CTX) and cholesterolesters (in TD), which are likely to underlie the myelin pathology [81]. In SLOS myelin defects occur due to reduced cholesterol levels and are reported to involve absence of myelin [82] and demyelination [83]. In spite of significant progress in understanding the effects of altered sterol metabolism, there remains no clearly effective treatment for the most debilitating symptoms of SLOS and other sterol disorders. Cholesterol supplementation, statin treatment, and similar pharmacologic approaches have each shown some promise for improved outcomes [84].

Optic nerve involvement in CTX has been reported, including a case of optic neuropathy with features suggestive of optic neuritis [85]. The exact mechanism underlying this phenomenon remains unclear. However, due to the similarities in clinical presentation and imaging findings between this CTX patient and those observed in Leber's Hereditary Optic Neuropathy (LHON), it is possible that mitochondrial dysfunction—known to play a role in LHON—may also be implicated in CTX-related optic neuropathy.

(d) *Summary*

CTX can be manifested as juvenile cataract at variable age of occurrence as well as other ocular disorders in the retina and posterior segment. The concomitant presence of even one associated symptom to bilateral juvenile cataract should prompt the evaluation for CTX to support early definitive therapy and prevent systemic gastrointestinal, dermal (xanthomas) disturbances, and especially devastating neurological damage. Therefore, ophthalmologists, including pediatric ophthalmologists, have an important role in promoting early diagnosis of CTX by recommending testing for this disease in patients with idiopathic bilateral early-onset cataracts.

References

1. Berginer VM, Salen G, Shefer S. Cerebrotendinous xanthomatosis. Neurol Clin. 1989;7(1):55–74.
2. Berginer VM, Gross B, Morad K, Kfir N, Morkos S, Aaref S, Falik-Zaccai TC. Chronic diarrhea and juvenile cataracts: think cerebrotendinous xanthomatosis and treat. Pediatrics. 2009;123(1):143–7.
3. Salen G, Steiner RD. Epidemiology, diagnosis, and treatment of cerebrotendinous xanthomatosis (CTX). J Inherit Metab Dis. 2017;40(6):771–81.
4. Freedman SF, Del Monte MA, Diva U, Donahue SP, Drack AV, Dutta R, Fung SSM, Imperiale M, Jordan CO, Lenhart PD, Lim ME, McCourt EA, Nihalani BR, Sabahi T, Stahl ED, Miraldi Utz VA, Wilson ME Jr, Yen KG, VanderVeen DK. Prevalence of cerebrotendinous xanthomatosis among patients diagnosed with early-onset idiopathic bilateral cataracts: final analysis. J AAPOS. 2023;27(4):208–11.
5. Cruysberg JR. Cerebrotendinous xanthomatosis: juvenile cataract and chronic diarrhea before the onset of neurologic disease. Arch Neurol. 2002;59(12):1975.
6. Balkhadir H, Tahiri L, Fathi I, Bardouni A, Zouaidia F, Rkain H, Karkouri S, Allali F. Cerebrotendinous xanthomatosis: a Moroccan case report and review of literature. Ann Indian Acad Neurol. 2021;24(5):841–3.
7. Verrips A, van Engelen BG, Wevers RA, van Geel BM, Cruysberg JR, van den Heuvel LP, Keyser A, Gabreëls FJ. Presence of diarrhea and absence of tendon xanthomas in patients with cerebrotendinous xanthomatosis. Arch Neurol. 2000;57(4):520–4.
8. Berginer VM, Salen G, Shefer S. Long-term treatment of cerebrotendinous xanthomatosis with chenodeoxycholic acid. N Engl J Med. 1984;311(26):1649–52.
9. Abdel-Hamid MS, Issa MY, Otaify GA, Zaki MS. A novel frameshift mutation in the sterol 27-hydroxylase gene in an Egyptian family with cerebrotendinous xanthomatosis without cataract. Metab Brain Dis. 2017;32(2):311–5.
10. National Eye Institute: Cataracts. 2023. https://www.nei.nih.gov/learn-about-eye-health/eye-conditions-and-diseases/cataracts. Accessed 25 June 2024.
11. American Academy of Ophthalmology: Cataract. 2024. https://eyewiki.aao.org/Cataract. Accessed 25 June 2024.
12. Yi J, Yun J, Li ZK, Xu CT, Pan BR. Epidemiology and molecular genetics of congenital cataracts. Int J Ophthalmol. 2011;4(4):422–32.
13. Berzelius JJ. Lehrbuch der Chemie ... Nach des Verfassers schwedischer Bearbeitung der Blöde-Palmstedt'schen Auflage übersetzt von F. Wöhler. Dresden & Leipzig; 1825–1831.
14. Feldman GL, Feldman LS. New concepts of human lenticular lipids and their possible role in cataracts. Investig Ophthalmol. 1965;4:162–6.
15. Li LK, So L, Spector A. Membrane cholesterol and phospholipid in consecutive concentric sections of human lenses. J Lipid Res. 1985;26(5):600–9.
16. Kapourchali FR, Surendiran G, Goulet A, Moghadasian MH. The role of dietary cholesterol in lipoprotein metabolism and related metabolic abnormalities: a mini-review. Crit Rev Food Sci Nutr. 2016;56(14):2408–15.
17. Cenedella RJ. Sterol synthesis by the ocular lens of the rat during postnatal development. J Lipid Res. 1982;23(4):619–26.
18. Zelenka PS. Lens lipids. Curr Eye Res. 1984;3(11):1337–59.
19. Cenedella RJ. Cholesterol and cataracts. Surv Ophthalmol. 1996;40(4):320–37.
20. Van Meer G, Voelker DR, Feigenson GW. Membrane lipids: where they are and how they behave. Nat Rev Mol Cell Biol. 2008;9(2):112–24.

21. Pól J, Vidová V, Hyötyläinen T, Volný M, Novák P, Strohalm M, Kostiainen R, Havlíček V, Wiedmer SK, Holopainen JM. Spatial distribution of glycerophospholipids in the ocular lens. PLoS One. 2011;6(4):e19441.
22. Borchman D, Yappert MC. Lipids and the ocular lens. J Lipid Res. 2010;51(9):2473–88.
23. Mohanty BP, Bhattacharjee S, Paria P, Mahanty A, Sharma AP. Lipid biomarkers of lens aging. Appl Biochem Biotechnol. 2013;169(1):192–200.
24. Nita M, Grzybowski A. The role of the reactive oxygen species and oxidative stress in the pathomechanism of the age-related ocular diseases and other pathologies of the anterior and posterior eye segments in adults. Oxidative Med Cell Longev. 2016;1:3164734.
25. Beatty S, Koh H, Phil M, Henson D, Boulton M. The role of oxidative stress in the pathogenesis of age-related macular degeneration. Surv Ophthalmol. 2000;45(2):115–34.
26. Williams DL. Oxidative stress and the eye. Vet Clin North Am Small Anim Pract. 2008;38(1):179–92. vii
27. Sunkireddy P, Jha SN, Kanwar JR, Yadav SC. Natural antioxidant biomolecules promises future nanomedicine based therapy for cataract. Colloids Surf B Biointerfaces. 2013;112:554–62.
28. Spector A. Review: oxidative stress and disease. J Ocul Pharmacol Ther. 2000;16(2):193–201.
29. Widomska J, Raguz M, Subczynski WK. Oxygen permeability of the lipid bilayer membrane made of calf lens lipids. Biochim Biophys Acta. 2007;1768(10):2635–45.
30. McNulty R, Wang H, Mathias RT, Ortwerth BJ, Truscott RJ, Bassnett S. Regulation of tissue oxygen levels in the mammalian lens. J Physiol. 2004;559(Pt 3):883–98.
31. Babizhayev MA. Analysis of lipid peroxidation and electron microscopic survey of maturation stages during human cataractogenesis: pharmacokinetic assay of Can-C N-acetylcarnosine prodrug lubricant eye drops for cataract prevention. Drugs R D. 2005;6(6):345–69.
32. Kisic B, Miric D, Zoric L, Ilic A. Role of lipid peroxidation in the pathogenesis of age-related cataract. In: Lipid peroxidation. Rijeka: IntechOpen; 2012.
33. Miric DJ, Kisic BM, Zoric LD, Miric BM, Mirkovic M, Mitic R. Influence of cataract maturity on aqueous humor lipid peroxidation markers and antioxidant enzymes. Eye (Lond). 2014;28(1):72–7.
34. Zhou YF, Guo B, Ye MJ, Liao RF, Li SL. Protective effect of Rutin against H2O2-induced oxidative stress and apoptosis in human lens epithelial cells. Curr Eye Res. 2016;41:933–42.
35. Delamere NA, Tamiya S. Expression, regulation and function of Na,K-ATPase in the lens. Prog Retin Eye Res. 2004;23:593–615.
36. Kim JY, Park JH, Kang SS, Hwang SB, Tchah H. Topical nerve growth factor attenuates streptozotocin-induced diabetic cataracts via polyol pathway inhibition and Na+/K+-ATPase upregulation. Exp Eye Res. 2021;202:108319.
37. Chiang JY. Bile acid metabolism and signaling. Compr Physiol. 2013;3:1191–212.
38. McMillin M, DeMorrow S. Effects of bile acids on neurological function and disease. FASEB J. 2016;30:3658–68.
39. Mertens KL, Kalsbeek A, Soeters MR, Eggink HM. Bile acid signaling pathways from the enterohepatic circulation to the central nervous system. Front Neurosci. 2017;11:617.
40. Li T, Chiang JY. Bile acid signaling in liver metabolism and diseases. J Lipids. 2012;2012:754067.
41. Schwarz M, Russell DW, Dietschy JM, Turley SD. Alternate pathways of bile acid synthesis in the cholesterol 7alpha-hydroxylase knockout mouse are not upregulated by either cholesterol or cholestyramine feeding. J Lipid Res. 2001;42:1594–603.
42. Bjorkhem I, Hansson M. Cerebrotendinous xanthomatosis: an inborn error in bile acid synthesis with defined mutations but still a challenge. Biochem Biophys Res Commun. 2010;396:46–9. https://doi.org/10.1016/j.bbrc.2010.02.140.
43. Skrede S, Bjorkhem I, Buchmann MS, Hopen G, Fausa O. A novel pathway for biosynthesis of cholestanol with 7 alpha-hydroxylated C27-steroids as intermediates, and its importance for the accumulation of cholestanol in cerebrotendinous xanthomatosis. J Clin Invest. 1985;75:448–55.

44. Panzenboeck U, Andersson U, Hansson M, Sattler W, Meaney S, Bjorkhem I. On the mechanism of cerebral accumulation of cholestanol in patients with cerebrotendinous xanthomatosis. J Lipid Res. 2007;48:1167–74.
45. Koyama S, Sekijima Y, Ogura M, Hori M, Matsuki K, Miida T, Harada-Shiba M. Cerebrotendinous xanthomatosis: molecular pathogenesis, clinical spectrum, diagnosis, and disease-modifying treatments. J Atheroscler Thromb. 2021;28(9):905–25.
46. McKenna P, Morgan SJ, Bosanquet RC. Laker MF: a case of cerebrotendinous xanthomatosis. II: The sterol content of a cataractous lens. Br J Ophthalmol. 1990;74:629–30.
47. Van Heijst AF, Verrips A, Wevers RA, Cruysberg JR, Renier WO, Tolboom JJ. Treatment and follow-up of children with cerebrotendinous xanthomatosis. Eur J Pediatr. 1998;157:313–6.
48. Tibrewal S, Duell PB, DeBarber AE, Loh AR. Cerebrotendinous xanthomatosis: early diagnosis on the basis of juvenile cataracts. J AAPOS. 2017;21:505–7.
49. Verrips A, van Engelen BG, ter Laak H, Gabreëls-Festen A, Janssen A, Zwarts M, Wevers RA, Gabreëls FJ. Cerebrotendinous xanthomatosis. Controversies about nerve and muscle: observations in ten patients. Neuromuscul Disord. 2000;10(6):407–14.
50. Wong JC, Walsh K, Hayden D, Eichler FS. Natural history of neurological abnormalities in cerebrotendinous xanthomatosis. J Inherit Metab Dis. 2018;41(4):647–56.
51. Mignarri A, Gallus GN, Dotti MT, Federico A. A suspicion index for early diagnosis and treatment of cerebrotendinous xanthomatosis. J Inherit Metab Dis. 2014;37(3):421–9.
52. Fernández-Eulate G, Martin GC, Dureau P, Speeg-Spatz C, Brassier A, Gillard P, Bremond-Gignac D, Thouvenin D, Pagan C, Lamari F, Nadjar Y. Prospective cholesteanol screening of cerebrotendinous xanthomatosis among patients with juvenile-onset unexplained bilateral cataracts. Orphanet J Rare Dis. 2022;17(1):434.
53. Atilla H, Coskun T, Elibol B, Kadayifcilar S, Altinel S, GEN-EYE-I Working Group. Prevalence of cerebrotendinous xanthomatosis in cases with idiopathic bilateral juvenile cataract in ophthalmology clinics in Turkey. JAAPOS. 2021;25(5):269.e1–6.
54. Gillespie RL, Urquhart J, Anderson B, Williams S, Waller S, Ashworth J, Biswas S, Jones S, Stewart F, Lloyd IC, Clayton-Smith J, Black GC. Next-generation sequencing in the diagnosis of metabolic disease marked by pediatric cataract. Ophthalmology. 2016;123(1):217–20.
55. Musleh M, Hall G, Lloyd IC, Gillespie RL, Waller S, Douzgou S, Clayton-Smith J, Kehdi E, Black GC, Ashworth J. Diagnosing the cause of bilateral paediatric cataracts: comparison of standard testing with a next-generation sequencing approach. Eye (Lond). 2016;30(9):1175–81.
56. Sheeladevi S, Lawrenson JG, Fielder AR, Suttle CM. Global prevalence of childhood cataract: a systematic review. Eye (Lond). 2016;30(9):1160–9.
57. Freedman SF, Brennand C, Chiang J, DeBarber A, Del Monte MA, Duell PB, Fiorito J, Marshall R. Prevalence of cerebrotendinous xanthomatosis among patients diagnosed with acquired juvenile-onset idiopathic bilateral cataracts. JAMA Ophthalmol. 2019;137(11):1312–6.
58. Khan AO, Aldahmesh MA, Mohamed JY, Alkuraya FS. Juvenile cataract morphology in 3 siblings not yet diagnosed with cerebrotendinous xanthomatosis. Ophthalmology. 2013;120(5):956–60.
59. Pagoulatos D, Kapsala Z, Makri OE, Georgakopoulos CD. Christmas tree cataract and myotonic dystrophy type 1. Eye. 2018;32(11):1794–5.
60. Beutler E, Matsumoto F, Kuhl W, Krill A, Levy N, Sparkes R, Degnan M. Galactokinase deficiency as a cause of cataracts. N Engl J Med. 1973;288(23):1203–6.
61. Bosch AM, Bakker HD, van Gennip AH, van Kempen JV, Wanders RJ, Wijburg FA. Clinical features of galactokinase deficiency: a review of the literature. J Inherit Metab Dis. 2002;25(8):629–34.
62. Stambolian D. Galactose and cataract. Surv Ophthalmol. 1988;32(5):333–49.
63. Kretzer FL, Hittner HM, Mehta RS. Ocular manifestations of the Smith-Lemli-Opitz syndrome. Arch Ophthalmol. 1981;99(11):2000–6.

64. Curcio CA, Johnson M, Huang JD, Rudolf M. Aging, age-related macular degeneration, and the response-to-retention of apolipoprotein B-containing lipoproteins. Prog Retin Eye Res. 2009;28(6):393–422.
65. Dotti MT, Rufa A, Federico A. Cerebrotendinous xanthomatosis: heterogeneity of clinical phenotype with evidence of previously undescribed ophthalmological findings. J Inherit Metab Dis. 2001;24(7):696–706.
66. Tserentsoodol N, Sztein J, Campos M, Gordiyenko NV, Fariss RN, Lee JW, Fliesler SJ, Rodriguez IR. Uptake of cholesterol by the retina occurs primarily via a low density lipoprotein receptor-mediated process. Mol Vis. 2006;12:1306–18.
67. Fliesler SJ, Bretillon L. The ins and outs of cholesterol in the vertebrate retina. J Lipid Res. 2010;51(12):3399–413. https://doi.org/10.1194/jlr.R010538.
68. Lee JW, Fuda H, Javitt NB, Strott CA, Rodriguez IR. Expression and localization of sterol 27-hydroxylase (CYP27A1) in monkey retina. Exp Eye Res. 2006;83(2):465–9.
69. Mast N, Reem R, Bederman I, Huang S, DiPatre PL, Bjorkhem I, Pikuleva IA. Cholestenoic acid is an important elimination product of cholesterol in the retina: comparison of retinal cholesterol metabolism with that in the brain. Invest Ophthalmol Vis Sci. 2011;52(1):594–603.
70. Babiker A, Andersson O, Lund E, Xiu RJ, Deeb S, Reshef A, Leitersdorf E, Diczfalusy U, Björkhem I. Elimination of cholesterol in macrophages and endothelial cells by the sterol 27-hydroxylase mechanism. Comparison with high density lipoprotein-mediated reverse cholesterol transport. J Biol Chem. 1997;272(42):26253–61.
71. Murtazina DA, Andersson U, Hahn IS, Bjorkhem I, Ansari GA, Pikuleva IA. Phospholipids modify substrate binding and enzyme activity of human cytochrome P450 27A1. J Lipid Res. 2004;45(12):2345–53.
72. Omarova S, Charvet CD, Reem RE, Mast N, Zheng W, Huang S, Peachey NS, Pikuleva IA. Abnormal vascularization in mouse retina with dysregulated retinal cholesterol homeostasis. J Clin Invest. 2012;122:3012–23.
73. Saadane A, Mast N, Charvet CD, Omarova S, Zheng W, Huang SS, Kern TS, Peachey NS, Pikuleva IA. Retinal and nonocular abnormalities in Cyp27a1(−/−)Cyp46a1(−/−) mice with dysfunctional metabolism of cholesterol. Am J Pathol. 2014;184:2403–19.
74. Kuzmanovic M, Dudley VJ, Sarthy VP. GFAP promoter drives Müller cell-specific expression in transgenic mice. Invest Ophthalmol Vis Sci. 2003;44(8):3606–13.
75. Curcio CA, Johnson M, Rudolf M, Huang JD. The oil spill in ageing Bruch membrane. Br J Ophthalmol. 2011;95(12):1638–45.
76. Cruysberg JR, Wevers RA, van Engelen BG, Pinckers A, van Spreeken A, Tolboom JJ. Ocular and systemic manifestations of cerebrotendinous xanthomatosis. Am J Ophthalmol. 1995;120(5):597–604.
77. Mondelli M, Rossi A, Scarpini C, Dotti MT, Federico A. Evoked potentials in cerebrotendinous xanthomatosis and effect induced by chenodeoxycholic acid. Arch Neurol. 1992;49(5):469–75.
78. Rizzo JF 3rd, Andreoli CM, Rabinov JD. Use of magnetic resonance imaging to differentiate optic neuritis and nonarteritic anterior ischemic optic neuropathy. Ophthalmology. 2002;109(9):1679–84.
79. Norton WT, Poduslo SE. Myelination in rat brain: method of myelin isolation. J Neurochem. 1973;21(4):749–57.
80. Wanders RJ, Ferdinandusse S, Brites P, Kemp S. Peroxisomes, lipid metabolism and lipotoxicity. Biochim Biophys Acta. 2010;1801(3):272–80.
81. Hörster F, Surtees R, Hoffmann GF. Disorders of intermediary metabolism: toxic leukoencephalopathies. J Inherit Metab Dis. 2005;28(3):345–56.
82. Pollock M, Nukada H, Frith RW, Simcock JP, Allpress S. Peripheral neuropathy in Tangier disease. Brain. 1983;106(Pt 4):911–28.
83. Ness GC, Lopez D, Borrego O, Gilbert-Barness E. Increased expression of low-density lipoprotein receptors in a Smith-Lemli-Opitz infant with elevated bilirubin levels. Am J Med Genet. 1997;68(3):294–9.

84. Svoboda MD, Christie JM, Eroglu Y, Freeman KA, Steiner RD. Treatment of Smith-Lemli-Opitz syndrome and other sterol disorders. Am J Med Genet C Semin Med Genet. 2012;160C(4):285–94.
85. Miyamoto M, Ishii N, Mochizuki H, Shiomi K, Kaida T, Chuman H, Nakazato M. Optic neuropathy with features suggestive of optic neuritis in cerebrotendinous xanthomatosis. Case Rep Neurol Med. 2019;2019:2576826.

Part VIII

Newborn Screening and Early Treatment in Cerebrotendinous Xanthomatosis (CTX)

Update on Newborn Screening for Cerebrotendinous Xanthomatosis (CTX)

25

Andrea E. DeBarber, Michael H. Gelb, Monica Martin, Hannah McNeight, Joseph Orsini, Nicolas Szabo-Fresnais, Frederic M. Vaz, Melissa Wasserstein, and Zitao Zhou

Abbreviations

CTX	Cerebrotendinous xanthomatosis
GlcA-tetrol	5β-cholestane-3α,7α,12α,25-tetrol glucuronide
DBS	Dried blood spot
NBS	Newborn screening
t-CDCA	Tauro-chenodeoxycholic acid

A. E. DeBarber
School of Medicine, Oregon Health and Science University, Portland, OR, USA
e-mail: debarber@ohsu.edu

M. H. Gelb (✉) · Z. Zhou
Department of Chemistry, University of Washington, Seattle, WA, USA
e-mail: gelb@uw.edu

M. Martin · H. McNeight · J. Orsini
Wadsworth Center, New York State Department of Health, Newborn Screening Program, David Axelrod Institute, Albany, NY, USA
e-mail: monica.martin@health.ny.gov; hannah.mcneight@health.ny.gov; joseph.orsini@health.ny.gov

N. Szabo-Fresnais
Utah Department of Health and Human Services, Salt Lake City, UT, USA
e-mail: nszabo@utah.gov

F. M. Vaz
Department of Laboratory Medicine and Pediatrics, Laboratory Genetic Metabolic Diseases, Emma Children's Hospital, Amsterdam UMC, Amsterdam, The Netherlands
e-mail: f.m.vaz@amsterdamumc.nl

M. Wasserstein
Department of Pediatrics, Albert Einstein College of Medicine and Children's Hospital at Montefiore, Bronx, NY, USA
e-mail: mwassers@montefiore.org

A. Federico et al. (eds.), *Cerebrotendinous Xanthomatosis*,
https://doi.org/10.1007/978-3-031-92526-9_25

t-THCA	Tauro-trihydroxycholestanoic acid
(7α12αC4)	7α,12α-dihydroxy-4-cholesten-3-one
(LC-MS/MS)	Liquid chromatography-tandem mass spectrometry

Introduction

Cerebrotendinous xanthomatosis (CTX; OMIM #213700) is a rare autosomal recessive disorder associated with the deficiency of sterol 27-hydroxylase, encoded by the *CYP27A1* gene, which is involved in the biosynthesis of the primary bile acids, cholic acid, and chenodeoxycholic acid, from cholesterol [1]. Replenishment of chenodeoxycholic acid in CTX downregulates bile acid synthesis through a negative feedback mechanism, thereby preventing the accumulation of cholestanol and bile alcohols [1]. The prognosis of CTX is good when treatment is started early, but is less favorable when initiated at a later age [2]. Thus, CTX has become of recent interest for newborn screening (NBS) [3].

The top performing biomarker for NBS of CTX is the bile alcohol 5β-cholestane-3α,7α,12α,25-tetrol glucuronide (GlcA-tetrol) [3, 4]. The rationale for the use of this marker in the context of the bile acid biosynthetic pathway and CYP27A1 deficiency has been presented previously [3]. It is also necessary to monitor the additional biomarkers tauro-chenodeoxycholic acid (t-CDCA) and tauro-trihydroxycholestanoic acid (t-THCA) to distinguish CTX patients from those who present with neonatal cholestasis or Zellweger syndrome [3]. These three biomarkers can be measured in dried blood spots (DBS) using either flow-injection-tandem mass spectrometry [5] or liquid chromatography-tandem mass spectrometry (LC-MS/MS) [4, 5].

A population-size pilot NBS study for CTX on ~30,000 newborns made use of LC-MS/MS to quantify GlcA-tetrol in the presence of a deuterated, chemically identical internal standard [4]. Measurement of the auxiliary biomarkers t-CDCA and t-THCA can be done in the same LC-MS/MS run that requires ~2 min per newborn [4] or run as a second-tier test when GlcA-tetrol is elevated in the first-tier analysis. In this pilot study, a single newborn with GlcA-tetrol elevated above the cutoff and with auxiliary markers t-CDCA and t-THCA all suggestive of CTX was found. Genotyping from the same DBS confirmed a biochemical diagnosis of CTX [4]. This provides an initial estimate of the false positive rate of 0 per 30,000 showing that this NBS method works exceptionally well. The false negative rate is suggested to be zero by setting the GlcA-tetrol cutoff low enough such that several DBS from patients with CTX were detected by this LC-MS/MS method [4].

A second pilot study on ~20,000 newborn DBS was carried out with both flow-injection-MS/MS and LC-MS/MS done in parallel for comparison [5]. In this study, no CTX-affected newborns were identified, but the false positive rate was also likely to be zero using both the flow-injection and LC-MS/MS options. Considering the low incidence of CTX and the excellent test performance, it's likely that no CTX cases were missed, but more likely that no newborns with CTX were included in the modest sized study. Using flow injection-MS/MS, complete separation of the CTX group from the random newborn DBS (reference range) was achieved by measuring the auxiliary bile metabolites along with tetrol in every run so that the ratio of metabolites could be used. The same was true for the LC-MS/MS version. With LC-MS/MS only, measurement of GlcA-tetrol alone led to a large separation of CTX patients from the reference range. It's recommended that for LC-MS/MS, any newborn displaying elevated GlcA-tetrol when measured alone should still be submitted to second-tier LC-MS/MS quantification of t-CDCA and t-THCA to rule out cholestasis and Zellwegger syndrome. Alternatively, all three bile metabolite biomarkers can be measured in the same first-tier LC-MS/MS run. In summary, two different MS/MS assay variations can be used for extremely high precision NBS for CTX. DeBarber and colleagues have discovered that the bile acid pathway metabolite 7α,12α-dihydroxy-4-cholesten-3-one (7α12αC4) is an additional powerful biomarker of CTX detectable in CTX newborn DBS [6]. For practical reasons as discussed previously, this biomarker is most suitable for additional second-tier analysis [4].

Assay Improvement by Additional Multiplexing

The above pilot studies were carried out with de-identified DBS. More recently, the ScreenPlus prospective pilot program was initiated that uses LC-MS/MS to screen for 14 treatable diseases including CTX [7]. In this program, two parallel LC-MS/MS assays are currently run per newborn using two separate 3 mm punches per DBS. The first LC-MS/MS requires about 2 min per newborn and measures newborn screening analytes for 11 disorders (mucopolysaccharidosis types II, IIIB, IVA, VI, and VII, GM1-gangliosidosis, ceroid lipofuscinosis type 2, lysosomal acid lipase deficiency, Fabry disease, Gaucher disease, and Niemann-Pick-A/B disease). Positive-mode electrospray ionization is used for this analysis. A second LC-MS/MS run, also about 2 min per newborn, is used to detect biomarkers for NBS of CTX, Niemann-Pick-C, and metachromatic leukodystrophy where detection is by electrospray ionization in negative mode. More recently, we have updated this platform to reduce the method to a single LC-MS/MS run with ionization mode switching, and in this report, we show how the biomarkers for NBS of CTX can easily be incorporated into the first LC-MS/MS run (11-plex). We are also able to add the biomarkers for Niemann-Pick-C and metachromatic leukodystrophy to this single LC-MS/MS (not shown here). In the near future, we plan to modify the ScreenPlus pilot method by screening for all 14 disorders with a single LC-MS/MS run per newborn.

Focusing on CTX, the only requirement for adding the biomarkers to the ScreenPlus 11-plex is that the CTX analytes elute from the LC column in a time window where analytes for the other 11 disorders do not elute. This enables polarity switching whereby the mass spectrometer starts out in positive mode, then is switched into negative ionization mode during the time period in which the CTX analytes elute, and then the machine is switched back to positive mode for detection of the remaining analytes. As shown in Fig. 25.1, this is easily feasible for the CTX analytes. The CTX biomarker GlcA-tetrol elutes at 1.29 min. In the ScreenPlus multiplex, the closest analyte that elutes earlier than GlcA-tetrol is the product for Pompe disease at 1.13 min. The closest peak to GlcA-tetrol that elutes after is the product for Gaucher disease at 1.73 min. The secondary biomarkers for CTX, t-CDCA, and t-THDA are not shown in Fig. 25.1, but they elute within a few seconds of GlcA-tetrol [4]. These results show that CTX can be included in the ScreenPlus multiplex simply by automated switching the electrospray source polarity to negative mode during the time window in which GlcA-tetrol elutes, while using positive mode for all other times regions.

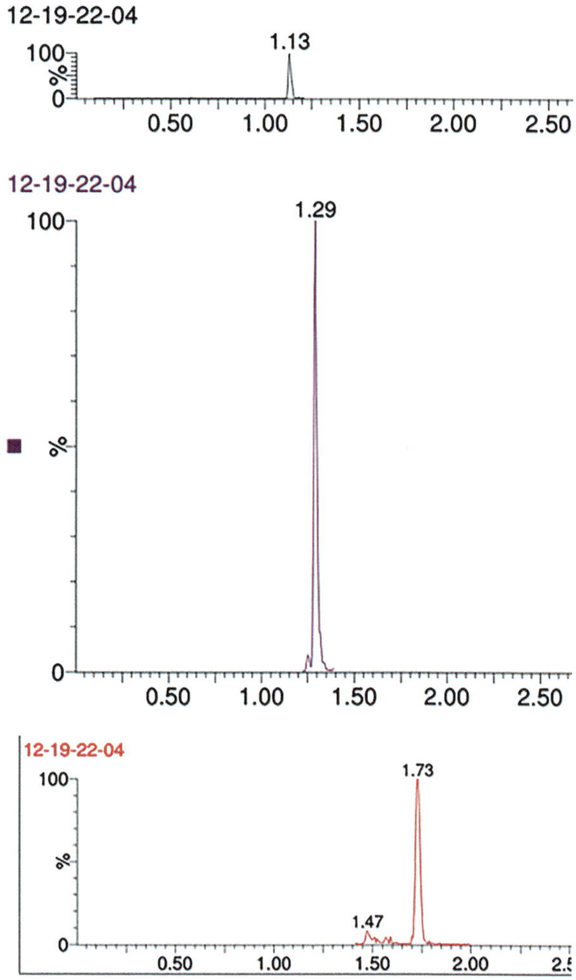

Fig. 25.1 UPLC-MS/MS chromatograms for specific analytes in the ScreenPlus pilot program. The *Y*-axes show the multiple reaction monitoring ion intensity (as a percentage of the maximum signal in the chromatogram) for Pompe disease enzymatic product (top panel, 1.13 min), GlcA-tetrol CTX biomarker (middle panel, 1.29 min), and Gaucher disease enzymatic product (bottom panel, 1.73 min). The UPLC solvent program is as published [4]

Assay Improvement by Reducing the Number of DBS Punches Required

As noted above, our ongoing ScreenPlus pilot program makes use of two 3 mm punches per newborn from the same DBS. Since DBS punches are limited, it is always advantageous to reduce the number of required punches. This also reduces the number of pre-LC-MS/MS liquid transfers. This is easily accomplished for the CTX biomarkers by first incubating the DBS punch with aqueous buffer and enzyme substrates for 11 disorders (see above) overnight to allow for enzymatic conversion of substrates to products and then to quench the reaction mixture with methanol containing internal standard (deuterated GlcA-tetrol). Extraction of a DBS punch with methanol is the method previously used for capture of the biomarkers for CTX, Niemann-Pick-C, and metachromatic leukodystropy [8]. Therefore, the update is simply to do the methanol extraction after the enzymatic assay incubation leading to recovery of the CTX biomarkers and quenching of the enzymatic reactions. After methanol quenching, the 96-well sample plate is centrifuged for a few minutes to pellet insoluble material. A portion of the supernatant is transferred to the autosampler plate, and 10 uL is injected for LC-MS/MS analysis. Studies with DBS extract and spiking with authentic biomarkers (GlcA-tetrol and t-CDCA) show no difference in MS/MS signal compared to using the original processing method for CTX with a separate punch (data not shown). Spiking with t-THCA is not possible because the biomarker is not available in pure form, but we already determined that this auxiliary marker is extracted out of DBS with methanol [4, 5]. In this variation of the workflow, the original liquid-liquid extraction of the 11-plex with ethyl acetate is replaced by quenching with methanol. Insoluble material in the methanol quench is removed by centrifugation. Salts and other highly polar components of the mixture are normally not carried into the ethyl acetate layer, and rather some of them remain dissolved in methanol. However, these elute in the void volume of the LC-MS/MS run and are shunted away from the mass spectrometer by a diversion value that sends the early eluting material to waste. Detergent present in the 11-plex buffer remains soluble in methanol, but it elutes as a well-defined peak in the LC-MS/MS and does not cause interference. In the original 11-plex method with ethyl acetate liquid-liquid extraction, some of the detergent partitions into the ethyl acetate layer and is also injected onto the LC column [8]. It may also be noted that the Illinois NBS laboratory originally carried out a 6-plex LC-MS/MS assay for six lysosomal storage diseases by skipping the liquid-liquid extraction with ethyl acetate and replacing it with an organic solvent quench step followed by centrifugation. Again, detergent was found to elute as a sharp peak in the LC-MS/MS run and does not cause interference. This method was run on several hundred thousand samples and was found to be robust (UPLC column replacement every 10,000–20,000 runs and routine MS/MS source cleaning every 1–2 weeks [9]).

Identification of the First CTX Patient in a Prospective Pilot Study

The ScreenPlus program has adopted a cutoff for the primary CTX screening biomarker GlcA-tetrol of ≥100 nM in dried blood spots, which is based on the value of 100 nM determined for the lowest concentration CTX newborn dried blood spot identified to date (stored by California Newborn Screening laboratory for >two decades, provided by A. DeBarber, Oregon Health and Science University). The program now uses a second biomarker t-CDCA and reports out newborns who display GlcA-tetrol ≥100 nM and a multiple-of-the-daily-median (MoDM) t-CDCA of <0.3. t-CDCA is measured in the same LC-MS/MS run as GlcA-tetrol. The median value of GlcA-tetrol across ~30,000 newborn DBS was 67 nM [4].

Using GlcA-tetrol concentration as an initial screen has resulted in 85 positives out of 27,391 samples screened for the ScreenPlus study. Thus far, of the samples with GlcA-tetrol ≥100 nM identified, only five samples had a t-CDCA MoDM of <0.3, one of which was a confirmed positive CTX newborn sample (with GlcA-tetrol of 237 nM and t-CDCA MoDM of 0.1081). The newborn CTX patient identified in the ScreenPlus study went on to receive a clinical and genetic diagnosis of CTX and CDCA treatment was initiated. The false positive rate for the ScreenPlus study is 5 in 27,391 (0.018%). This is certainly an acceptably low false positive rate for newborn screening. Newborns that test positive with this two part screening algorithm would receive genotype analysis of *CYP27A1* and testing for other blood biomarkers of CTX (e.g., 7α12αC4) either as part of newborn screening or during post-newborn screening follow-up.

Conclusions and Future Prospects

NBS laboratories screening for lysosomal storage diseases (MPS-I, Pompe, and others) typically use flow injection-MS/MS to analyze for enzymatic products. A subset of these laboratories use LC-MS/MS, and extensive studies show that both MS/MS methods are sufficiently rapid and robust for high-throughput NBS [9]. MPS-II has recently been added to the Recommended Uniform Screening Panel by the Secretary's Advisory Committee on Heritable Disorders in Newborns and Children, and addition of this disorder requires upgrading the flow injection-MS/MS assay to the LC-MS/MS platform. With LC-MS/MS in place for widespread NBS for lysosomal storage diseases (and other diseases), it would be a simple matter to add the biomarkers for NBS of CTX as shown in this chapter.

Addition of a condition to the Recommended Uniform Screening Panel requires a prospective pilot study with the identification of at least one newborn confirmed to have the condition. This has now been accomplished for CTX as part of the ScreenPlus prospective pilot program. Efforts are underway to generate quality-control DBS material and commercially available CTX NBS assay reagents (mainly deuterium-labeled GlcA-tetrol internal standard) to help support implementation of NBS for CTX should this condition be added to NBS panels.

References

1. DeBarber AE, Duell PB. Update on cerebrotendinous xanthomatosis. Curr Opin Lipidol. 2021;32:123–31. https://doi.org/10.1097/MOL.0000000000000740.
2. Stelten BML, Huidekoper HH, van de Warrenburg BPC, Brilstra EH, Hollak CEM, Haak HR, Kluijtmans LAJ, Wevers RA, Verrips A. Long-term treatment effect in cerebrotendinous xanthomatosis depends on age at treatment start. Neurology. 2019;92:e83–95. https://doi.org/10.1212/WNL.0000000000006731.
3. Vaz FM, Bootsma AH, Kulik W, Verrips A, Wevers RA, Schielen PC, DeBarber AE, Huidekoper HH. A newborn screening method for cerebrotendinous xanthomatosis using bile alcohol glucuronides and metabolite ratios. J Lipid Res. 2017;58:1002–7.
4. Hong X, Daiker J, Sadilek M, DeBarber AE, Chiang J, Duan J, Bootsma AH, Huidekoper HH, Vaz FM, Gelb MH. Toward newborn screening of cerebrotendinous xanthomatosis: results of a biomarker research study using 32,000 newborn dried blood spots. Genet Med. 2020;22:1606–12.
5. Vaz FM, Jamal Y, Barto R, Gelb MH, DeBarber AE, Wevers RA, Nelen MR, Verrips A, Bootsma AH, Bouva MJ, Kleise N, van der Zee W, He T, Salomons GS, Huidekoper HH. Newborn screening for cerebrotendinous xanthomatosis: a retrospective biomarker study using both flow-injection and UPLC-MS/MS analysis in 20,000 newborns. Clin Chim Acta Int J Clin Chem. 2023;539:170–4. https://doi.org/10.1016/j.cca.2022.12.011.
6. DeBarber AE, Kalfon L, Fedida A, Fleisher Sheffer V, Ben Haroush S, Chasnyk N, Shuster Biton E, Mandel H, Jeffries K, Shinwell ES, Falik-Zaccai TC. Newborn screening for cerebrotendinous xanthomatosis is the solution for early identification and treatment. J Lipid Res. 2018;59:2214–22. https://doi.org/10.1194/jlr.M087999.
7. Kelly NR, Orsini JJ, Goldenberg AJ, Mulrooney NS, Boychuk NA, Clarke MJ, Paleologos K, Martin MM, McNeight H, Caggana M, Bailey SM, Eiland LR, Ganesh J, Kupchik G, Lumba R, Nafday S, Stroustrup A, Gelb MH, Wasserstein MP. ScreenPlus: a comprehensive, multi-disorder newborn screening program. Mol Genet Metab Rep. 2024;38:101037. https://doi.org/10.1016/j.ymgmr.2023.101037.
8. Hong X, Sadilek M, Gelb MH. A highly multiplexable biochemical assay for analytes in dried blood spots: application to newborn screening and diagnosis of lysosomal storage disorders and other inborn errors of metabolism. Genet Med. 2020;22(7):1262–8.
9. Gelb MH, Basheeruddin K, Burlina A, Chen H-J, Chien Y-H, Dizikes G, Dorley C, Giugliani R, Hietala A, Hong X, Kao S-M, Khaledi H, Klug T, Kubaski F, Liao H-C, Martin M, Manning A, Orsini J, Peng Y, Ranieri E, Rohrwasser A, Szabo-Fresnais N, Turgeon CT, Vaz FM, Wang L-Y, Matern D. Liquid chromatography-tandem mass spectrometry in newborn screening laboratories. Int J Neonatal Screen. 2022;8:62. https://doi.org/10.3390/ijns8040062.

Early Treatment Improves Outcomes for Patients with Cerebrotendinous Xanthomatosis (CTX)

26

Aviv Mesika, Andrea E. DeBarber, and Tzipora C. Falik-Zaccai

Introduction

Cerebrotendinous xanthomatosis (CTX) is a rare and severe genetic disorder characterized by a spectrum of debilitating signs and symptoms that can manifest beginning early in life [1–6]. Often overlooked, CTX can lead to severe complications, including liver disease, juvenile cataracts, tendon xanthomas, developmental delays, intellectual disabilities, and neurological impairments if left untreated [5–8]. The complexity of its clinical presentation frequently results in diagnostic delays [5], sometimes extending beyond two decades. Recent studies reveal a significant underdiagnosis of CTX [9, 10], highlighting the urgent need for increased awareness among healthcare providers and the implementation of effective screening measures. This chapter explores the clinical manifestations of CTX, particularly during infancy and childhood, the critical importance of early diagnosis and intervention, and the promising outcomes associated with timely treatment. By examining the latest research and case studies, we underscore the necessity for universal newborn screening to ensure that affected infants receive the care they need to improve their long-term health outcomes and quality of life.

A. Mesika · T. C. Falik-Zaccai (✉)
Azrieli Faculty of Medicine, Bar Ilan University, Safed, Israel

A. E. DeBarber
School of Medicine, Oregon Health and Science University, Portland, OR, USA

A. Federico et al. (eds.), *Cerebrotendinous Xanthomatosis*,
https://doi.org/10.1007/978-3-031-92526-9_26

Delay in Diagnosis

A recent study by Pramparo et al. [10] estimated the prevalence of CTX to range from 1 in 44,000 to 1 in 3,400,000 across different global populations, based on allele frequencies derived from large genomic databases. However, the actual number of diagnosed cases is significantly lower than these prevalence predictions, suggesting that CTX is most likely underdiagnosed [9, 10]. The rarity of the condition, along with its diverse clinical presentations, complicates the diagnostic process, often resulting in delayed diagnosis in adulthood, despite symptom onset during childhood [5]. Data from larger patient cohorts worldwide suggest that the typical age of diagnosis in CTX is between 25 and 41 years old [5, 6, 11–15]. Patients who are diagnosed with CTX frequently remain undiagnosed for 16–20 years after onset of initial symptoms [11–15]. Additionally, misdiagnosis is common due to the overlap of CTX symptoms with more prevalent conditions [5].

To address these challenges, increasing awareness among healthcare providers, improving access to sensitive genetic and biochemical tests, and implementing newborn screening programs are essential. For instance, to increase awareness among healthcare providers and assist in earlier diagnosis, Mignarri et al. [5] developed a clinical suspicion index that serves as a straightforward and cost-effective tool to decrease diagnostic delay. This index allows earlier diagnosis and treatment of CTX, ideally before significant neurological impairment occurs. It identifies early systemic signs such as juvenile bilateral cataracts, chronic diarrhea, and neonatal cholestatic jaundice as strong indicators in younger age CTX patients, alongside neurological symptoms like intellectual disabilities, psychiatric issues, ataxia, spastic paraparesis, and dentate nucleus abnormalities on MRI at later ages. Tendon xanthomas and having an affected sibling are also considered very strong indicators. The findings revealed that the average age at diagnosis improved from 35.5 ± 11.8 years to 10.6 ± 9.8 years with the use of this clinical diagnostic tool ($p < 0.01$). Nevertheless, further research is needed to enhance diagnostic methods and facilitate earlier detection and treatment of CTX, which would lead to better treatment outcomes and management of the disease [16, 17], improving patients' quality of life and preventing reduced life expectancy.

Early Treatment

Timely diagnosis and initiation of oral primary bile acid treatment are essential for improving long-term outcomes and preventing serious neurological decline in patients with CTX. Considering the increasing evidence supporting the efficacy of treatment with chenodeoxycholic acid (CDCA), therapeutic intervention in patients is typically initiated with CDCA. Standard treatment for adult patients with CTX is CDCA at a dosage of 750 mg per day, usually divided into three, for adults [18, 19]. Bile acid therapy inhibits abnormal bile acid synthesis, lowers cholestanol and bile alcohol levels, and helps stabilize or improve clinical symptoms while preventing disease progression [18]. A recent multicenter study suggested that cholic acid (CA) may be a suitable alternative therapy for adults with CTX [20], especially in patients with side effects and hepatotoxicity related to CDCA. CA is also an alternative therapy for neonates with CTX and has been shown to been effective in the treatment of other genetic defects in bile acid synthesis [21]. Our experience has been that CA is a safe and effective option for treating CTX patients especially at a younger age and when they suffer side effects of CDCA or hepatotoxicity. The bile acid dosage for infants and children is calculated according to their weight with an average of 10–15 mg per kg body weight per day (mg/kg/day) divided into three [22]. However, infants may rarely experience hepatotoxicity at 15 mg/kg/day CDCA [23], which can be managed by reducing the dosage to 5–10 mg/kg/day.

A recent observational study in a large cohort of older patients by Yahalom et al. [16] revealed that Israeli patients who commenced CDCA treatment after the age of 25 had poorer ambulation and cognitive outcomes. The study involved 18 patients (10 men) from 11 families, with 16 included in the analysis due to treatment adherence issues. The mean age at the last evaluation was 35.0 years (range 16–45 years). All patients began treatment at an average age of 22.6 years. Those starting after 25 years experienced significantly worse ambulation ($P = 0.004$) and cognitive impairment ($P = 0.047$). Five patients starting treatment later continued to deteriorate despite CDCA. The study concluded that early initiation of CDCA is critical in preventing neurological damage in CTX patients, as established and advanced pathology limits the effectiveness of treatment [16].

Another retrospective larger cohort study in older patients by Stelten et al. [17] reported for 56 Dutch patients with CTX (age 6 months–31.5 years) that those diagnosed and treated before age 24 had significantly better outcomes. In the subset of patients with good treatment adherence ($n = 43$), neurologic symptoms were not present in all patients diagnosed and treated early, with no new symptoms developing during follow-up. Conversely, 61% of patients diagnosed and treated after age 24 showed worsening neurological symptoms, particularly treatment-resistant parkinsonism. This further emphasizes the importance of early treatment in preventing neurological symptoms in CTX [17].

There is no data available from a larger patient cohort study assessing the effect of early treatment in infants or young children with CTX. The earliest signs of CTX can include chronic diarrhea from birth onward, intellectual disability in childhood, juvenile bilateral cataracts, and hepatic jaundice/cholestasis in the neonatal period that can resolve or can progress to severe liver disease, which may necessitate a liver transplant or that can be fatal [24–27]. In one study CTX was determined to be the cause of severe cholestasis in eight infants, of which five died from, or were transplanted for, liver failure (only one patient was treated with CDCA and for only 1 month prior to death) [27].

A number of case reports describing treatment in infants and children with CTX indicate that long-term bile acid treatment is safe and can prevent symptom development in CTX.

Berginer et al. [28] presented a family where two young sisters began CDCA treatment in childhood (one was treated from age 2 and the other from age 7) prior to clinical signs/symptoms of CTX, while their two older uncles, who had already developed CTX manifestations in their teenage years, served as a control group. During 14 years of treatment, cholestanol levels normalized and remained normal in all four patients (<6 microg/mL), with the sisters remaining asymptomatic on 750 mg of CDCA daily, while only moderate symptom improvement occurred in their uncles who started treatment at age 16 years and 27 years at the daily dose of 750–1000 mg CDCA, but with partial compliance. Both uncles presented with developmental delay, cataracts, xanthomas, and intellectual disability. This underscores the benefit of early CDCA administration in preventing the CTX phenotype [28].

Degrassi et al. [29] reported long-term treatment of an infant diagnosed with CTX presenting with neonatal cholestasis that resolved after treatment with 10–15 mg/kg/day of CDCA therapy, beginning at 7 months of age and remained under follow-up for 13 years, with no additional early signs of CTX observed and no neurological impairment.

Lipinski et al. [30] reported on two infant CTX patients; one presented with cholestatic jaundice at 10 weeks of age and developed end-stage liver disease, necessitating a liver transplant at 8 months old. However, the patient passed away 3 years post-transplant. The second patient, a sibling, also presented with cholestatic jaundice from birth and treatment with CDCA (5 mg/kg/day) was initiated at 4 months of age, following diagnosis. A 1 year follow-up was normal.

Alsaleem et al. [31] reported on three infants diagnosed with CTX presenting with diarrhea that were treated with 250 mg/day of CDCA therapy (plus sodium bicarbonate); patients were monitored from between 1 and 8.5 years of treatment, diarrhea resolved in two cases after treatment, no additional early signs of CTX were observed and no neurological impairment.

Huidekoper et al. [23] reported on an infant diagnosed with CTX initially treated with 15 mg/kg/day of CDCA therapy. Therapy was discontinued when patient's liver enzyme values increased. Lower dose of 5 mg/kg/day was sufficient to maintain metabolic control of serum cholestanol. Patient was monitored for 3 years, no additional early signs of CTX were observed and no neurological impairment.

CA is a less hepatotoxic alternative for treatment of CTX in infancy. Pierre et al. [25] reported on CA treatment at 15 mg/kg/day in two infant siblings affected with CTX. One patient had low average development and one had delayed verbal skills but normal brain MRI after 7 years of follow-up.

Despite the evidence supporting the benefit of early bile acid treatment in CTX, outside of case reports, no comprehensive larger patient cohort studies have specifically evaluated the health outcomes of CDCA or CA treatment initiated in infancy for CTX patients. However, a recent study by Kalfon, Falik-Zaccai et al. (unpublished data) has begun to fill in this gap. Their study assessed health outcomes for eight affected newborns with biallelic pathogenic variants in the *CYP27A1* gene, all treated with CDCA or CA from infancy (0–6 months).

Kalfon, Falik-Zaccai et al. found that administering CDCA or CA within the first 6 months of life significantly alleviates many CTX symptoms in infants affected with CTX compared to those treated later in childhood or adulthood and enhanced health outcomes (unpublished data).

The researchers stratified 28 patients, 26 of Druze origin and 2 of Moroccan Jewish origin. Each ethnic group represents a homogeneous genetic background, with the results more likely to be a consequence of early treatment with CDCA and less influenced by the clinical and genetic heterogeneity observed in CTX patients, especially those from different genetic backgrounds. The patients were grouped into three cohorts based on the age at which treatment was initiated: [1] infancy (<2 years) [2], childhood and adolescence (2–18 years), and [3] adulthood (>18 years). Of note, in the eight patients included in the infancy group, treatment was initiated before the age of 6 months.

The findings demonstrated that treatment initiation within the first 6 months of life was associated with significantly improved health outcomes, particularly in relation to early clinical manifestations of CTX, including chronic diarrhea juvenile cataracts, cognitive impairment, and intellectual disability. Among patients who commenced treatment before the age of 6 months and were followed for an average duration of 9.8 years (range: 2–17 years), disease progression and early CTX symptom burden (chronic diarrhea juvenile cataracts, cognitive impairment, and intellectual disability) were actually absent, in comparison to those who initiated therapy between 2 and 8 years of age (average follow-up: 10.1 years, range: 2–18 years).

Furthermore, neurobehavioral manifestations—such as attention-deficit/hyperactivity disorder (ADHD), and depression—were not observed in the infancy-treated group; however, one patient had behavioral changes and agitation aggression. The same patient also had seizures pre- and post-treatment, suggesting these symptoms may not have been due to CTX. It is crucial to note that these individuals had not yet reached adulthood at the time of this analysis, precluding definitive conclusions regarding age-related neurological outcomes.

Patients who initiated treatment in childhood (mean age of diagnosis: 8.9 years, range: 2–14 years) also exhibited significant symptomatic improvements relative to those treated in adulthood. Specifically, childhood-treated patients demonstrated amelioration of gait disturbances and intellectual disabilities, as well as a lower prevalence of additional CTX-related symptoms, including cataracts, tendon xanthomas, seizures, and developmental delays. By contrast, patients who commenced treatment in adulthood (mean age of diagnosis: 26.1 years, range: 19–46 years) exhibited a more severe disease trajectory with persistent symptomatology. It is important to emphasize that the pediatric cohort had not yet transitioned into adulthood at the time of this analysis, thereby necessitating extended follow-up to accurately assess the long-term neurological outcomes in this population.

Initiation of treatment before 6 months of age conferred protection against both neurological and non-neurological manifestations of CTX. Moreover, significant and clinically meaningful differences in growth parameters were observed, with substantial improvements in growth trajectories among individuals who received early intervention during infancy. Specifically, patients treated from infancy demonstrated significantly higher height percentiles in childhood compared to those diagnosed and treated during childhood. Additionally, both height and weight percentiles were markedly higher in the infancy-treated cohort relative to individuals diagnosed and treated in adulthood. These findings underscore the profound impact of early therapeutic intervention on overall growth and developmental outcomes in CTX.

The cohort analyzed by Kalfon, Falik-Zaccai et al. comprised 26 patients of Druze ancestry who were homozygous for the c.355del variant in the *CYP27A1* gene [32–34], as well as two patients of Jewish Moroccan descent harboring known pathogenic variants [35]. A potential limitation in assessing the clinical efficacy of CDCA or alternative bile acid therapies in this study is the limited genetic heterogeneity within the cohort. This genetic homogeneity raises the possibility that disease progression, biochemical profiles, and therapeutic responses may differ in patients with other *CYP27A1* genotypes [36, 37]. On the other hand, the genetic homogeneity of our cohort can be considered a strength of the study as it decreases the possibility that results may have been influenced by clinical presentation heterogeneity seen in CTX irrespective of treatment. However, it is important to note that no definitive genotype-phenotype correlation has been established for CTX to date [38–40].

In summary, the data from Kalfon, Falik-Zaccai et al. (unpublished data) demonstrate that initiating treatment during infancy significantly improves health outcomes for CTX patients compared to starting treatment later in childhood or adulthood (unpublished data). While there is concern regarding CDCA-induced hepatotoxicity in infants identified through newborn screening, evidence suggests this risk can be managed by either lowering the CDCA dose or by switching the patient to CA [41]. Close monitoring of liver enzymes, as well as the effectiveness of CDCA or CA in suppressing abnormal bile acid synthesis and reducing CTX biomarkers should occur regularly. We recommend monthly testing of transaminases during the initial phase of treatment with CDCA in infants during the first 6–12 months post-treatment initiation (and at least annually thereafter [4]).

Conclusions

The real-world data from Kalfon, Falik-Zaccai et al. indicate that treating CTX with bile acids in the early months of life is safe with careful clinical monitoring and that patients treated early in life experience better health outcomes compared to those treated later in childhood or adulthood. Based on this data, as well as a review of the latest literature, and in accordance with CTX expert consensus guidelines [4] that recommend to initiate treatment from birth onward to prevent the accumulation of harmful metabolic intermediates, we advise initiating treatment within the first few months of life for patients identified in infancy identified through family history, genetic testing, or newborn screening for CTX.

Multiple reports support that early identification and treatment are crucial to optimizing outcomes for patients with CTX, ideally treatment beginning in infancy. More efficient identification of CTX in the newborn period can best be achieved through pre- or post-natal genetic screening programs, such as we have deployed in a high-risk population in Northern Israel [34], or through universal newborn screening for CTX. Newborn screening for CTX has not yet been implemented, although highly effective tandem mass spectrometry methods with a zero false-positive rate

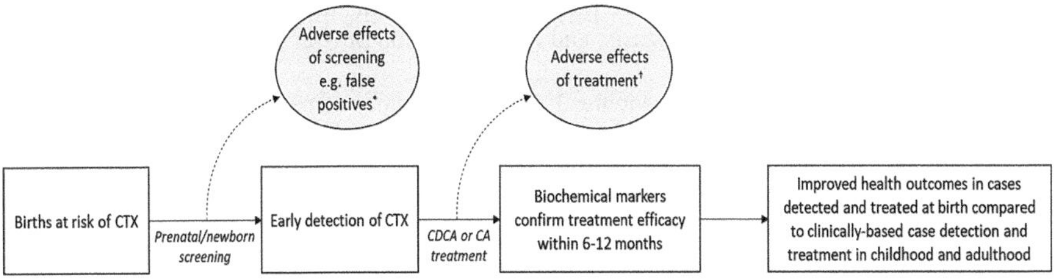

Fig. 26.1 Potential benefits/harms of identification of CTX through prenatal/newborn screening and early treatment. CA cholic acid, CDCA chenodeoxycholic acid, CTX cerebrotendinous xanthomatosis. *Zero false-positive rate for MS/MS newborn screening methods. †2 of 8 patients of Kalfon, Falik-Zaccai et al.'s study had CDCA-induced hepatotoxicity that improved with CA treatment

are available for screening newborn dried blood spots for CTX [42–45]. Identification of CTX through newborn screening will greatly benefit CTX-affected individuals and their families, allowing early access to treatment and providing better health outcomes for CTX patients (see Fig. 26.1). The potential harms of identification of CTX through newborn screening and early treatment include screening harms, for example false-positive results, which will be minimal as published screening methods have a zero false-positive rate [42–45]. The potential harms of early treatment (hepatotoxicity from CDCA therapy) can be managed safely with careful clinical monitoring as we have described in this chapter.

We believe that the evidence compiled here will enhance the timing of optimal treatment for this condition, particularly for affected infants who may be identified in the future. Furthermore, the implementation of universal newborn screening for CTX will be critical to facilitate early identification and intervention during infancy, leading to improved health outcomes for affected patients and a reduction in the morbidity and mortality associated with the untreated progression of this serious disease.

References

1. DeBarber AE, Duell PB. Update on cerebrotendinous xanthomatosis. Curr Opin Lipidol. 2021;32(2):123–31.
2. Salen G, Steiner RD. Epidemiology, diagnosis, and treatment of cerebrotendinous xanthomatosis (CTX). J Inherit Metab Dis. 2017;40(6):771–81.
3. Federico A, Gallus GN. Cerebrotendinous xanthomatosis. GeneReviews®. Seattle: University of Washington, Seattle; 2022.
4. Stelten BML, Dotti MT, Verrips A, et al. Expert opinion on diagnosing, treating and managing patients with cerebrotendinous xanthomatosis (CTX): a modified Delphi study. Orphanet J Rare Dis. 2021;16(1):353.
5. Mignarri A, Gallus GN, Dotti MT, Federico A. A suspicion index for early diagnosis and treatment of cerebrotendinous xanthomatosis. J Inherit Metab Dis. 2014;37(3):421–9.
6. Duell PB, Salen G, Eichler FS, et al. Diagnosis, treatment, and clinical outcomes in 43 cases with cerebrotendinous xanthomatosis. J Clin Lipidol. 2018;12(5):1169–78.

7. Pietrobattista A, Spada M, Candusso M, et al. Liver transplantation in an infant with cerebrotendinous xanthomatosis, cholestasis, and rapid evolution of liver failure. Pediatr Transplant. 2022;26(6):e14318.
8. Wong JC, Walsh K, Hayden D, Eichler FS. Natural history of neurological abnormalities in cerebrotendinous xanthomatosis. J Inherit Metab Dis. 2018;41(4):647–56.
9. Appadurai V, DeBarber A, Chiang PW, et al. Apparent underdiagnosis of cerebrotendinous xanthomatosis revealed by analysis of ~60,000 human exomes. Mol Genet Metab. 2015;116(4):298–304.
10. Pramparo T, Steiner RD, Rodems S, Jenkinson C. Allelic prevalence and geographic distribution of cerebrotendinous xanthomatosis. Orphanet J Rare Dis. 2023;18(1):13.
11. Zubarioglu, et al. Clinical, biochemical, and molecular insights into cerebrotendinous xanthomatosis: a nationwide study of 100 Turkish individuals. Mol Genet Metab. 2024;142(2):108493.
12. Verrips A, Hoefsloot LH, Steenbergen GC, et al. Clinical and molecular genetic characteristics of patients with cerebrotendinous xanthomatosis. Brain. 2000;123(pt 5):908–19.
13. Pilo-de-la-Fuente B, Jimenez-Escrig A, Lorenzo JR, Pardo J, Arias M, Ares-Luque A, Duarte J, Muñiz-Pérez S, Sobrido MJ. Cerebrotendinous xanthomatosis in Spain: clinical, prognostic, and genetic survey. Eur J Neurol. 2011;18(10):1203–11.
14. Fussiger H, Lima PLGSB, Souza PVS, Freua F, Husny ASE, Leão EKEA, Braga-Neto P, Kok F, Lynch DS, Saute JAM, Nóbrega PR. Clinicogenetic characterization of cerebrotendinous xanthomatosis in Brazil. Clin Genet. 2024;106(6):721–32.
15. Sekijima Y, Koyama S, Yoshinaga T, Koinuma M, Inaba Y. Nationwide survey on cerebrotendinous xanthomatosis in Japan. J Hum Genet. 2018;63(3):271–80.
16. Yahalom G, Tsabari R, Molshatzki N, Ephraty L, Cohen H, Hassin-Baer S. Neurological outcome in cerebrotendinous xanthomatosis treated with chenodeoxycholic acid: early versus late diagnosis. Clin Neuropharmacol. 2013;36(3):78–83.
17. Stelten BML, Huidekoper HH, van de Warrenburg BPC, et al. Long-term treatment effect in cerebrotendinous xanthomatosis depends on age at treatment start. Neurology. 2019;92(2):e83–95.
18. Berginer VM, Salen G, Shefer S. Long-term treatment of cerebrotendinous xanthomatosis with chenodeoxycholic acid. N Engl J Med. 1984;311(26):1649–52.
19. Verrips A, Dotti MT, Mignarri A, Stelten BML, Verma S, Federico A. The safety and effectiveness of chenodeoxycholic acid treatment in patients with cerebrotendinous xanthomatosis: two retrospective cohort studies. Neurol Sci. 2020;41(4):943–9.
20. Mandia D, Chaussenot A, Besson G, Lamari F, Castelnovo G, Curot J, Duval F, Giral P, Lecerf JM, Roland D, Pierdet H, Douillard C, Nadjar Y. Cholic acid as a treatment for cerebrotendinous xanthomatosis in adults. J Neurol. 2019;266(8):2043–50.
21. Setchell KD, Heubi JE. Defects in bile acid biosynthesis-diagnosis and treatment. J Pediatr Gastroenterol Nutr. 2006;43(Suppl 1):S17–22.
22. Van Heijst AF, Verrips A, Wevers RA, Cruysberg JR, Renier WO, Tolboom JJ. Treatment and follow-up of children with cerebrotendinous xanthomatosis. Eur J Pediatr. 1998;157(4):313–6.
23. Huidekoper HH, Vaz FM, Verrips A, Bosch AM. Hepatotoxicity due to chenodeoxycholic acid supplementation in an infant with cerebrotendinous xanthomatosis: implications for treatment. Eur J Pediatr. 2016;175(1):143–6.
24. Von Bahr S, Björkhem I, Van't Hooft F, Alvelius G, Nemeth A, Sjövall J, Fischler B. Mutation in the sterol 27-hydroxylase gene associated with fatal cholestasis in infancy. J Pediatr Gastroenterol Nutr. 2005;40(4):481–6.
25. Pierre G, Setchell K, Blyth J, Preece MA, Chakrapani A, McKiernan P. Prospective treatment of cerebrotendinous xanthomatosis with cholic acid therapy. J Inherit Metab Dis. 2008;31:S241–5.
26. Clayton PT, Verrips A, Sistermans E, Mann A, Mieli-Vergani G, Wevers R. Mutations in the sterol 27-hydroxylase gene (CYP27A) cause hepatitis of infancy as well as cerebrotendinous xanthomatosis. J Inherit Metab Dis. 2002;25(6):501–13.

27. Gong JY, Setchell KDR, Zhao J, Zhang W, Wolfe B, Lu Y, Lackner K, Knisely AS, Wang NL, Hao CZ, Zhang MH, Wang JS. Severe neonatal cholestasis in cerebrotendinous xanthomatosis: genetics, immunostaining, mass spectrometry. J Pediatr Gastroenterol Nutr. 2017;65(5):561–8.
28. Berginer VM, Gross B, Morad K, et al. Chronic diarrhea and juvenile cataracts: think cerebrotendinous xanthomatosis and treat. Pediatrics. 2009;123(1):143–7.
29. Degrassi I, Amoruso C, Giordano G, et al. Case report: early treatment with chenodeoxycholic acid in cerebrotendinous xanthomatosis presenting as neonatal cholestasis. Front Pediatr. 2020;8:382.
30. Lipiński P, Klaudel-Dreszler M, Ciara E, Jurkiewicz D, Płoski R, Cielecka-Kuszyk J, Socha P, Jankowska I. Sterol 27-hydroxylase deficiency as a cause of neonatal cholestasis: report of 2 cases and review of the literature. Front Pediatr. 2021;8:616582.
31. Alsaleem BM, Ahmed AB, Alruwaithi MM, Alamery TY, Alrajhi NN. Early diagnosis and follow-up of cerebrotendinous xanthomatosis in infant siblings presenting with congenital diarrhea: a case study from Saudi Arabia. Mol Genet Metab Rep. 2025;42:101188.
32. Gallus GN, Dotti MT, Federico A. Clinical and molecular diagnosis of cerebrotendinous xanthomatosis with a review of the mutations in the CYP27A1 gene. Neurol Sci. 2006;27(2):143–9.
33. Leitersdorf E, Safadi R, Meiner V, et al. Cerebrotendinous xanthomatosis in the Israeli Druze: molecular genetics and phenotypic characteristics. Am J Hum Genet. 1994;55(5):907–15.
34. Falik-Zaccai TC, Kfir N, Frenkel P, et al. Population screening in a Druze community: the challenge and the reward. Genet Med. 2008;10(12):903–9.
35. Leitersdorf E, Reshef A, Meiner V, et al. Frameshift and splice-junction mutations in the sterol 27-hydroxylase gene cause cerebrotendinous xanthomatosis in Jews of Moroccan origin. J Clin Invest. 1993;91(6):2488–96.
36. Guenzel AJ, DeBarber A, Raymond K, Dhamija R. Familial variability of cerebrotendinous xanthomatosis lacking typical biochemical findings. JIMD Rep. 2021;59(1):3–9.
37. DeBarber AE, Schaefer EJ, Do J, et al. Genetically and clinically confirmed atypical cerebrotendinous xanthomatosis with normal cholestanol and marked elevations of bile acid precursors and bile alcohols. J Clin Lipidol. 2024; [Epub ahead of print];18:e465.
38. Zadori D, Szpisjak L, Madar L, et al. Different phenotypes in identical twins with cerebrotendinous xanthomatosis: case series. Neurol Sci. 2017;38(3):481–3.
39. Taboada M, Martínez D, Pilo B, et al. Querying phenotype-genotype relationships on patient datasets using semantic web technology: the example of cerebrotendinous xanthomatosis. BMC Med Inform Decis Mak. 2012;12:78.
40. Stelten BML, Raal FJ, Marais AD, Riksen NP, Roeters van Lennep JE, Duell PB, van der Graaf M, Kluijtmans LAJ, Wevers RA, Verrips A. Cerebrotendinous xanthomatosis without neurological involvement. J Intern Med. 2021;290(5):1039–47.
41. Heubi JE, Bove KE, Setchell KDR. Oral cholic acid is efficacious and well tolerated in patients with bile acid synthesis and Zellweger spectrum disorders. J Pediatr Gastroenterol Nutr. 2017;65(3):321–6.
42. DeBarber AE, Kalfon L, Fedida A, et al. Newborn screening for cerebrotendinous xanthomatosis is the solution for early identification and treatment. J Lipid Res. 2018;59(11):2214–22.
43. Vaz FM, Bootsma AH, Kulik W, et al. A newborn screening method for cerebrotendinous xanthomatosis using bile alcohol glucuronides and metabolite ratios. J Lipid Res. 2017;58(5):1002–7.
44. Vaz FM, Jamal Y, Barto R, et al. Newborn screening for Cerebrotendinous Xanthomatosis: a retrospective biomarker study using both flow-injection and UPLC-MS/MS analysis in 20,000 newborns. Clin Chim Acta. 2023;539:170–4.
45. Hong X, Daiker J, Sadilek M, et al. Toward newborn screening of cerebrotendinous xanthomatosis: results of a biomarker research study using 32,000 newborn dried blood spots. Genet Med. 2020;22(10):1606–12.

Part IX

Cerebrotendinous Xanthomatosis (CTX): Patient and Family Experiences and Patient Advocacy

Cerebrotendinous Xanthomatosis (CTX) Patient and Family Opinions and International CTX Patient Advocacy

27

Jean R. Pickford, Robert D. Steiner, Shosh Benyaish, Neel Odedara, Rubén Hernández-Alcoceba, and Hanka Dekker

Introduction

Several patient advocacy groups worldwide are dedicated to supporting individuals and families affected by cerebrotendinous xanthomatosis (CTX) within their communities. These groups facilitate education, peer-to-peer connections, patient resources, and advocacy for early detection and screening. Despite CTX's classification as a rare disease, it is likely underdiagnosed. Recent studies using advanced genetic and bioinformatic methods have revealed a higher incidence of CTX in various populations than previously estimated: 1 in 135,000 to 1 in 460,000 for White populations, 1 in 260,000 to 1 in 470,000 for Black populations, and 1 in 64,000 to 1 in 75,000 for Asian populations [1]. More recently, a study using comparable but updated techniques came to similar conclusions [2]. Improved identification of CTX patients is crucial for early treatment, a focal point for most CTX advocacy groups.

J. R. Pickford (✉) · N. Odedara
CTX Alliance, Kulpsville, PA, USA
e-mail: info@ctxalliance.org

R. D. Steiner
Division of Genetics and Metabolism at University of Wisconsin, Madison, WI, USA
e-mail: rsteiner3@wisc.edu

S. Benyaish
CTX Magen, Jerusalem, Israel

R. Hernández-Alcoceba
Gene Therapy Program, University of Navarra, Pamplona, Spain
e-mail: rubenh@unav.es

H. Dekker
VKS, Stofwisselingsziekten, Zwolle Area, The Netherlands
e-mail: h.dekker@stofwisselingsziekten.nl

A. Federico et al. (eds.), *Cerebrotendinous Xanthomatosis*,
https://doi.org/10.1007/978-3-031-92526-9_27

Established CTX patient groups globally welcome individuals seeking support or interested in replicating their programs. Representatives from established patient advocacy groups convened prior to the International CTX Scientific Meeting on August 27, 2023, including the following:

- The CTX Alliance in the United States, established in 2021, is a prominent advocacy group dedicated to improving the lives of CTX patients and their families through education, support, and advocacy efforts. Through programs of patient and caregiver education and advocacy for newborn screening panel inclusion, the CTX Alliance provides comprehensive support and resources for patients and healthcare professionals.
- CTX Magen in Israel focuses on addressing the needs of CTX patients and their families within the Israeli community through advocacy and support initiatives. Operating independently, CTX Magen relies on member contributions to raise awareness and secure medication reimbursement, successfully advocating for CTX treatment with CDCA to be included in medical services.
- VKS in the Netherlands supports patients with metabolic diseases like CTX by providing information, assistance, and collaboration opportunities. Employing a unique approach, the Netherlands fosters collaboration between patient communities and clinical experts to address medication-related challenges. With potential breakthroughs in newborn screening, the Netherlands exemplifies proactive disease management.
- Established in 2012, AEXCT is a support network for individuals and families affected by CTX in Spain. It aims to enhance disease recognition for early diagnosis and address delayed diagnoses leading to advanced symptoms. Despite pharmacologic treatment coverage under the Spanish health system, AEXCT continues efforts to expand its advocacy reach.

Perspectives from Around the World

Patient adherence to treatment presents a significant challenge in CTX treatment, with individuals often initiating but subsequently discontinuing their medication regimen. Mass spectrometry laboratory monitoring in the Netherlands reveals a non-adherence rate of approximately 10%, highlighting the complexity of maintaining treatment adherence, particularly as children transition to independent medical care. Education, particularly targeting teenagers, is essential to address this issue and emphasize the importance of continuous CDCA intake.

Improving patient identification at a younger age and promoting adherence through educational initiatives, including impactful visuals and supportive meetings, can enhance adherence. At the International Meeting, challenges in neuro and cognitive rehabilitation were addressed. It was acknowledged that while these therapies may not cure CTX, they contribute to stabilization. An integrated approach encompassing cognitive, physio, and social therapies is crucial, alongside medication. Comprehensive care also involves raising awareness about potential complications such as xanthomas and cataracts, which may not be immediately linked to CTX and can lead to misdiagnosis. Improved search engine optimization for accurate information retrieval is necessary to aid patient understanding and self-management.

Prior to the International CTX Scientific Meeting in Jerusalem, Israel on August 27, 2023, the CTX Alliance conducted an anonymous online survey among organized CTX patient advocacy groups in Israel, the Netherlands, Spain, and the USA. The survey aimed to gather aggregate data directly from CTX patients and representatives to identify areas for improving patient outcomes. Administered through the CTX Alliance's Google account, the survey was overseen by an Organizing Committee comprising clinicians, scientists, and a patient advocate. Approved by the North Star Review Board, the survey collected data for descriptive statistical analysis and was exempt from a requirement for informed consent. Participants, aged 18 and above with a CTX diagnosis or parents/guardians of patients under 18, were provided with a document explaining the study's purpose and anonymity assurance. Available in English and Hebrew, the survey was disseminated through email communications to reach respective patient communities. Participation was voluntary, with no costs or compensations involved. The survey garnered responses from 54 anonymous participants, revealing a median patient age of 12 years, ranging from infants to 59-year-olds.

Survey section	Key findings
Patient diagnosis	Chronic diarrhea (28%), bilateral cataracts (22%), and neurologic issues (21%) were the most frequently reported first noticeable symptoms of CTX. Tendon xanthomas were reported as a first noticeable symptom in 14% of cases. Autism spectrum disorder, family history, and psychiatric issues were each reported as the first noticeable symptom in 5% of cases.
Time to diagnosis	39% of respondents experienced an interval of 10–29 years from the first symptom to a confirmed CTX diagnosis. 18% each experienced intervals of 6–10 years and less than 1 year. 9% each experienced intervals of 1–2 years, 3–5 years, and 30+ years.
Diagnostic methods	35% of respondents had their CTX diagnosis confirmed through genetic testing for *CYP27A1* pathogenic variants. 23% were diagnosed using increased cholestanol biomarker through biochemical testing. 21% reported being diagnosed through a combination of genetic and biochemical testing. 21% were unsure of the diagnostic method for their CTX.
Medical care and treatment	Neurologists (81%) were the most consulted specialists for CTX symptoms, followed by ophthalmologists (65%). 63% of respondents received assistance from their general practitioner or family medicine doctor. 35% reported visits to both a psychiatrist and an endocrinologist. Physical therapists and cardiologists were consulted by 26% of respondents each. Other specialists mentioned included gastroenterologists, occupational therapists, orthopedics, physiatrists, rehabilitators, sleep specialists, and urologists.

(continued)

Survey section	Key findings
CDCA therapy	96% of respondents were regularly prescribed and consumed CDCA therapy without any reported side effects. Reasons for not being on CDCA therapy included concerns about cost, lack of awareness of CDCA as a treatment option, satisfaction with cholic acid treatment, side effects, and fear.
Cholic acid therapy	Only 7% of respondents received a prescription for cholic acid therapy. Of these patients, 75% expressed satisfaction with its effectiveness. Among those who hadn't been prescribed cholic acid therapy, reasons included considering it unnecessary, lack of awareness of cholic acid as a treatment option, satisfaction with CDCA therapy, side effects, access issues, and high cost.
Most challenging symptoms	Neurologic issues (40%) were the most challenging symptoms reported, followed by psychiatric issues (18%) and tendon xanthomas (14%). Other reported challenging symptoms included bilateral cataracts (11%) and chronic diarrhea (7%).
Family symptoms	Among respondents, 42% indicated that neither a parent nor a sibling exhibited any of the mentioned symptoms. Psychiatric issues (31%), early cataracts (28%), and mental decline (25%) were the most commonly reported symptoms among family members. Peripheral neuropathy, gallstones, osteoporosis, xanthomas/lipomas, atherosclerosis, heart disorders, nephrolithiasis, and Parkinson's disease were also reported to varying extents.

This encouraging participation of responders (54) led the group to consider that a future survey might yield greater success with the input of all patient advocacy group leaders, contributing to the design, clarity, and content of questions tailored to their respective communities. Moreover, there was a recommendation to have more targeted questions that can delve deeper into the neurology section, addressing more detailed and specific aspects.

In addition to the statistical data collected from the 2023 survey, the insights shared in the 2021 Voice of the Patient Report further highlight the urgent need for international collaborative patient advocacy efforts (https://ctxalliance.org/wp-content/uploads/2022/04/Unlock-CTX-meeting-report-FINAL-digital-file.pdf).

On September 14, 2021, members of the global cerebrotendinous xanthomatosis (CTX) community convened for a meeting with the US Food and Drug Administration as part of their Patient-Focused Drug Development program. Seventeen community members from the USA, England, Norway, and Spain, representing various roles within the CTX community, participated in this event. Their collective aim was to share personal experiences and expectations regarding CTX, including individuals diagnosed with CTX, parents of affected children, adolescents, and adults, as well as spouses, siblings, caregivers, and dedicated professionals advocating for the CTX community.

The diagnostic journey for those with CTX proved to be prolonged and challenging, often with significant implications for their lives. Symptoms were observed shortly after birth in some cases, but diagnosis was frequently delayed by years or even decades. For others, symptoms emerged in early adulthood, marked by the unexpected appearance of xanthomas. Additionally, some individuals experienced escalating gastrointestinal, neurological, behavioral, or mobility issues during their teenage or adult years, ultimately leading to a CTX diagnosis. Sadly, severe and irreversible disease progression was often observed by the time of diagnosis. Many participants identified missed opportunities for earlier detection, particularly those with a history of early-onset cataracts.

CTX symptoms affect various body systems and manifest at different life stages. Initial indicators prompting medical attention included cataracts, chronic diarrhea, failure to thrive, and developmental delays. Participants also highlighted challenges with cognition, communication, mobility, balance, and coordination, along with immediate difficulties such as tremors, seizures, joint pain, musculoskeletal abnormalities, osteoporosis, bone fractures, and xanthomas on the tendons of the hand and ankle. Some described autism-like complications, including severe communication and intellectual challenges from an early age, leading to significant functional impairments. Depression, anxiety, and behavioral issues further compounded the burden for both patients and caregivers.

The profound impact of these symptoms was evident, affecting physical, intellectual, and emotional well-being. While some individuals diagnosed early reported milder impacts, caregivers and families were deeply affected by the CTX experience. Emotional, social, and financial challenges were vividly described, including feelings of fear, helplessness, guilt, anxiety, depression, strains on relationships, and negative impacts on work, education, career attainment, and family dynamics. The testing of other blood relatives for CTX presented additional challenges for some families. These collective narratives underscore the complex challenges associated with CTX, emphasizing the urgent need for increased awareness, early detection, and comprehensive support for affected individuals and their families.

Access to the Voice of the Patient Report is available on the CTX Alliance website, www.ctxalliance.org.

Conclusion

Living with or caring for someone with CTX poses significant physical, emotional, and financial challenges for patients and their families. International patient advocacy groups are uniting around four key initiatives: advocating for earlier diagnosis, promoting physician and patient education, ensuring access to treatment, and providing support and connections for those affected by CTX.

Advocating for Earlier Diagnosis

International patient groups collaborate on development and implementation of CTX newborn screening efforts to share information, advocate for policy changes, conduct joint awareness campaigns, engage with healthcare professionals, support research, establish guidelines, leverage global partnerships, work with regulatory authorities, promote public awareness, and monitor and evaluate screening programs. This collaborative effort seeks to ensure early diagnosis globally for CTX, improving outcomes and promoting consistent screening practices.

Physician and Patient Education

Enhancing clinical suspicion among healthcare providers is crucial to intervene before debilitating neurologic and non-neurologic symptoms emerge. Coordination among various specialists and health-allied professionals is essential, along with enhanced education for residents and fellows to improve detection and treatment. Patient education focused on the impact of treatment non-adherence is necessary to mitigate long-term debilitating symptoms that may occur without consistent therapy.

International collaboration allows for comprehensive and culturally sensitive educational materials about CTX to be created, including brochures, videos, and online resources designed to educate both patients and healthcare professionals. These materials can be translated and localized into different languages and adapted to various cultural contexts, ensuring accessibility and relevance to diverse populations worldwide. Personal narratives can be powerful tools to raise awareness and demonstrate the positive impact of early identification and treatment.

Access to Treatment

International collaboration between patient advocacy organizations can significantly contribute to improving access to affordable treatments for CTX by addressing common challenges and advocating for global standards. Sharing best practices and negotiating with pharmaceutical companies to address medication pricing disparities can make a difference. The exchange of knowledge and promotion of research collaboration, including an international patient registry of well-characterized CTX patients, will significantly contribute to the research landscape.

Providing Patient Support and Connections

International collaboration involves sharing resources through online platforms and participation in international conferences where patients can meet and learn from each other. The creation of shared online support communities and joint educational initiatives could help build a framework for a CTX toolkit for existing and newly diagnosed individuals. Establishing cross-border patient assistance programs and other patient-centered initiatives can amplify the impact, foster a global support network, and enhance the well-being of individuals affected by CTX.

In summary, international collaboration among patient advocacy organizations creates a powerful force that can address systemic challenges, advocate for global standards, and ultimately improve access to screening, diagnosis, and affordable treatments for individuals affected by CTX. The recent international meeting in Jerusalem marked a significant commitment to the CTX patient community, embodying the motto "Nothing about you, without you."

References

1. Appadurai V, DeBarber A, Chiang PW, Patel SB, Steiner RD, Tyler C, Bonnen PE. Apparent underdiagnosis of Cerebrotendinous Xanthomatosis revealed by analysis of ~60,000 human exomes. Mol Genet Metab. 2015;116(4):298–304. https://doi.org/10.1016/j.ymgme.2015.10.010. Epub 2015 Oct 26. PMID: 26643207; PMCID: PMC4767010
2. Pramparo T, Steiner RD, Rodems S, Jenkinson C. Allelic prevalence and geographic distribution of cerebrotendinous xanthomatosis. Orphanet J Rare Dis. 2023;18(1):13. https://doi.org/10.1186/s13023-022-02578-1. PMID: 36650582; PMCID: PMC9843874

Index

A. Federico et al. (eds.), *Cerebrotendinous Xanthomatosis*, https://doi.org/10.1007/978-3-031-92526-9

GPSR Compliance

The European Union's (EU) General Product Safety Regulation (GPSR) is a set of rules that requires consumer products to be safe and our obligations to ensure this.

If you have any concerns about our products, you can contact us on ProductSafety@springernature.com

In case Publisher is established outside the EU, the EU authorized representative is:

Springer Nature Customer Service Center GmbH
Europaplatz 3
69115 Heidelberg, Germany

Batch number: 10726060

Printed by Printforce, the Netherlands